DISRUPTIVE BEHAVIOR DISORDERS

Evidence-Based Practice for
Assessment and Intervention

FRANK M. GRESHAM

THE GUILFORD PRESS

New York   London

Library of Congress Cataloging-in-Publication Data

Gresham, Frank M.
  Disruptive behavior disorders : evidence-based practice for assessment and
intervention / Frank M. Gresham.
    pages cm
  Includes bibliographical references and index.
  ISBN 978-1-4625-2129-6 (hardcover : acid-free paper)
  1. Problem children—Education.   2. Problem children—Behavior modification.
3. School mental health services.   4. Behavioral assessment.   5. Behavior
disorders in children.   I. Title.
  LC4801.G74 2015
  371.93—dc23
                                                                    2015018100

To Hill M. Walker, whose untiring dedication to children and youth with emotional and behavioral disorders over the past 50 years has been a continuing source of inspiration to me and my career in the field

About the Author

Frank M. Gresham, PhD, is Professor in the Department of Psychology at Louisiana State University. He is a Fellow of the American Psychological Association (APA) and of APA Divisions 16 (School Psychology), 5 (Quantitative and Qualitative Methods), and 53 (Society for Clinical Child and Adolescent Psychology), and is one of the few psychologists to be awarded Fellow status in the American Association for the Advancement of Science. Dr. Gresham is a recipient of the Lightner Witmer Award and the Senior Scientist Award from APA Division 16. His research and more than 250 publications address topics including social skills assessment and training, response to intervention, and assessment and intervention for students with emotional and behavioral disorders.

Preface

Disruptive behavior disorders have been the subject of intense interest by researchers and practitioners in various disciplines, including school psychology, clinical psychology, psychiatry, social work, counseling, and special education. The field of psychology especially has developed a powerful empirical literature around disruptive behavior disorders that can be used to assist families and schools in coping with these behavior challenges.

Disruptive behavior disorders account for approximately 10% of any given school population. Thus, in a school of 500 students, one might expect at least 50 children to exhibit some type of disruptive behavior disorder. Unfortunately, schools are often at a loss as to how best to handle this population. A major goal of this book is to communicate and adapt a knowledge base for effective use by families and educators who must cope with the rising tide of disruptive behavior disorders in home and school settings.

Disruptive behavior disorders can be characterized by problems in self-control of emotions and behaviors that create adjustment difficulties in personal and interpersonal domains. These disorders consist of two fundamental types: (1) antisocial behavior pattern and (2) defiant/disrespectful behavior pattern. An antisocial behavior pattern involves the repeated violation of social norms across a range of contexts such as home, school, and community. It ranks as the most frequently cited reason for referral of young people to mental health services and accounts for nearly half of all such referrals. A defiant/disrespectful behavior pattern involves negative and resistant social interactions, especially with adults (teachers and parents). It is primarily a problem in noncompliance with adult commands or directives.

This book is organized into 10 chapters:

- Chapter 1 deals with the characteristics, correlates, causes, and outcomes of disruptive behavior disorders.
- Chapter 2 provides information on how to evaluate the evidence base for these disorders.
- Chapter 3 describes evidence-based assessment strategies.
- Chapter 4 discusses issues, guidelines, and resources for implementing interventions.
- Chapter 5 describes evidence-based school interventions.
- Chapter 6 reviews evidence-based home interventions.
- Chapter 7 discusses evidence-based multicomponent interventions.
- Chapter 8 summarizes primary prevention strategies.
- Chapter 9 describes replacement behavior training strategies.
- Chapter 10 provides detailed case study applications for best practices. Case studies of children with defiant/disrespectful and antisocial behavior patterns are presented for illustrative purposes.

This book focuses on children and youth who develop challenging, disruptive behavior patterns at home and subsequently bring these behavior patterns to school. These behavior patterns create considerable problems for family members and school personnel. They not only produce chaotic home and school environments, but also disrupt the learning and achievement of others. This book provides parents and school personnel with evidence-based assessment and intervention procedures to deal with the approximately 10% of the school population who demonstrate these behavior patterns.

Contents

DISRUPTIVE BEHAVIOR DISORDERS

Characteristics, Correlates, Causes, and Outcomes of Disruptive Behavior Disorders in Children and Youth

This chapter examines disruptive behavior disorders (DBDs) in terms of their characteristics, correlates, causes, and outcomes. I describe the negative impact that DBDs have on the children and youth who display them, their peers, family members, teachers, and school administrators. DBDs are just one class of problems that schools are called upon to solve that often are not of their own making. These problems include youth violence, school dropout, bullying, academic failure, and a host of mental health issues.

Schools and families are charged with raising and educating an increasingly diverse child population in terms of predominant attitudes and beliefs, behavioral styles, racial–ethnic backgrounds, socioeconomic levels, and risk status. Children and youth who develop challenging, disruptive behavior patterns at home and subsequently bring these behavior patterns to school can create considerable trouble for family members *and* school personnel. These behavior patterns not only create chaotic home and school environments, but also disrupt the learning and achievement of others. These children and youth can be extremely difficult to discipline and teach because many parents and school personnel often do not have a thorough understanding of the origins, characteristics, and developmental course of disruptive behavior patterns, which further complicates their appropriate reactions.

Despite this rather bleak picture of the pernicious effects of disruptive behavior patterns, there is reason for optimism based on the progress that has been made in understanding and developing solutions for them. Over the past 10 years, we have made enormous strides in the assessment and intervention of DBDs, particularly early in their developmental course. Research based on randomized controlled trials, single case experimental designs, and longitudinal research designs has generated a wealth of knowledge regarding the most appropriate means of screening, assessing, and intervening upon DBDs (Dunlap & Fox, 2014; Leff, Waanders, Waasdorp, & Paskewich, 2014; Reid, Patterson, & Snyder, 2002; Seeley, Severson, & Fixen, 2014).

DBDs have been the subject of intense interest by researchers and practitioners in various disciplines and fields including school psychology, clinical psychology, psychiatry, social work, counseling, and education. The field of psychology especially has developed a powerful empirical literature around DBDs that can be used to assist families and schools in coping with these problematic behaviors. Unfortunately, this knowledge base has been adopted into child rearing and educational practices in only a limited fashion. A major goal of this book is to communicate and adapt this knowledge base for effective use by families and educators who must cope with the rising tide of DBDs in home and school settings.

DBDs Defined

DBDs can be characterized by problems in self-control of emotions and behaviors that create adjustment difficulties in personal and interpersonal domains. These disorders are manifested in behavioral forms or types that violate the rights of others (e.g., aggression, property damage, relational aggression) and/or bring individuals into significant conflict with societal norms and authority figures. The underlying causes of these problems in self-control of emotions and behaviors vary greatly among individuals, and no single intervention will be universally successful for all individuals.

Types of DBDs

DBDs consist of two fundamental types: (1) antisocial behavior pattern and (2) defiant/disrespectful behavior pattern. An antisocial behavior pattern involves the repeated violation of social norms across a range of contexts such as home, school, and community. This behavior patterns also entails hostility and aggression toward others, a willingness to break rules, and defiance of adult authority. This behavior pattern is one of the most common forms of psychopathology among children and youth. It ranks as the most frequently cited reason for the referral of young people to mental health services, and accounts for nearly half of all such referrals. This behavior pattern also tends to be highly persistent over time, resistant to interventions, and frequently leads to rejection by peers, teachers, and caregivers. The long-term prognosis for youth with well-established conduct disorders is extremely bleak, and schools and families do not perform well in either buffering or reducing the social impact of DBDs (Cottle, Lee, & Heilbrun, 2001; Crews et al., 2007).

A defiant/disrespectful behavior pattern involves negative and resistant social interactions, especially with adults (teachers and parents). It is primarily a problem in *noncompliance* with adult commands or directives. Noncompliance refers to a failure to comply with a specific directive and is noted if (1) no response is forthcoming, (2) no response is produced or initiated within a prescribed time period (usually 10 seconds), or (3) some alternative, nonrequested behavior is performed instead (McMahon & Forehand, 2003). Noncompliance can assume four basic forms: (1) simple refusal, (2) direct defiance, (3) passive noncompliance, and (4) attempts to renegotiate the form or terms of the directive. High levels of noncompliance early in life often lead to much more serious behavioral issues later in life.

Tables 1.1 and 1.2 depict the behavioral characteristics of antisocial behavior pattern and defiant/disrespectful behavior pattern, respectively. Antisocial behavior pattern consists of two fundamental types based on age of onset: *childhood onset* (typically prior to 10 years of age) and *adolescent onset* (typically no behavioral characteristics prior to age 10). Individuals with an antisocial behavior pattern often display a lack of remorse or guilt, are unconcerned about others' feelings, are poorly motivated about their school performance, and show shallow or deficient affect. An antisocial behavior pattern can range from mild (two to three antisocial behavior problems), to moderate (four to six antisocial behavior problems), or severe (seven or more antisocial behavior problems). The defiant/disrespectful behavior pattern consists of three basic forms of behavior: (1) angry/irritable mood, (2) argumentative/defiant behavior, and (3) vindictiveness. This disorder can be *mild* (behaviors are confined to one setting such as home or school), *moderate* (behaviors expressed in at least two settings), or *pervasive* (behaviors exhibited in three or more settings).

TABLE 1.1. Antisocial Behavior Problems

- Bullies others.
- Fights with others.
- Uses weapons to harm others.
- Is cruel to others.
- Steals from others.
- Sets fires.
- Burglarizes homes.
- Shoplifts.
- Is truant.
- Cheats in games or activities.
- Lies.
- Intimidates others.
- Forces others to act against their will.

Prevalence of DBDs

There are varying estimates with regard to the prevalence rates of antisocial behavior pattern and defiant/disrespectful behavior pattern. One-year population prevalence estimates for antisocial behavior pattern range from 2% to more than 10% with a median prevalence estimate of about 4%. Prevalence rates of antisocial behavior increase from childhood to adolescence and are higher among males than among females (American Psychiatric Association, 2013).

The prevalence rate of defiant/disrespectful behavior pattern ranges from 1 to 11% with a median prevalence rate of about 5%. This prevalence rate varies depending on age and gender, with the disorder being more prevalent in males prior to adolescence.

TABLE 1.2. Defiant/Disrespectful Behavior Problems

- Frequently loses temper.
- Is resentful.
- Argues excessively with parents, teachers, and peers.
- Is noncompliant.
- Provokes others.
- Accuses others for own mistakes.
- Defies parents and teachers.
- Yells or talks out.
- Complains.

Based on the above prevalence estimates, it appears that about 9 or 10% of the school-age population would qualify for a diagnosis of DBDs with about equal numbers of individuals having antisocial behavior pattern and defiant/disrespectful behavior pattern. This would indicate that in a school population of 500 students, approximately 50 of them would be at risk for having a DBD. Schools that do not have identification and intervention plans to deal with these children will almost certainly have chaotic school and classroom environments. It is important to note that more than half of all school office disciplinary referrals are typically accounted for by this relatively small percentage of the school's total student population. This finding is similar to that for delinquency, wherein a majority of delinquent acts are accounted for by approximately 6% of the juvenile population. Thus, the social impact is extremely disruptive of school routines, severely stresses the management and teaching skills of school staff, and is disproportionate to the relatively small number of students with DBDs accounting for it.

The functional consequences of antisocial behavior pattern often lead to school suspensions and expulsions, contact with the juvenile justice system, sexually transmitted diseases, and physical injury from fights (Patterson, Reid, & Dishion, 1992). These problems may prevent attendance in ordinary schools or living in a parental or foster home. The functional consequences of oppositional defiant disorder leads individuals into frequent conflicts with parents, teachers, peers, and romantic partners. These problems often result in substantial impairments in an individual's emotional, social, and academic adjustment (Moffitt, 2003).

DBDs and Comorbidity

Comorbidity refers to the fact that individuals with a single disorder (e.g., conduct disorder or oppositional defiant disorder) may be at increased risk for a second disorder or multiple disorders, which may in turn negatively affect their developmental course (Eyberg, Nelson, & Boggs, 2008). Comorbidity represents perhaps the highest risk status for pernicious outcomes because the existence of multiple disorders (e.g., conduct disorder and depression or oppositional defiant disorder and attention-deficit/hyperactivity disorder [ADHD]) often produces a negative "multiplier effect."

An excellent example of the deleterious effects of comorbidity was highlighted and illustrated by Lynam (1996), who developed a theoretical formulation for future chronic offenders. Lynam reviewed and synthesized empirical evidence that points to at-risk youth who fit the profile of conduct disorder mixed with ADHD. He argues that the presence of ADHD and conduct disorder dramatically increases risk for later, seriously destructive outcomes (e.g., school failure and social behavior problems) and that this combination of disorders produces a virulent strain of conduct disorder that is strongly associated with chronic offending.

Gresham and colleagues (Gresham, Lane, et al., 2001; Gresham, Lane, & Lambros, 2000; Gresham, MacMillan, Bocian, Ward, & Forness, 1998) have replicated Lynam's findings on comorbidity with a longitudinal sample of at-risk elementary-age students. These investigators found that those students who were comorbid for ADHD *and* conduct disorder were also at elevated risk on a host of social-behavioral measures compared with samples of students who manifested only one disorder or problem.

Both ADHD and oppositional defiant disorders are common in individuals with conduct disorders, and this comorbid pattern predicts worse outcomes for these individuals. Conduct disorders may also co-occur with one or more of the following disorders: *specific learning disabilities, anxiety disorders, depressive or bipolar disorders, and substance-related disorders* (American Psychiatric Association, 2013).

Oppositional defiant disorder is much higher in samples of children and adolescents with ADHD. Oppositional defiant disorder often precedes the development of conduct disorder—particularly in individuals with childhood-onset conduct disorder. Individuals with oppositional defiant disorder are also at increased risk for major depressive disorder and anxiety disorders due primarily to angry-irritable mood symptoms (American Psychiatric Association, 2013).

Developmental Pathways of DBDs

Much research conducted in the field of developmental psychopathology has enlightened our understanding of how DBDs develop over time. Longitudinal and descriptive studies in the United States and other countries have contributed enormously to our knowledge and understanding of the developmental course of DBDs (Lynam, 1996; Patterson, 2002; Reid, 1993; Reid et al., 2002). Loeber and his colleagues have identified three different pathways to the development of DBDs: (1) covert path, (2) overt path, and (3) defiant/disobedience path. Individuals on a *covert path* are characterized by stealth and concealment and typically direct their deviant behavior toward property (vandalism, theft, arson), toward themselves (substance abuse), or both (Loeber, 1988; Loeber & Dishion, 1983) The dishonesty involved in the covert path (lying, cheating, stealing) is strongly objectionable to parents, teachers, and peers and often leads to social rejection.

In contrast, individuals on an *overt path* tend to direct their problem behavior toward other persons by confronting and victimizing them, acting aggressively, and using coercive tactics to get their way or to force their submission. Behaviors such as bullying, coercion, aggression, and physical fighting are strongly associated with this path. Individuals following the *defiance/disobedience path* display strong opposition to adult-imposed rules and expectations. This path is most common among individuals with or at risk for oppositional defiant disorder. Behaviors characterizing this path include arguing with adults, defiance, noncompliance, and an angry, resentful mood. Table 1.3 depicts behavioral examples of each of these three developmental pathways.

With respect to antisocial behavior problems, there are two fundamental types: (1) *childhood onset* (onset prior to age 10) and (2) *adolescent onset* (no symptoms prior to age 10). Although the onset of antisocial behavior may occur as early as the preschool years, typically the behavioral indicators of antisocial behavior emerge during mid-childhood through mid-adolescence. In terms of prognosis, the childhood-onset type of antisocial behavior has a much worse prognosis

TABLE 1.3. Developmental Pathways to DBDs

Covert pathway
- Stealing
- Lying
- Burglary
- Drug and alcohol involvement
- Vandalism
- Relational aggression

Overt pathway
- Aggression
- Coercion
- Manipulation of others

Defiance/disobedience pathway
- Noncompliance
- Oppositional defiant behavior
- Resistance to adult influence
- Deliberate annoyance of others

than the adolescent-onset type (Kazdin, 1987; Loeber, 1988). Individuals with childhood-onset antisocial behavior predict an increased risk of criminal behavior and substance abuse in adulthood. This type of antisocial behavior is also called the *aggressive/versatile pathway* and is characterized by the most severe antisocial behavior pattern. It is thought to begin in early childhood with the development of defiant/disrespectful behavioral problems (e.g., defiance, disobedience, noncompliance) which progresses toward early features of antisocial behavior (e.g., lying, stealing, fighting). Most children diagnosed with antisocial behavior also meet the diagnostic criteria for defiant/disrespectful behavior pattern (Lahey et al., 1990). It should be noted that there are wide differences among individuals with antisocial behavior pattern, with some engaging in more serious behaviors early in life (predictive of a worse prognosis) while other individuals develop this behavior pattern later in adolescence (predictive of a better prognosis).

The best predictor of the long-term persistence of antisocial behavior and aggression is early onset (Kazdin, 1987; Loeber & Dishion, 1983). Many children exhibiting this behavior pattern display aggression, hostility, and violation of social norms. This behavior pattern is highly resistant to intervention. As Kazdin (1987) has suggested, after about age 8 (grade 3), conduct disorders should be viewed as a chronic condition that cannot be "cured," but rather controlled and managed (e.g., diabetes) with appropriate interventions and supports.

The defiant/disrespectful behavior pattern is a common precursor to the childhood-onset antisocial behavior pattern, and children having it often display symptoms of ADHD as well. Lynam (1996) has described three models that explain the development of conduct problems: (1) a risk-factor model, (2) a stepping-stone model, and (3) a subtype model. Each of these models is briefly described in the following sections.

Risk-Factor Model

Symptoms of ADHD (hyperactivity/impulsivity/inattention, or HIA) are involved with the development of conduct problems in two ways. These symptoms may operate as risk factors that accelerate the development within a pathway or may act as stepping stones by serving as a first step along a developmental pathway (Lynam, 1996). HIA leads to situations that create problems for children that often escalate into antisocial behavior. HIA combined with defiant/disrespectful behavior pattern most certainly produces stress on parents and families that often leads them into a coercive style of parenting, which, in turn, frequently produces antisocial behavior (Patterson, 2002). School entry for these children often leads to academic failure that can result in frustration, which increases the risk of aggressive behavior (Hinshaw, 1992). This behavior pattern frequently leads to peer rejection, social isolation, and peer conflicts that have deleterious long-term consequences on a child's social development (Parker & Asher, 1987).

HIA is one risk factor among many that is associated with this behavior pattern. Long-term exposure to such risk factors such as poor parenting, low academic achievement, peer rejection, and social isolation operate synergistically as powerful influences leading to the development of conduct disorders. This risk-factor model suggests several evidence-based intervention strategies. Parent management training based on the coercive family process model of Patterson (2002—to be described in detail later in this book) helps parents and children control behavior in the home. Another strategy would be to teach these children social problem-solving strategies that feature nonaggressive means of solving interpersonal problems (Kazdin, 1993). A third strategy might focus on academic interventions, particularly in reading, to counter the effects of school failure (Denton & Vaughn, 2010). A final strategy could focus on appropriate peer-group entry strategies that would teach the child to enter social networks from which they have been excluded (Coie, Dodge, & Kupersmidt, 1990).

Stepping-Stone Model

The stepping-stone model argues that HIA behaviors lead to the development of oppositional defiant disorder that subsequently evolves into an antisocial behavior pattern. Moffitt (1993) suggests that these children are born with difficult temperamental characteristics that prompt a series of problematic parent–child encounters, which in turn can create chaotic home environments. One implication of the stepping-stone model is that if one provides early treatment of HIA, then it can prevent the development of antisocial behavior pattern later. These early treatments would typically involve stimulant medication and behavioral parent training that have been shown to ameliorate the symptoms of HIA. One caveat, however, is that not all children who have HIA go on to develop antisocial behavior problems, and evidence suggests that stimulant medication shows little effect on the development of antisocial behavior in adolescence (Blouin, Bornstein, & Trites, 1978; Weiss, Kruger, Danielson, & Elman, 1975). Moreover, stimulant medication in childhood has not been shown to affect later peer rejection or academic achievement (Jacobvitz, Sroufe, Stewart, & Leffert, 1990; MTA Cooperative Group, 2004).

It appears that the stepping-stone model provides an adequate explanation for some, but certainly not all, children who subsequently develop antisocial behavior problems. Some studies have shown that children with HIA and conduct problems have worse home/parenting environments than children with HIA-only behavior pattern in terms of family conflicts, harsh and inconsistent discipline, and lower socioeconomic status (Anderson, Williams, McGee, & Silva, 1987; Lahey et al., 1987; Moffitt, 1990). Based on the extant empirical evidence, it appears that neither the risk-factor model nor the stepping-stone model provides an adequate explanation for the development of conduct disorder, which suggests that a third model is required.

Subtype Model

Lynam (1996) has proposed an interesting third model, the subtype model, to explain the development of HIA and conduct disorder in some children. This model postulates that individuals showing symptoms of both HIA and conduct problems constitute a unique subtype of antisocial behavior problems that he calls "fledgling psychopaths." These children have what is called a "psychopathic deficit" that plays out in different behavior patterns as the child develops from early childhood into adolescence. According to Lynam (1996), this psychopathic deficit results in a failure to inhibit a dominant response (e.g., impulsivity or aggression) in the presence of changing environmental contingencies. These individuals are less likely to pause and incorporate new information when engaging in goal-directed behavior (Newman & Wallace, 1993).

Individuals with these behavioral deficits are low in what is called *constraint* (Tellegen, 1985). Persons high in constraint would describe themselves as cautious, restrained, and accepting of conventional social norms and mores of society. In contrast, persons low in constraint would describe themselves as being impulsive, adventurous, and inclined to reject the conventional social mores and norms of society.

Children with this psychopathic deficit begin life with low constraint levels that created difficulties in incorporating information and feedback from the environment to control their behavior. In early childhood, these individuals will show signs of the HIA behavioral complex in terms of impulsivity, hyperactivity, and inattention. Typically, a child will not respond to disciplinary overtures from parents due to inattentiveness and will demand immediate gratification of their wants or desires (impulsivity). As the child develops and becomes more verbal, he or she will be less able to control anger, use obscene language, inhibit active avoidance responses, refrain from blaming others for mistakes, and avoid coercive behavior patterns with family members. Finally, in adulthood, these individuals will more likely show the signs and symptoms of psychopathy and will lie, manipulate, and blame others. Very often they will exhibit poor behavioral control and will engage in a variety of criminal activities (Lynam, 1996).

This subtype model of conduct problems would argue for the early identification and intervention with these individuals prior to the development of serious antisocial behavior patterns later in life. Early identification and assessment activities should seek to distinguish between individuals with the HIA–conduct problems complex from those individuals with HIA-only behavior pattern. For example, the subtype version of children with HIA–conduct problems should show more signs of impulsivity whereas HIA-only children should show more signs of inattention. Early intervention efforts for the conduct problems subtype should focus on behavioral parent training, social problem solving, early literacy interventions, and stimulant medication. It should be noted that empirical evidence for the validity of the subtype model of conduct disorder is incomplete and somewhat speculative at this point. Despite this reality, this explanation provides some valuable guidance for early identification, assessment, and intervention.

Origins and Development of DBDs

Historically, the origins of disruptive patterns of behavior among children in general, and among acting-out children in particular have been a subject of continuing debate and controversy. However, today we have a much better understanding of how this behavior pattern is acquired and evolves. Understanding why some children have an apparent immunity to the negative impact of high-risk family and socioeconomic conditions would provide important keys to prevention. For example, the quality of mother–child interactions, the availability of social support networks, and school-related academic competence appear to be three important factors in buffering the effects of stressful conditions that put children at risk for developing disruptive behavior patterns.

The most prominently mentioned causal theories of DBDs involve *temperamental factors, neurological factors,* and *environmental factors.* It is well established that problems with temperament serve as a precursor to a host of social-behavioral adjustment problems later in a child's development. Restlessness, fussiness, irritability, and crying among infants and young children have been consistently identified as antecedents for later behavior problems, including ADHD, defiant/disrespectful behavior, and antisocial behavior. Children born with difficult temperaments are a challenge to parents and may negatively condition parents to avoid, neglect, suppress, and/or punish them. These temperamental difficulties are strongly related to low birth weight, maternal substance abuse, pregnancy complications, and prematurity. Anything that disrupts normal parenting practices is likely to put a child at risk for later adjustment problems. If severe enough, these disruptive influences can lay the foundation for the development of a disruptive, acting-out behavior pattern. Despite the predictive validity of poor temperament on the subsequent development of DBDs, there is no way to effectively intervene upon or change a poor temperament. In other words, a poor temperament is important as a predictor, but is also an unalterable variable in the development of DBDs.

Neurological factors are frequently cited as structural antecedents to social-behavioral adjustment problems. ADHD is an example of a neurodevelopmental disorder that has powerful social, behavioral, and learning manifestations and is considered to have a neurological basis (Barkley, 2006). Approximately 40% of children with ADHD have antisocial behavior patterns, and approximately 20% of these children have a specific learning disability (DuPaul, Laracy, & Gormley, 2014). Drug-affected babies present a huge, looming problem in our society because of the long-term negative impact of prenatal drug and alcohol exposure. Such exposed children suffer from severe attentional problems, agitated states, and hyperactivity that present difficulties for parents and schools to manage.

At present, we do not have the ability to precisely identify and differentially weight the causal factors that influence the development of DBDs. The role of these factors probably varies from case to case. In addition, we do not have the means to substantially affect or attenuate the causal roles of neurological factors on the development of DBDs. This suggests that we will enjoy the greatest success targeting environmental factors that clearly contribute to the development of DBDs.

There is a broad consensus in our society that environmental factors, including social and economic conditions that place children and families at risk for DBDs, are potent breeding grounds for the development of acting-out behaviors. These risk factors commonly include poverty, neglect, abuse (physical and sexual), family dysfunction, criminal behavior of family members, and an unstable home environment. These conditions place great stress on a family and can severely disrupt normal parenting. Disrupted parenting often results in harsh discipline; weak monitoring of children's activities, their whereabouts, and whom they affiliate with; limited parental involvement with the child; and incompetent problem-solving and conflict resolution skills (Patterson, 2002; Synder & Stoolmiller, 2002).

It is clear that DBDs are associated with a host of temperamental, neurological, and environmental risk factors. It is also apparent that a child's behavior pattern is the result of a complex interaction of (1) temperamental predisposition to DBDs; (2) neurological causal mechanisms within the child; and (3) environmental risk factors such as poverty, abuse, neglect, and poor parenting. Trying to determine in what proportion of the child's behavior pattern is attributable to each of these sources is a futile and unnecessary task. DBDs can be changed very effectively without knowing the specific, original causes for their acquisition and development. Furthermore, these causal factors may no longer play a role in the maintenance of disruptive behavior patterns. A major purpose of this book is to present a set of practical strategies for use by parents, caregivers, and school personnel in effectively identifying, assessing, and remediating acting-out behavior patterns displayed by children and youth with DBDs.

The Role of Coercive Family Process in the Development of DBDs

Much to the dismay of parents/caregivers, classroom teachers, and school administrators, these adults often learn that behavior management procedures that have worked so well with typical students do not work well with students displaying DBDs, particularly for students with antisocial behavior patterns (Reid et al., 2002; Walker, Ramsey, & Gresham, 2004). In fact, many tried and true behavior management procedures often make the behaviors of antisocial students much worse! Do these students learn differently than typical students? Do they require interventions based on a completely different set of learning principles? Not really! As we shall see in the following sections and subsequent chapters, the contingencies and principles by which this behavior pattern is acquired and maintained are quite lawful and predictable.

A DBD behavior pattern is learned primarily through the process of behavioral *coercion*. That is, at-risk children learn to control their environment(s) and the individuals in it through the skillful use of extremely forceful *coercive behavioral tactics*. Once learned, these tactics are highly resistant to change because they are powerfully reinforced and supported naturally by the social environment. Typically developing children, as a general rule, learn through the processes of modeling, positive reinforcement, and encouragement. Positive reinforcement, such as social praise, use of rewards, recognition, and access to preferred activities, easily influence the behavior pattern of the typically developing child. Children with DBDs, however, learn primarily through the process of *negative reinforcement*. That is, by using coercive tactics, they learn to escape, avoid, delay, or reduce aversive demands placed on them by others. They are very skilled in using coercion to escape or avoid undesired demands, tasks, or activities. Remember, a negative reinforcement contingency is one in which a behavior produces the removal, termination, reduction, or postponement of an aversive stimulus, which leads to an increase in that behavior (Cooper, Heron, & Heward, 2007). For example, engaging in disruptive behavior to escape academic task demands, having a temper tantrum in response to parental demands to engage an activity (e.g., clean your room or do your homework), or defying the teacher in order to escape the classroom and be sent to the office are all examples of behaviors maintained by negative reinforcement.

Patterson and colleagues (1982, 2002; Patterson et al., 1992) have contributed the most complete, detailed, and empirically supported explanations of the causal events and processes that account for the development of DBDs. They present a causal model in which a host of stressors (e.g., poverty, divorce, drug/alcohol abuse, and the abuse of family members) pressure the family dynamics very severely. Under the influence of these stressors, normal parenting practices are disrupted and family routines become chaotic, negative, and unpredictable. Disrupted parenting practices, in turn, lead to escalated social interactions among family members that involve the use of coercive techniques to force the submission of others. Over time, such conditions provide a fertile breeding ground for the development of DBDs. Children from these homes come to school with negative attitudes toward schooling, a limited repertoire of cooperative behavioral skills, and a strong predilection to use coercive tactics to control and manipulate others. They are usually deficient in the school success skills that teachers expect and reinforce (e.g., cooperation, sharing, focusing on assigned tasks, complying with teacher directives, accepting criticism and feedback).

The coercive process that helps explain the development of DBDs can be characterized as the outcome of a five-step interaction between parent and child wherein (1) the child applies coercive tactics in order to achieve a social goal (e.g., control, dominance) or responds aversively to a parental directive; (2) the parent reacts negatively to the child's behavior; (3) the child then escalates the aversiveness and/or intensity of coercive tactics; (4) the parent "gives in" and allows child to have his way in order to reduce aversiveness and eliminate the coercion; and (5) the child in turn reduces the level of aversiveness and terminates the coercion. In this interaction, both parent and child are powerfully reinforced but through differing variations of the same reinforcement principle. That is, the parent succeeds in reducing the child's aversiveness and use of coercive tactics by giving in or by withdrawing or changing the directive (i.e., negative reinforcement) and the child is positively reinforced by getting his way (i.e., parent gives in).

In family contexts that produce antisocial children, this sequence is repeated literally thousands of times over the course of a DBP child's development, becomes a routine habit, and is frequently observed in public spaces such as grocery stores. The following example illustrates the point. A mother and her 4-year-old son enter a grocery store where the mother is stressed by her long grocery list and insufficient time to get through it. Within 5 minutes of entering the store, her son begins issuing a loud series of "I want" requests (called mands) to which she answers a consistent "no." This manding is highly disruptive and becomes more frequent and intense until the mother grants the most recent request in order to terminate this aversive process. Thus, in a very brief exchange, while managing to terminate an aversive interaction, the parent has taught and strengthened a class of child behaviors that will be more, rather than less difficult to manage over time—an example of winning the battle and losing the war! Through this coercive family process, the child learns to control and manipulate his or her environment very efficiently in order to achieve desired social goals, and/or to escape or avoid unwanted task demands and activities. As we have noted earlier, this set of coercive tactics accompanies the child to school where it can be at least as effective with peers and teachers as it is with family members (Walker, Colvin, & Ramsey, 1994). This transfer of learning process is described and illustrated in a later section of this book.

The Matching Law and Coercive Behavior

One of the most conceptually powerful learning principles used to explain behavior is known formally as the *matching law* (Herrnstein,

1970). In his original formulation, Herrnstein (1961) stated that the rate or frequency of any behavior matches the rate or frequency of reinforcement for that behavior. In other words, response rate matches reinforcement rate. Matching is studied in what are known as concurrent schedules of reinforcement. A concurrent schedule of reinforcement refers to the delivery of reinforcement for two or more different behaviors as related to two simultaneous, but different, schedules of reinforcement (i.e., concurrently). For example, if aggressive behavior is reinforced, on average, every third time it occurs and prosocial behavior is reinforced, on average, every fifteenth time it occurs, then the matching law would predict that, on average, aggressive behavior will be chosen 5 times more frequently than prosocial behavior (15÷3 = 5). Empirical research has consistently shown that behavior under concurrent schedules of reinforcement closely follows or tracks the matching law (Synder & Stoolmiller, 2002).

With respect to DBDs, the matching law involves a choice between engaging in coercive behaviors (e.g., threatening, hitting, bullying) that force the submission of others or engaging in prosocial forms of behavior (e.g., sharing, cooperating, asking questions, negotiating conflicts, solving problems) that are maintained by positive reinforcement from key social agents (i.e., parents, teachers, peers). Thus the probability that a child will engage in either of these behaviors depends directly on the relative rate of reinforcement for each type of behavior. Synder and Stoolmiller (2002) suggest that the utility of a given behavior can be calculated by counting how often the target behavior results in conflict termination divided by the frequency with which it occurs in conflict sequences. For example, if defiant and aggressive behavior results in conflict termination 8 out of 10 times, then defiance/aggression has a *utility index* of 80%.

By comparison, prosocial behaviors for children with DBDs are relatively ineffective in terminating conflict social interaction sequences (i.e., they have a low utility index). This means that parents and teachers dealing with such behavior have the odds stacked against them in trying to divert children from this well-established and highly effective pattern of coercion. Coercive interaction between children with DBDs and adults as well as peers is an important engine that drives a child's social development. Their use of highly aversive, coercive tactics that force the submission of others as a behavioral requirement for them to be terminated or withdrawn is a highly efficient behavior pattern that is richly rewarded by the natural social environment. Negative reinforcement, occurring on such strong schedules of reinforcement for terminating conflicts, is an insidious process that leads to the development of conduct problems, delinquency, and criminality later in life. Results from research on the matching law have numerous implications for implementation of preventive and educational interventions. These implications and recommendations are fully described in subsequent chapters of this book.

Chapter Summary Points

- DBDs consist of two fundamental types: *conduct disorders* and *oppositional defiant disorder.*

- Antisocial behavior patterns are primarily a problem in *aggressive behavior* and is one of the most common forms of psychopathology in children and adolescents.

- Defiant/disrespectful behavior patterns are primarily a problem in *noncompliance* to adult commands, instructions, or directives.

- High levels of noncompliance early in life often leads to more serious behavior problems later in a child's development.

- Antisocial behavior pattern consist of two types: *childhood onset* (onset prior to age 10) and *adolescent onset* (onset after age 10).

- Childhood-onset antisocial behavior patterns have a much poorer lifetime prognosis than adolescent-onset conduct disorders.

- The median prevalence rate for antisocial behavior pattern is around 5% and the median prevalence rate for defiant/disrespectful behavior pattern is around 5%.

- Approximately 9–10% of the school-age population would qualify for a diagnosis of a DBD.

- Comorbidity (presence of more than one disorder in an individual) is quite common for DBDs.

- The defiant/disrespectful behavior pattern and ADHD have a high comorbidity rate in the school-age population.

- ADHD often co-occurs with antisocial behavior problems.

- Three developmental pathways have been identified for the development of DBDs: the covert pathway, the overt pathway, and the defiance/disobedience pathway.

- Three models have been identified to explain the comorbid presence of ADHD and conduct problems: (1) the risk-factor model, (2) the stepping-stone model, and (3) the subtype model.

- Three causal theories have been prominently mentioned for the development of DBDs: (1) temperamental causality, (2) neurological causality, and (3) environmental causality.

- DBDs can be changed effectively without knowing the specific, original causes of these disorders.
- DBDs are learned primarily through the process of behavioral coercion.
- Typically developing children learn through the process of positive reinforcement and encouragement.
- Children with DBDs learn primarily through the process in which aversive interactions with adults and peers are terminated by the target victim's submission or giving in to reduce the aversiveness of the child's coercive behavior.
- The matching law explains the presence of coercive behaviors maintained by negative reinforcement and the low frequency of prosocial behaviors maintained by positive reinforcement.

Evaluating, Selecting, and Implementing Evidence-Based Practices in School Contexts

Key Issues and Recommendations

Program evaluation is the systematic process of studying a program or practice to determine how well it works to achieve a set of intended goals. This form of evaluation serves three major purposes: (1) program assessment—for documenting or verifying program activities and their effects; (2) program improvement—for finding out where a program may be failing or needs improvement; and (3) strategic management—for providing information that can help an agency or organization to make decisions about how resources should be applied to better serve its mission or goals (Substance Abuse and Mental Health Services Administration, 2012).

The overarching goal of this chapter is to present information that help assist school professionals to make wise and strategic investments regarding effective practices and increasingly scarce resources. To this end, I focus particularly on the third purpose of program evaluation in terms of the strategic management of decisions around the selection, adoption, and use of practices that are more likely to improve the social-behavioral adjustment and school success of students with disruptive behavior problems. Step 1 in this process is to identify a pool of practices that have proven to have an acceptable evidence base undergirding them. Step 2 is to select from among these identified practices in a way that matches the problem and solves it better than what is currently being used. Step 3 is to then apply this practice with high treatment integrity so that its chance of success is maximized. I view this as a consumer protection issue that can be addressed successfully with the tools provided by systematic program evaluation. The sections that follow address each of these major topics.

Evaluation of the Evidence Base for Intervening with Students Having DBDs

Over the past two decades, there has been a widespread focus on evidence-based approaches to assessment and intervention across a range of disciplines (Flay et al., 2005). This development has stimulated creation of standards and criteria that can be applied in judging the efficacy and effectiveness of such approaches. A corollary development, also stimulated by this emphasis, has been the creation of vetted lists of recommended programs that are promoted by federal and state agencies as being acceptable because of their purported evidence base. The Institute of Education Sciences, the Office for Safe and Drug-Free Schools, and the Office of Juvenile Justice and Delinquency Prevention are all examples of federal agencies that have published lists of recommended programs. Private foundations, such as the Annie E. Casey Foundation, have also produced such lists.

Although these lists are convenient for consumers and have proven valuable at some level in the selection process, we have no assurances that they are based on similar criteria and standards. The review and selection procedures used in this vetting process can also differ markedly across agencies. Smolkowski, Strycker, and Seeley (2014) have recently addressed this issue by contributing an informative analysis of tools and procedures for evaluating research on school-related behavior disorders. Their work and the material presented here allow professional consumers to become more proficient in gauging the efficacy or effectiveness of an intervention. Given the increasing pressures on schools to accommodate a more diverse and difficult student population and, at the same time, to be more accountable for improving outcomes, these procedures may allow school gatekeepers to make more cost-effective decisions about allocating diminishing resources.

Defining what constitutes *evidence* and basing our actions on the resulting definition is sometimes a challenging task. Some professionals accept what they consider to be evidence only if it fits their preexisting belief systems and they reject any evidence that does not conform to these beliefs. This is a well-established phenomenon from the field of social psychology called *cognitive dissonance*. Cognitive dissonance describes the tendency of individuals to strive for consistency among their beliefs, attitudes, and behaviors, and any inconsistency among them is rejected out of hand, even in the face of overwhelming disconfirming evidence. For example, if you purchase an expensive new car and it turns out to be a lemon, you may tend to maintain that it is a good car despite its numerous imperfections. In many ways, scientific evidence for or against phenomena operates in much the same way. Kauffman (2014) eloquently captured this notion as follows:

> Science is a cruel mistress. It demands doubt and brooks no choice to believe an alternative explanation when the evidence served up by fidelity to its method undermines faith in that alternative. This is a bitter pill for many to swallow, so it is not at all surprising that many politicians and educators—even many special educators, including those who study emotional and behavioral disorders (EBD)—find science unpalatable. (p. 1)

Kauffman goes on to say that it is unsurprising that many individuals have trouble accepting the verdict of scientific evidence since, in order to do so, they first must reject long-held, cherished beliefs and values.

An excellent example of this is *facilitated communication*, which maintains that individuals with autism and intellectual disability have hidden or undiscovered levels of communicative ability that must be "facilitated" by an expert. However, most controlled studies of this technique have unequivocally shown that facilitators were unintentionally cuing the target participant, thus reflecting the facilitator's expectations rather than the actual communicative skills of the individual being assisted (Myles & Simpson, 1996). On the surface, this method seems harmless, but it has actually ruined the lives of innocent persons. For example, a number of individuals have served prison sentences based on flawed convictions supported by false evidence of victimization generated by facilitated communication.

What Is Evidence?

To be a sophisticated consumer of scientific knowledge, one must understand the criteria and standards used to identify and establish what constitutes acceptable levels of evidence. Different fields have varying standards that are used to judge evidence. In physics, scientists provide evidence about the laws of nature from either quantum theory or the theory of relativity. Quantum theory is concerned with the discrete rather than continuous nature of phenomena at the atomic and subatomic level, whereas relativity is concerned with the description of phenomena that take place from the perspective of an observer. Each theory in physics uses somewhat different standards for what each considers admissible evidence (Issacson, 2007). In contrast, the law relies on several types of evidence that are used to establish an individual's guilt or innocence. There is direct evidence (e.g., physical evidence, eyewitness testimony, confession) and circumstantial evidence (e.g., past behavior, character testimony, expert witness). Each of these types of evidence is weighed differently by juries and judges. Finally, in paleontology, different types of evidence are used to support the theory of evolution. These types of evidence might include fossil evidence, genetic evidence (DNA), or distributional evidence (i.e., species are not randomly distributed across different geographic regions). Charles Darwin's remarkable work on the origins of species comes to mind in this context regarding his ability to make discrete observations of natural events and then synthesize them in ways that supported his theory of evolution.

Some individuals and organizations falsely dichotomize interventions and practices into evidence-based and non-evidence-based categories. In our view, research evidence does not fall neatly into these two categories. Rather, research evidence is best thought of as existing on a continuum anchored by evidence-based and non-evidence-based poles. This requires that we think in terms of levels or strata of evidence demonstrating stronger or weaker forms of scientific support. Kazdin (2004) distinguished between an absolute threshold versus a hierarchical approach to evaluating evidence. The *threshold method* is an absolute standard, whereas the *hierarchical method* is a relative standard that considers a range of evidence generated by different research methods. We subscribe to the hierarchical method for establishing an evidence base for certain practices and procedures. Determining whether a particular treatment or practice is evidence based requires that we evaluate the research methodology used. That is, to what extent does the methodology control for various threats to internal validity, external validity, construct validity, and statistical conclusion validity (Shadish, Cook, & Campbell, 2002)?

It is important to distinguish between the terms *evidence-based treatments* and *evidence-based practices*. Evidence-based treatments are interventions that have been shown to be efficacious through rigorous research methods that have good internal validity. In contrast, evidence-based practices are intervention approaches rather than specific intervention(s) applied to an individual. Evidence-based treatments are used to make decisions about individual students (e.g., being classified as a responder or a nonresponder to a particular treatment). Evidence-based practices are grounded in scientific research that supports implementation of certain intervention approaches because across studies, implementation groups, sites, investigators, and contexts, they consistently produce positive outcomes. An example of an evidence-based practice is the response-to-intervention (RTI) paradigm that is applied in order to change, continue, or terminate an intervention for an individual student using sensitive progress monitoring procedures (Walker & Shinn, 2010).

Another important distinction is between *efficacy research* and *effectiveness research*. Efficacy research focuses on the measurable effects of specific interventions, with the randomized controlled trial being the prototypical example (Nathan, Stuart, & Dolan, 2000). Efficacy studies compare one or more experimental treatments with one or more control conditions (e.g., no-treatment controls, wait-list controls, or placebo). Efficacy studies have high internal validity, meaning they are carried out under tight experimental conditions that control for most potentially confounding factors and typically use short-term, targeted outcome measures.

Effectiveness research seeks to determine whether treatments have measurable beneficial effects across broad populations and in real-world settings (Nathan et al., 2000). Effectiveness research typically is high in external validity (generalizability) and is concerned with the extent to which a causal relationship is established and persists in the face of variations in settings, persons, treatments, and outcomes (Shadish et al., 2002). Effectiveness research typically uses broadly defined outcome measures rather than the specific, narrowly construed outcome measures that are typically used in efficacy research. As a rule, effect sizes are smaller for *effective* than *efficacious* interventions because effective interventions are (1) implemented in real-world, sometimes chaotic schooling conditions and (2) they are implemented in the absence of the supports, technical assistance, and trouble-shooting typically provided by their developers in the efficacy evaluation process. As a rule, interventions considered to be effective are preferred, as they have passed the difficult test of "real-world" application (i.e., they work under the normal conditions of schooling). However, such interventions are not always available for solving particular problems, so less robust intervention approaches may have to be considered.

Types of Research Evidence

Evidence-based practices have the goal of gathering the best research evidence related to intervention strategies to prevent or ameliorate the effects of disruptive behavior problems in children and youth. Multiple types of research evidence are used to support evidence-based practices, among them (1) efficacy studies, (2) effectiveness studies, (3) cost-effectiveness studies, (4) longitudinal intervention outcome(s) studies, and (5) epidemiological studies. Various types of research designs are better suited to answer certain questions than others (Smolkowski et al., 2014). These designs include the following:

- Observation of DBDs within target settings, including case studies, can be a valuable source of hypotheses generation concerning the behavioral challenges of children and youth, and their value is often underestimated.
- Qualitative research can be used to describe the subjective or "real-world" experiences of individuals undergoing an intervention procedure.
- Single-case experimental designs are useful in drawing causal inferences about the effectiveness of interventions for individuals in a controlled manner.
- Epidemiological research can be used to track the availability, utilization, and acceptance of various intervention procedures.
- Moderator/mediator studies can be used to identify correlates of intervention outcomes and to establish the mechanisms of change in specific intervention procedures.
- Randomized controlled trials (RCTs) or efficacy studies can provide the strongest types of research evidence that protects against most threats to the internal validity of a study.
- Effectiveness studies can be used to assess the outcomes of interventions in less controlled, real-world settings and to determine whether causal relationships persist across individuals, treatment agents, settings, and/or participants.
- Meta-analyses of the research literature provide a quantitative metric or index concerning the effects of multiple studies on various target populations, age groups, genders, and/or settings.

The types of research evidence developed by using the above methodologies can be rank ordered in terms of their strength based on research design logic. As such, observations can be used to formulate hypotheses and describe outcomes but cannot be used to draw causal inferences about a phenomenon. Single-case experimental designs can be used to draw causal inferences about the effect of an intervention on a given individual, but these effects cannot be generalized to other individuals with different types of problems. RCTs can be used to draw causal inferences about the efficacy of an intervention under tightly controlled conditions, but cannot be generalized to other populations, settings, therapists, or participants under less controlled conditions. Meta-analyses can provide estimates of the effect sizes of interventions, but cannot be used to draw causal inferences about the effects of specific interventions on specific individuals.

Threats to Valid Inference Making

All science depends on the validity of making inferences about phenomena under investigation. Validity refers to the truth of an inference or the extent to which evidence supports an inference being true or correct (Shadish et al., 2002). In the philosophy of science, *correspondence theory* states that a knowledge claim can only be true if it corresponds to what we know about the real world. However, what we think we know about the real world may have different interpretations. A good example of this can be found in quantum physics and the *uncertainty principle*. The uncertainty principle states that the very act of observing something affects the accuracy of that observation. This implies that no objective reality exists apart from our observations of this reality. This is at odds with what is assumed to be true in classical physics, which maintains that an objective reality exists apart from our ability to measure it. This disagreement between what is known to be "truth" about the universe by quantum physics and by classical physics created intense debates in the 1920s and 1930s between Niels Bohr and Albert Einstein regarding the nature of the universe (Issacson, 2007).

The goal of research methodology is to design studies that uncover relations among variables that might not otherwise be obvious from casual observation. Research designs help us simplify complex situations in which many variables are simultaneously operating and help researchers to control and/or isolate variables of interest, thus ruling out alternative, competing explanations for the data collected in a study. The degree to which any research design is successful in ruling out plausible rival hypotheses is not absolute, but rather one of degree. Four types of validity are typically considered in this context: internal validity, external validity, construct validity, and statistical conclusion validity (Shadish et al., 2002).

Internal Validity

Internal validity refers to the degree to which a researcher can attribute changes in a dependent or outcome variable to systematic, manipulated changes in an independent (intervention) variable while simultaneously ruling out alternative explanations. Threats to internal validity include history, maturation, instrumentation, statistical regression, selection biases, attrition, and the interaction of selection biases with other threats to internal validity (Shadish et al., 2002). The RCT is the gold standard for protection against virtually all threats to the internal validity of a research investigation. Single-case experimental designs also provide protection from many, but not all, threats to internal validity. Quasi-experimental designs, which do not involve random assignment, don't provide this level of protection against internal validity threats and can lead to erroneous conclusions.

External Validity

External validity refers to the generalizability of the results of a research study. It is concerned with the extent to which a study's results can be generalized to other populations, therapists/teachers, settings, treatment variables, and measurement variables. External validity is concerned with the boundary conditions or limitations of research findings. Whereas internal validity is concerned with attributing changes in a dependent variable to an independent variable, external validity is concerned with the extent to which the same effect would be obtained with other participants, other therapists, other settings, and with different methods for measuring outcomes.

Internal validity is the central concept in *efficacy studies* that investigate phenomena under rigidly controlled conditions, whereas external validity is the key concept in *effectiveness studies* that investigate phenomena in real-world settings or conditions. Several threats to external validity have been noted and are classified into four broad categories: sample, stimulus, contextual, and assessment characteristics (Bracht & Glass, 1968).

Construct Validity

Construct validity establishes the basis for interpreting the causal relation between an independent variable and a dependent variable. Shadish et al. (2002) have identified numerous threats to the construct validity of a study, which include inadequate explication of constructs, construct confounding, mono-operation bias, mono-method bias, and treatment diffusion. Each of these threats can compromise the interpretation or meaning of a particular research finding, thereby creating confusion about why treatments are successful or unsuccessful. In contrast, internal validity is concerned with whether an independent variable was responsible for changes in a dependent variable. Construct validity concentrates on the *reason* or *explanation* of a change in a dependent variable brought about by an independent variable. The construct validity of a study is based on two questions: What is the intervention? What explains the causal mechanism for change in a dependent variable?

For example, parent management training (PMT) has a long and well-established history as a treatment for disruptive behavior problems (Eyberg et al., 2008; Patterson, Reid, Jones, & Conger, 1975). PMT focuses on teaching parents basic behavioral principles to modify and monitor child behavior problems. The reason PMT brings about substantial changes in children's disruptive behavior patterns is that it substantially reduces coercive interactions between parents and children by eliminating negative reinforcement process that sustain and strengthen problem behaviors (Patterson, 1982).

Statistical Conclusion Validity

Statistical conclusion validity refers to threats in drawing valid inferences that result from random error and inappropriate selection of statistical analysis procedures. It deals with whether a presumed cause and effect covary and how strongly they covary. In the first case, statistical conclusion validity deals with commission of *Type I errors* (falsely concluding an effect exists when it does not) and *Type II errors* (falsely concluding there is no effect when in fact there is). In the second case, we may overestimate or underestimate the effects of an independent variable on a dependent variable.

Various threats to statistical conclusion validity exist and include low statistical power, violated assumptions of statistical tests, unreliability of measures, unreliability of treatment implementation (i.e., poor treatment integrity), and inaccurate effect size estimation. Although all of these threats are problematic, many studies of disruptive behavior problems suffer from low statistical power because they utilize too few participants or fail to control for heterogeneity in experimental conditions.

Standards for Establishing Evidence-Based Treatments

Several professional groups have developed and adopted differing but related criteria and nomenclatures for the levels of scientific evidence necessary for determining whether a treatment is evidence based. Division 12 (Clinical Psychology), Division 16 (School Psychology), Division 17 (Counseling Psychology), Division 53 (Clinical Child and Adolescent Psychology), and Division 54 (Pediatric Psychology) of the American Psychological Association all have published separate documents specifying criteria for classifying treatments based on the quality of research supporting those treatments. Although there is some variation among these divisions' documents, all have agreed on the criteria that should be in the classification of scientific evidence.

- *Criterion 1: Well-established treatment.* There must be two good group design experiments, conducted in at least two independent research settings, and by independent research teams, demonstrating efficacy by showing the intervention to be (1) statistically superior to a pill or psychological placebo or another treatment, *or* (2) equivalent (i.e., not statistically different) to an already established treatment in experiments with sufficient statistical power to detect moderate differences, *and* (3) treatment manuals or their logical equivalent were used for implementation of the treatment, conducted with a target population, treated for specific problems, for whom inclusion criteria have been delineated, reliable and valid outcome measures were selected, and appropriate data analyses were used.

- *Criterion 2: Probably efficacious treatment.* There must be at least two good experiments showing that the treatment is superior (statistically significant) to a wait-list control group, or one or more good experiments meeting the criteria for well-established treatments with the one exception of having been conducted in two independent research settings and by different investigatory teams.

- *Criterion 3: Possibly efficacious treatment.* There must be at least one good study showing the treatment to be efficacious in the absence of conflicting evidence.

- *Criterion 4: Experimental treatment.* The treatment has not yet been tested in trials meeting established criteria for methodology.

Nathan et al. (2000) developed a list of six types of treatment studies that vary along the levels of evidence each provides in support of a treatment. In their typology, *Type 1 studies* are the most rigorous and involved randomized, prospective clinical trial methodology. These types of studies include comparison groups with random assignment, blinded assessments, clear presentation of inclusion and exclusion criteria, state-of-the art diagnostic methods, adequate sample size with sufficient statistical power, and clearly described statistical methods. *Type 2 studies* are clinical trials in which an intervention is tested with at least one aspect of the Type 1 requirements missing. For example, a Type 2 study might not use blinded assessments or might not have adequate statistical power to detect a moderate effect. *Type 3 studies* are methodologically limited and involve open enrollment or trials aimed at collecting pilot data to determine whether more rigorous designs are warranted. *Type 4 studies* are reviews with secondary data analyses such as meta-analyses. *Type 5 studies* are literature reviews that do not use secondary data analyses. *Type 6 studies* are case studies, essays, and opinion/position papers.

Single-Case Experimental Designs

The guidelines for well-established, probably efficacious, possibly efficacious, and experimental treatments specified by the various divisions of the American Psychological Association only included group experimental designs and did not specify what criteria should be used to evaluate the quality of studies using single-case experimental designs. We consider this to be a glaring omission that ignores a huge body of excellent research on disruptive behavior problems using single-case experimental design methodology.

Single-case designs (SCDs) are interrupted time-series designs that provide a rigorous experimental evaluation of intervention effects (Kazdin, 1982; Kennedy, 2005; Kratochwill et al., 2010). SCDs have many variations, but always involve repeated, systematic measurement of a dependent variable before, during, and after the manipulation of an independent variable (i.e., a treatment). These designs provide a strong basis for establishing causal inferences and are widely used in clinical psychology, school psychology, special education, and applied behavior analysis. Experimental control in SCDs is established by replication of an intervention in an experiment using one of the following methods: (1) introduction, withdrawal, or reversal of the independent variable (e.g., ABAB designs); (2) iterative manipulation of the independent variable across different observational phases (e.g., multielement or alternating treatment designs); or (3) staggered introduction of the independent variable across different points in time or in different settings/contexts, such as morning, noon, and afternoon recess (e.g., multiple-baseline design) (Horner et al., 2005; Maggin, Briesch, & Chafouleas, 2013).

SCDs answer the following questions using variations in the experimental design:

- Does an intervention work? (withdrawal, multielement, multiple baseline, and changing criterion designs)
- Does one intervention work better than another? (reversal design with a simple phase change, multielement designs, multiple baseline designs)
- Do different intervention elements interact to produce behavior change? (reversal designs with complex phase changes, multielement designs, multiple baseline designs comparing different conditions)
- Do treatment effects maintain after treatment is withdrawn? (sequential withdrawal design, partial-withdrawal design, partial sequential withdrawal design, multiple baseline designs with withdrawal of treatment)

In SCD research, *replication* is a key mechanism for controlling threats to internal validity. Horner et al. (2005) stated that replication is established when the design documents *three demonstrations* of the experimental effect at *three different points in time* with a single case. Experimental control is established when the predicted changes in the dependent variable covary with manipulation of the independent variable.

Three major criteria are used to establish an experimental effect: level, trend, and variability. Level refers to the mean score for the data within a phase. Trend refers to the slope of the best-fitting straight line for the data within a phase. Variability refers to the fluctuation of the data around the mean (e.g., range or standard deviation). In addition to these three criteria, four other criteria are used to determine an experimental effect: immediacy of the effect, the proportion of overlap in the data, the consistency of the data across phases, and comparing observed and projected patterns of the outcome variable.

Kratochwill et al. (2010) established the following rules to determine whether a study's design meets evidence standards, meets evidence standards with reservations, or does not meet evidence standards. In order to meet evidence standards, the following design criteria must be present:

- The independent variable (i.e., the intervention) must be systematically manipulated with the researcher determining when and how the independent variable conditions change. If this standard is not met, the study does not meet evidence standards.

- Each outcome variable must be measured systematically over time by more than one observer, and the study needs to collect interobserver agreement (IOA) in each phase and on at least 20% of the data points in each condition. IOA must meet minimal standards of 80% for percentage agreement or .60 using Cohen's kappa. If these standards are not met, the study does not meet evidence standards.

The study must include at least three attempts to demonstrate an intervention effect at three different points in time or with three different phase repetitions. If this standard is not met, the study does not meet evidence standards. For a phase to qualify as an attempt to demonstrate an effect, the phase must have a minimum of three data points.

Quantification of Effect in SCDs

Visual inspection of graphed data is by far the most common way researchers using SCDs analyze their data (Horner et al., 2005; Kratochwill et al., 2010). Effects of intervention are determined by comparing baseline levels of performance to during and/or postintervention levels of performance to detect experimental treatment effects. Unlike statistical analyses, SCDs uses the "interocular" test of significance to determine an effect. Visual analysis typically takes place in four steps. First, a predictable baseline pattern is documented. Second, data within each phase are examined to assess within-phase patterns. Third, phase data are compared to data in the adjacent phases to assess whether manipulation of the independent variable is associated with an effect. Fourth, all information from all phases is integrated to determine whether there are at least three demonstrations of an effect at least three different points in time.

Kratochwill et al. (2010) made the following recommendations for combining studies using SCDs:

- A minimum of five SCD research papers examining the intervention that meet evidence standards or meet evidence standards with reservations.
- The SCD studies must be conducted by at least three different research teams at three different geographic locations.
- The combined number of experiments (i.e., SCD examples) across the papers totals at least 20.

Social Validation

Social validity deals with three fundamental questions in experimental research: What should we change? How should we change it? How will we know it was effective? Wolf (1978) is credited with originating the notion of social validity, and it has become common parlance among many researchers and practitioners. Social validity refers to the *social significance* of the intervention goals, the *social acceptability* of intervention procedures to accomplish these goals, and the *social importance* of the effects produced by an intervention. For purposes of this chapter, I will focus on this last aspect of social validation (social importance).

The social importance of the effects produced by an intervention establishes the clinical or practical importance of behavior change. That is, does the quality and quantity of behavior change make a difference in an individual's functioning? Is the behavior now in a "functional" range? The social importance of effects can be evaluated at several levels: the level of proximal effects, that of intermediate effects, and that of distal effects (Fawcett, 1991). Proximal effects represent changes in target behaviors as a function of an intervention (e.g., decreased disruptive behavior, decreased aggressive behavior). Intermediate effects represent concomitant, positive changes in collateral behaviors and outcomes as a function of changes in target behaviors (e.g., increased peer acceptance, reduction is disciplinary referrals, reduced school suspensions). Distal effects represent long-term changes in behavior or outcomes as a function of proximal and intermediate effects (e.g., increased friendships, high school graduation, reduced arrest rates).

Social importance can be determined by subjective judgments obtained from treatment consumers (e.g., teachers, parents), by social comparisons between treated and untreated participants, or by a combination of these two procedures (Kazdin, 1977). One could also socially validate a treatment on three levels: by specifying a priori *ideal* (best performance), *normative* (typical performance), and *deficient* (worst performance) levels (Fawcett, 1991). Thus interventions moving a child from deficient to normative or ideal levels of performance would be considered to have produced socially important changes in behavior.

The above material is designed to enhance one's understanding of how standards and criteria should be used to judge whether a practice or intervention is evidence based. The next section describes how school professionals can apply this information and program evaluation strategies to identify cost-effective approaches for remediating disruptive behavior problems and disorders in school.

Selecting Evidence-Based Approaches for DBDs

This section describes issues and strategies for the identification/selection of intervention approaches and practices that have an acceptable evidence base and that can actually address the problem(s) they are expected to solve. It is important to note that one does not always have to select the *most* efficacious or effective intervention when considering how to intervene with DBD students. Other dimensions are also quite important in this process. Key dimensions such as program–environment fit in relation to the applicable school context, the match between the intervention and the problem behavior types it has been proven to solve, and implementation site-related issues are also very important to consider in this regard. The material presented in the previous section will be particularly helpful in identifying a pool of evidence-based practices for DBDs by applying the provided standards and criteria for judging their efficacy and/or effectiveness. Guidelines for selecting from among a pool of identified emotional–behavioral disorders are provided below.

Substance Abuse and Mental Health Services Administration's Resource Guide for Evidence-Based Practices for DBDs

The U.S. Substance Abuse and Mental Health Services Administration (SAMHSA) has produced a comprehensive and valuable resource kit for professionals focused on interventions for DBDs. This guide to evidence-based practices for DBDs (within school, family, and community contexts) is available from SAMHSA (Center for Mental Health Services, SAMHSA, 1 Choke Cherry Road, Rockville, MD 20857). It can also be downloaded at no cost from *http://store.samhsa.gov/product/Interventions-for-Disruptive-BehaviorDisorders-Evidence-Based-Practices-EBP-KIT-SMA11-4634CD-DVD*. The kit consists of six booklets dealing with key topics such as characteristics and needs of children with DBDs and their families, how to select evidence-based practices, recommended interventions, and implementation issues. One of the kit's most important topics is factors to consider in decision making when selecting evidence-based practices for children with DBDs. Using a yes/no flowchart, this section of the kit guides the user through a six-step process for selecting evidence-based practices targeting disruptive behavior problems and disorders. The following questions must be answered in order to increase the likelihood of selecting an evidence-based practice more likely to work for students with DBDs:

- What is the intervention's level or degree of empirical support?
- Is the study population comparable to yours?
- Are the achieved outcomes meaningful?
- Is the intervention consistent with the agency's function(s)?
- Is the intervention judged acceptable and feasible by staff?
- Is it acceptable to clients (students, teachers and parents)?

Because of the aversive nature and strength of disruptive students' problem behavior, it is imperative that satisfactory answers be obtained for each of these questions. Later in this section, I provide additional questions and suggestions regarding this critical issue.

Types of School Interventions and Disruptiveness of School Routines

There are four types of intervention practices for influencing school performance, commonly applied to students with DBDs, and that vary significantly according to their disruptiveness of school operations and routines: (1) behavioral interventions applied within the school setting; (2) counseling and psychotherapy that are typically delivered in contexts external to the classroom and/or school setting; (3) psycho-pharmacological interventions for conditions such as ADHD, anxiety, and depression that are administered outside school but are designed to influence school behavior positively; and (4) hybrid interventions, such as the First Step to Success early intervention (Walker et al., 1998, 2009), that have multiple components and are applied simultaneously in school and home settings.

In selecting interventions and practices for DBP students in general, there are some generic factors to consider that should drive this decision making process. For example, Anderson and Borgmeier (2010) suggest analyzing office disciplinary referrals (ODRs) to detect which forms of unacceptable student behavior occur most frequently in a school. Teachers should be surveyed regularly to identify which students are engaging in what types of disruptive behavior and/or deficient academic performance and with what frequency. It is essential that the schools in which the practice is to be adopted have the infrastructure, capacity, and staff skills to support its implementation. Other practical issues concern the cost(s) of the intervention in materials and staff time, whether training is required to implement it with integrity, and whether it provides a prescriptive checklist or manual to guide implementation. All of these factors should enter into the practice selection process.

Selection of Interventions for Implementation Outside versus Inside the School Setting

Special contextual considerations are required in selecting intervention approaches and practices that are delivered *outside* versus *inside* the school setting. In addition to mental health-type interventions, psychopharmacological treatments and interventions are also administered outside the school setting, with the purpose of influencing student problem behavior within school, home, and community settings. Common targets of psychopharmacological interventions are conditions and disorders such as ADHD, depression, and stress and anxiety. The empirical literature associated with this intervention approach is highly robust and shows positive outcomes across a range of outcome measures and strong research designs (see Forness, Walker, & Serna, 2014; Konopasek & Forness, 2014).

Selection Considerations for Interventions and Practices Implemented outside the School Setting

There are some important points to consider when evaluating interventions designed to address in-school problems. These approaches are based on the assumption that intervention effects will transfer across settings and register their effects within problem contexts where they are *not* implemented. While psychopharmacological interventions do in fact produce such effects, this is by no means certain for behavioral and psychological treatments. The following questions should be asked of such interventions:

- Do they have an acceptable evidence base?
- How well do they match or potentially solve the problem(s) they are being selected to address?
- Have they been demonstrated efficacious or effective for use with the target student population under consideration (i.e., students with DBDs)?
- Have they produced acceptable effects within the target setting(s) where you plan to implement the practice?
- Is there evidence that practices, such as counseling or psychotherapy, can demonstrably address the problem, and/or its context, even though they are not implemented in the setting where the problem of concern occurs?

Each of these considerations should be evaluated carefully, as any one of them could influence the intervention's potential magnitude of effect. All of the above questions, except the last one, also apply to interventions or practices that are implemented *within* the setting or context in which the problem(s) occurs. However, there are some additional factors that must be considered in the selection and adoption of interventions for delivery within the problem setting. Below I offer some considerations and questions related to interventions of this type.

Selection Considerations for Interventions Implemented within the School Setting and Problem Context

Two issues of particular concern in this regard are (1) whether the achieved effects persist over time within the problem setting in the absence of the practice that produced them (i.e., after its termination or withdrawal), and 2) whether implementation agents (e.g., teachers, behavioral coaches) have the motivation and skills necessary to deliver and implement it well. (See Herman, Reinke, Frey, & Shepard, 2014, for information on applications of motivational interviewing and engagement in school settings.) Regardless of their skill level, if implementation agents in these settings are philosophically opposed to the intervention or object to the ratio they perceive of the *required effort to apply it* versus the *perceived benefits that can be derived from its implementation*, it is likely doomed to failure no matter how robust its evidence base. These factors can be grouped under the rubric of program–environment fit (see Horner, Sugai & Todd, 1994). They are of critical importance in the intervention selection process, as they can be key determinants of an intervention's likely success in solving the targeted problem(s).

In addition to careful consideration of the above issues, the questions below should be asked of interventions or practices that are geared for implementation in the context or situation(s) where the problem actually occurs.

- Can the practice or intervention be implemented seamlessly without disrupting existing classroom or school routines or at least doing so within acceptable disruptive levels? (See Burns & Hoagwood, 2002.)
- Are they consistent with the values and expectations that teachers hold for managing classroom environments (i.e., students should not derive any special benefits for engaging in problem behavior or in attempts to solve it; all students should be treated fairly and equitably; intractable problems that exceed teachers' skill levels and available resources should be someone else's responsibility)?

- If the intervention being considered is universal, are its promoters able to assemble a majority of staff stakeholders in the site to support and participate in it? The schoolwide positive behavioral interventions and supports (SWPBIS) system, for example, requires an 80% buy-in by a school's staff for a 2-year period in order to qualify for SWPBIS adoption and implementation (Sugai & Horner, 2009). This requirement no doubt accounts for some of the remarkable implementation success of this intervention approach and its having been adopted to date by more than 20,000 schools in the United States.
- Can a local champion be identified who is influential among likely implementation agents and can advocate for and promote the intervention or practice once it is adopted?
- Are there adequate resources and administrative supports available to help ensure the implementation process does not fail for this reason?
- Is there evidence that key implementation agents are open to receiving technical assistance and necessary supervision associated with the practice or intervention?

Can the implementation be classified as addressing "teacher-owned" student problems (e.g., teacher defiance, classroom disruption) versus "peer-owned" problems (e.g., bullying, peer harassment and relational aggression)? Students with DBDs present severe challenges for teachers in managing their classroom behavior and for peers in less structured settings such as the playground. However, general education teachers, as a rule, are much more motivated to address teacher-owned than peer-owned problems. This is an important fact to know in selecting DBD interventions.

Considerations of Program–Environment Fit

The careful review and consideration of program–environment fit variables should be a major factor in the selection of evidence-based interventions and practices for use with students with DBDs in school contexts. Together with solid treatment integrity, adequate resources, and administrative support, program–environment fit can exert a major influence on a school's ability to solve many of the problems presented by students with DBDs. The next section presents tips and recommendations for achieving high-quality implementation of evidence-based interventions and best practices.

Key Issues, Tips, and Recommendations for Achieving High-Quality Implementation of DBD Strategies in School Contexts

The interventions and practices to be described in subsequent chapters are organized around the following dimensions: (1) coverage of the K–12 age–grade span but with a primary emphasis on early intervention in the preschool and elementary developmental-grade levels; (2) use of proven strategies and tactics for DBPs; and (3) addressing home-only, school-only, and multicomponent interventions that are implemented across home and school contexts. In using this organizing framework, our goal is to contextualize evidence-based interventions and practices so that professional consumers are better able to match their needs with available intervention resources for use with students with DBDs. We will give special emphasis to secondary (Tier 2) intervention approaches within this framework, as advocated by SWPBIS professionals, since the behavior problems of students with DBDs are generally not easily solved by universal intervention approaches alone due to their severity and intractability. Our purpose in this section is (1) to provide access to some websites that list evidence-based interventions and practices that are targeted for students with disruptive behavior problems and disorders and (2) to provide some essential recommendations regarding the generic implementation of evidence-based practices in school contexts and settings that we believe improve their outcomes. This information should help determine whether they can be implemented with integrity in a particular context.

As noted earlier, we give special attention to secondary or Tier 2 interventions and practices for students with DBDs. We do so because (1) students with DBDs have problem behavior repertoires that are often resistant to tactics of adult influence; (2) they are expert at training school staff to avoid, punish, and inadvertently reinforce their problem behavior as illustrated in Chapter 1; (3) their investment in problem behavior often has a long history and is frequently reinforced and supported outside the school setting; and (4) Tier 2 approaches have received much less attention in the professional literature than Tier 1 or Tier 3 interventions (Seeley et al., 2014).

Some websites, available to school professionals, are useful in accessing pools of previously vetted interventions and practices that can be implemented for DBDs. The following websites are available to school professionals for this purpose:

- Social Programs That Work (*www.evidencebasedprograms. org*)
- Blueprints for Violence Prevention: (*www.colorado.edu/cspv/ blueprints/index.html*)
- The What Works Clearinghouse (*www.whatworks.ed.gov*)
- Campbell Collaboration (*www.campbellcollaboration.org*)

Sometimes these online resources also (1) identify which interventions are manualized and (2) indicate whether training and technical assistance is available for assisting with implementation. Settings that adopt the Blueprint series empirically based interventions, for example, can apply for resources, supported by federal grants, to support implementation.

There are numerous such websites available with recommended lists of intervention programs and vetted practices. However, when dealing with disruptive students, I *highly* recommend accessing the SAMHSA website on DBDs described above since (1) it profiles 18 evidence-based interventions that have been specifically developed for and tested with students having DBDs on a series of relevant variables, and (2) it provides recommended guidelines on how to implement these interventions with integrity. I have also found the federally funded School Mental Health Project at UCLA, directed by Howard S. Adelman and Linda Taylor, to be an excellent resource on school interventions for challenging behavior and academic performance problems. This center also develops and disseminates important information on school ecology and how it affects the way schools accommodate marginalized students. Their resources can be accessed at *www.smhp.psych.ucla.edu*.

While general education, and often special education teachers, are the primary implementers of DBD interventions, it is important that they not be expected to do so alone. At a minimum, the teacher needs to be the focus of some sort of school-based support structure such as a schoolwide teacher assistance team (SWAT) or a behavioral coach who has the time and skills to supervise the delivery process and to troubleshoot it in collaboration with the teacher. Teachers often feel abandoned in this process and then blamed when the intervention or practice doesn't produce the expected effects. As noted earlier, regular monitoring of the implementing teacher's motivation and ongoing view of the intervention's success is extremely important and should be the focus of problem-solving efforts at the earliest sign of trouble (see Herman et al., 2014).

Planning for Implementation of Evidence-Based Practices for Students with DBDs

Anderson and Borgmeier (2010) have addressed the issue of careful planning by a coach-teacher or a support team for implementation of a Tier 2 intervention. Table 2.1 lays out essential information about the Check-In/Check-Out intervention in terms of what it will accomplish and how it will do so. This sort of preplanning is essential to implementing evidence-based practices in general education settings.

Following are recommended procedures that should be adhered to in planning and implementing evidence-based interventions for students with DBDs. They are based on: (1) my experience in designing, implementing, and reporting on interventions for DBDs in schools; (2) the Coalition for Evidence-Based Policy (Gorman-Smith, 2006); (3) the specific works of Anderson and Borgmeier (2010), Hawken, Vincent, and Schumann (2008), and Sugai and Horner (2009); and (4) SAMHSA's (2012) *Non-Researcher's Guide for Implementing Evidence-Based Practices.*

Intervene with the Problem Behavior in the Setting(s) Where the Problem Occurs

I recommend assessing and analyzing the student's problem behavior in all settings where it is reported to be unacceptable or destructive and using this information to determine intervention sites. *I strongly recommend that the problem be dealt with where it occurs.* The adage, "What you teach is what you get and where you teach it is where you get it!" applies here. So, for example, trying to solve a bullying problem on the playground by intervening with the student in the classroom is generally not a good idea. One needs to intervene with the student on the playground and/or with peers (where the problem can be dealt with directly) in order to have a chance of addressing this problem. Counseling and mental health therapies can be used to supplement this approach, but they are unlikely to produce detectable behavioral changes and should not be used to try solving this problem in isolation.

Identify the Key Features of the Intervention That Account for Positive Outcomes

Most interventions for students with DBDs have more than one simple feature or essential procedure due to the difficulties involved in solving their behavior problems. Often, the more severe the problem behavior,

TABLE 2.1. Guiding Questions for the Check-In/Check-Out Intervention

1. Determine personnel needs and logistics.
   - Who will be the BEP coordinator?
   - Who will supervise the BEP coordinator?
   - Who will check the students in and out when coordinator is absent? Name at least two people who can substitute for the coordinator.
   - Where will check-in and check-out occur?
   - How many students can be served on the BEP at one time?

2. Develop a daily progress report.
   - What will the behavioral expectations be?
   - Are the expectations positively stated?
   - Is the DPR teacher-friendly? How often will teachers be asked to complete the DPR?
   - Is the DPR age-appropriate, and does it include a range of scores?
   - Are the data easy to summarize?

3. Develop a reinforcement system for students on the BEP.
   - What will the students daily point goal be?
   - What reinforcers will students receive for checking in?
   - What reinforcers will students receive for check-in and check-out and meeting their daily point goal?
   - How will you ensure students do not become bored with the reinforcers?
   - What are the consequences for students who receive major and minor referrals?

4. Develop a referral system.
   - How will students be referred to the BEP? What are the criteria for placing students on the BEP?
   - What does the parental consent form look like for students participating in the BEP?
   - What is the process for screening students who transfer into the school?
   - What is the process for determining whether students will begin the next school year on the BEP?

5. Develop a system for managing the daily data.
   - Which computer program will be used to summarize the data?
   - Which team in the school will examine the daily BEP data, and how frequently will it be examined?
   - Who is responsible for summarizing the data and bringing it to team meetings?
   - How frequently will data be shared with the whole staff?
   - How frequently will data be shared with parents?

6. Plan to fade students off the intervention.
   - What are the criteria for fading students off the BEP?
   - How will the BEP be faded, and who will be in charge of fading students off the BEP?
   - How will graduation from the BEP be celebrated?
   - What incentives and supports will be put in place for students who graduate from the BEP?

(continued)

TABLE 2.1. (*continued*)

7. Plan for staff training.
   - Who will train the staff on the BEP?
   - Who will provide teachers with individual coaching if the BEP is not being implemented as planned?
   - Who will provide yearly booster sessions about the purposes and key features in implementing the BEP?

8. Plan for student and parent training.
   - Who will meet with students to train them on the BEP?
   - How will parents be trained on the BEP?

Based on Crone, Hawken, and Horner (2010). *Note.* BEP, behavior education program; DPR, daily progress report.

the more complex the intervention or practice has to be. It is extremely important that these critical features be identified and fidelity monitoring procedures be used to monitor the quality and dosage with which they are applied. For example, in applying the First Step to Success early intervention program for students with DBDs, developed by my colleagues and I, we have identified the following as critical program features: (1) providing continuous feedback for the student on the appropriateness of his behavior using a red and green card; (2) maintaining a 4:1 ratio of praise to reprimands by the teacher *and* parents; and (3) arranging for the delivery of group activity rewards at school and individual rewards at home based on the student's school performance (see Walker, et al., 2009, 2014). Often, applied interventions fail in schools because of low dosage problems; that is, the practice is not fully implemented with sufficient frequency. However, failing to monitor and troubleshoot the intervention's critical features is also a frequent reason for such failure.

Match the Intervention's Strength to the Intractability or Severity of the Student's Problem Behavior

While it is very important to carefully match the intervention with the problem type(s) displayed by the student, it is also important to attend to the relationship between the strength of the intervention and the strength of the student's problem behavior. Admittedly, this can be an imprecise process. However, common sense dictates that some approximations be made in this regard in both the selection and implementation of interventions. For example, it makes little sense to try solving a severe problem of relational aggression among peers by using group self-esteem training or to use teacher praise to cope with a student's habit of defying the teacher's directives. We do not know of any scientific methods for addressing this issue, but it is important and should be a part of any planning process for students with DBDs in school.

Assess and Carefully Monitor Implementation Fidelity

I have long been identified as an expert on implementation fidelity, which refers to the extent to which an intervention or practice is applied according to the guidelines essential for ensuring its success (see Gresham, Mac-Millan, 2000). This topic, sometimes referred to as treatment integrity, has emerged as the sine qua non of research on the efficacy and effectiveness of applied school interventions. Research shows that it is a frequently identified reason for why interventions fail (Anderson & Borgmeier, 2010). It has been said the 20th century was about demonstrating that treatments worked and that the 21st will be about analyzing why and how they do or don't work. Investigations of implementation fidelity will be one of the most fruitful avenues for examining this question. It is essential that this variable be monitored directly, carefully and often, as the intervention or practice is applied using checklists and observations.

Plan for the Intervention's Effects to Be Sustained and Extended to Other Settings as Necessary

Research has clearly shown that social-behavioral gains produced by applied interventions in schools rarely are sustained within intervention settings, and generalization to nonintervention settings is even more rare (Gresham, 2002; Horner & Billingsley, 1988; Walker et al., 2014). As a rule, such effects must be carefully engineered by behavioral specialists. As a matter of course, one should not *expect* intervention effects to be sustained when a practice that produced them is abruptly terminated or withdrawn. For example, it often is necessary to provide a list of "maintenance" strategies for school staff who implement the First Step Program in order to ensure sustainability of achieved effects in the period between the program's completion until the end of the school year. Often, we have been called back to address a student's problem behavior at the beginning of the next school year who had received the First Step Program the pervious year (Walker et al., 2014).

Aside from the "behavioral laws" that control the durability and transfer of such effects, a change in teachers and a new mix of peers in the following school year can work strongly against the maintenance of behavioral gains. Barkley (2007) has provided a perceptive analysis of the decay of an intervention's effects following its withdrawal. He argues that behavioral interventions alter the natural social-behavioral contingencies operating in a classroom between and among teachers and students. When the intervention is abruptly withdrawn or terminated, those contingency arrangements are likely to revert to their form and status prior to the intervention. Taking the above two factors into account (i.e., changes in teachers and peers and alteration of a setting's natural contingencies) in planning for sustainability is crucial and should be addressed by any team of school support personnel charged with solving the problems of students with DBDs.

Concluding Remarks

This chapter has focused on three important factors regarding DBDs in schools: (1) criteria and standards for judging evidence-based interventions and practices, (2) recommendations for identifying and selecting evidence-based practices, and (3) tips and guidelines for planning and implementing evidence-based practices in school settings. In the chapters that follow, I apply this information to the presentation of strategies and tactics that can make a clear difference in the school success and social-behavioral adjustment of students with DBDs. Illustrating their effective application in this context will be a high priority for our efforts.

Chapter Summary Points

- What constitutes evidence and how it is classified varies across fields such as physics, law, education, and psychology.

- Evidence does not fall neatly into a dichotomy of evidence-based and non-evidence-based categories.

- Evidence exists on a continuum anchored by poles of strong support and no support and considers a broad range of evidence generated by different research methods.

- Evidence-based treatments are interventions that have been shown to be efficacious through rigorous research methods that have good internal validity. Evidence-based practices are approaches to intervention rather than specific interventions.

- Efficacy research involves a focus on measurable effects of specific interventions with the randomized controlled trial being the prototypical example. Effectiveness research seeks to determine whether treatments have measurable beneficial effects in real-world settings.

- Multiple types of research evidence are used to support evidence-based practices, including: (1) efficacy studies, (2) effectiveness studies, (3) cost–benefit/cost-effectiveness studies, and (4) epidemiological studies.

- Various types of research designs or methods are used to establish evidence, including: observation, qualitative research, single-case experimental designs, epidemiological research, moderator/mediator studies, randomized controlled trials, effectiveness studies, and meta-analyses.

- Four threats to valid inference making have been identified: (1) internal validity threats, (2) external validity threats, (3) construct validity threats, and (4) statistical conclusion validity threats.

- Empirical evidence for various treatments include: (1) well-established treatments, (2) probably efficacious treatments, (3) possibly efficacious treatments, and (4) experimental treatments.

- Six types of studies include: Type 1 studies that include randomized controlled trials; Type 2 studies that are missing at least one component of Type 1 studies; Type 3 studies that involve the collection of pilot data; Type 4 studies reviews with secondary data analyses such as meta-analyses; Type 5 studies that are literature reviews without secondary data analyses; and Type 6 studies that are case studies, essays, and opinion/position papers.

- Single-case experimental designs are interrupted time-series studies that provide a rigorous experimental evaluation of intervention effects.

- Single-case experimental designs include: (1) reversal or withdrawal designs; (2) iterative manipulation of the independent variables across different observation phases (multielement or alternating treatments designs); and (3) staggered introduction of the independent variable across different points in time (multiple baseline design).

- Single-case designs use replication as the key mechanism for controlling threats to internal validity.

- Replication involves documenting three demonstrations of an experimental effect at three different points in time.

- The criteria used to establish an experimental effect include: (1) level, (2) trend, (3) variability, (4) immediacy of effect, (5) proportion of overlap in data, (6) consistency of data across phases, and (7) comparison of observed and projected patterns in the outcome variable.

- Single-case experimental designs primarily use visual inspection of graphed data to analyze data.

- Single-case design researchers recommend the following for combining studies: (1) a minimum of five research papers that meet evidence standards or meet evidence standards with reservations; (2) studies must be conducted by at least three different research teams at three different geographic locations; and (3) there must be at least 20 experiments across papers.

- The social importance of the effects produced by a treatment establishes the clinical or applied importance of behavior change.

- Consider selecting interventions or practices for adoption that meet the relative rather than threshold standard of efficacy or effectiveness.

- Aside from demonstrated efficacy/effectiveness, a host of dimensions should be attended to in the selection process, including program–environment fit, the match between problem type and the intervention, and demonstration(s) that the intervention has been successful in settings similar to yours.

- It is important to ensure that the site or setting in which the intervention or practice is to be implemented can support a successful application.

- As the primary delivery agent for most school-based interventions, the classroom teacher usually ends up being responsible for implementation and must be fully supported in this role.

- When planning the implementation of a new or innovative practice, it is important to engage in a preplanning process that provides a roadmap for how to administer it.

- Implementation planning should include a process for withdrawing or reducing the intervention so that its effects can be sustained.

Evidence-Based Assessment Strategies

Screening, Identification, Progress Monitoring, and Outcomes

This chapter describes the types of assessment that are important for understanding and dealing effectively with DBDs. Reliable, valid, and accurate assessment of DBDs is an indispensible first step in intervening effectively with this behavior pattern. The main purpose of any assessment process is to collect information that will lead to correct decisions about the individuals involved. At least five types of decisions can be made in the assessment process: (1) screening, (2) identification and classification, (3) intervention, (4) progress monitoring, and (5) documentation of intervention outcomes.

Another way of conceptualizing the above types of decisions is to think of them as different types of "tests." For example, a *screening test* looks for a specific problem or disease. A hearing screening test detects hearing impairments. A *diagnostic test* looks for a disease. Biopsy of a lump on the breast determines whether an individual has breast cancer. A *treatment decision* test is designed to guide intervention decisions. A cholesterol panel guides prescription of anti-statin drugs. A *monitoring test* tracks the progress of a disease. For example, blood pressure monitoring tracks the progress of hypertension.

Decision Making in Assessment

Screening Decisions

Screening decisions are based on the evaluation of an entire population to determine whether they require more specialized, expensive,

47

and comprehensive assessments. For example, hearing screenings are routinely conducted in schools to determine which students should be referred for more comprehensive and expensive audiological examinations. Similarly, physicians screen for breast cancer in women using mammograms or for prostate cancer in males by analyzing prostate-specific antigen levels.

Screening tools are advantageous because they are brief and easy to administer and are typically effective in identifying children at risk for DBDs. Early screening for DBDs is essential for prevention. The longer these children go without effective interventions, the more intense and resistant their problem behavior will be later in their school careers (Kazdin, 1987).

There are two types of errors made in using screening tools: *false positive errors* and *false negative errors*. A false positive error occurs when a child is identified as having a DBD when, in fact, he or she does not have the problem. The cost of false positive errors is that a child might receive an expensive, labor-intensive intervention that he or she does not need. A false negative error is more costly and occurs when a student is not identified as having a DBD when in fact she or he does have one.

Note that we are willing to tolerate more false positive errors in making screening decisions than we would in making classification, intervention, or program evaluation decisions. In contrast, we are not willing to make too many false negative errors in the identification of DBDs. False negative errors in the identification of DBDs must be avoided because of the well-known developmental progression of this behavior pattern that intensifies and becomes more resistant to change over time. In fact, Kazdin (1987) reviews evidence showing that if these children are not identified by age 8, and their problems addressed, they are very likely to have a lifelong pattern of conduct problems and anti-social behavior.

Classification Decisions

Classification decisions are based on more comprehensive and expensive assessments than screening decisions. Information used in making classification decisions might include: (1) broadband norm-referenced behavior rating scales completed by parents, teaches, and students; (2) narrow-band focused behavior rating scales targeting specific types of problems (e.g., ADHD, oppositional defiant disorder, anxiety, depression); (3) interviews with parents, teachers, and students; and (4) school records, developmental histories, and systematic direct observations. Classification decisions are based on performance of children and adolescents that differ substantially from their normal or typical peers and correspond to the characteristics that define a condition or disorder. For example, research on antisocial behavior shows that it is desirable and necessary to identify and classify students who demonstrate characteristics of *both* ADHD and conduct disorder (Lynam, 1996; Waschbush, 2002).

Progress Monitoring Decisions

Progress monitoring of child and adolescent behaviors is crucial in determining whether an intervention is effective in changing behavior. Examples of progress monitoring tools are systematic direct observations in naturalistic environments (classrooms or homes), work samples of academic performance, school–home notes, brief behavior rating scales, and direct behavioral reports (Cook, Volpe, & Delport, 2014; Lane, Oakes, Menzies, & Germer, 2014). Progress monitoring uses individuals' baseline levels of performance as the criterion against which the effects of intervention are compared or evaluated.

Intervention Decisions

Intervention decisions are based on assessment information that relates directly to choices of interventions designed to change behavior. The most important criterion in making intervention decisions is *treatment validity*, which refers to the degree to which assessment information contributes to beneficial treatment outcomes (Hayes, Nelson, & Jarrett, 1987). The key in establishing treatment validity is to show a clear relationship between the assessment information collected and the treatment planning process. Specifically, for any assessment procedure to have treatment validity, it must lead to the identification of target behaviors, result in more effective treatments, and be useful in evaluating treatment outcomes (Gresham & Lambros, 1998). The practice of *functional behavioral assessment* is based on a treatment validity notion or standard. In functional behavioral assessment, interventions are selected and implemented based on systematic assessment of behavioral function or particular purpose that a behavior serves for an individual (Gresham, Watson, & Skinner, 2001).

Program Evaluation Decisions

Data concerning the effectiveness of intervention programs are important in making decisions about continuing, modifying, or discontinuing them. The concept of *response to intervention* (RTI) is based on the systematic making program intervention decisions using reliable, valid, and accurate assessment data. RTI assigns students to increasingly intensive intervention levels (universal, selected, and intensive) based on their unresponsiveness to less intensive levels of intervention (Gresham, Reschly, & Shinn, 2010). Program evaluation decisions can also be used to conduct cost–benefit analyses to support continued or increased resources for intervention programs.

Assumptions in Assessment

Central to the assessment process are the assumptions that underlie the use of procedures to make decisions about individuals. The rules by which we judge whether assessment procedures are reliable, accurate, and valid are well established. A particularly valuable heuristic to guide assessment practices was presented by Messick (1995), who argued that the validity of any assessment process must be based on (1) whether it accomplishes some clear purpose (identification, classification, intervention) and (2) whether the consequences of using it benefit the individuals involved. Consistent with our earlier definition, valid assessment leads to correct decisions about individuals. In turn, these decisions should lead to beneficial outcomes for individuals.

It is important to understand the assumptions on which assessment practices are based:

- *Assumption 1*: Individual differences among children and adolescents are relative rather than absolute.
- *Assumption 2*: Assessments are samples of behavior.
- *Assumption 3*: The primary reason for assessment is to improve intervention.
- *Assumption 4*: All types of assessment contain error.
- *Assumption 5*: Good assessment involves gathering information about the environment.

With regard to Assumption 1, children and adolescents often differ from their peers on at least one dimension. The key question is whether we should be concerned about such differences. Making this determination often depends on the expectations regarding a particular child's situation. Specific forms of behavior, for example, might be considered normal in one setting or situation and deviant or abnormal in another setting, depending on the context. For example, a boy engaging in disruptive and aggressive behavior might be considered to have a behavior problem if he attends a school in which most students are compliant and well-behaved. However, if that same boy attends a chaotic school where most students engage in disruptive and aggressive behavior, he would not be considered deviant or abnormal relative to the other students at the school.

According to Assumption 2 (assessments are samples of behavior), a single assessment procedure should not be used to make decisions about children. Rather, people should make decisions about children and youth based on a full consideration and analysis of all issues. For example, basing a decision about a child's antisocial behavior on a 10-minute playground observation would not be considered best practice because it would be based on an inadequate sample of behavior. Similarly, basing a decision about a child's behavior solely on the results of a brief behavior rating scale completed by a teacher would be inappropriate for the same reason. Collecting and integrating samples of behavior from multiple sources will help ensure that decisions are based on an adequate knowledge base that involves multimethod, multi-informant, and multisetting assessments.

With regard to Assumption 3 (the primary reason for assessment is to improve intervention), assessment can have many goals, ranging from determining the causes of problem behavior to determining whether the child is responding to an intervention program. However, the ultimate goal of assessment should be to guide the selection, implementation, and evaluation of intervention efforts. This requires that assessment procedures have adequate treatment validity, reliability, and sensitivity.

According to Assumption 4, error is present in any assessment activity, test, or evaluation procedure. For example, polygraph tests (lie detectors) are inadmissible in courts of law because they contain too much error (10–25%). Many tests used in schools and clinics by educators and psychologists contain even more error, but are often used to make important long-term decisions about students.

Measurement error is a direct reflection of the *unreliability* of test scores. Unreliability in test scores comes from a variety of sources. First, the items on a test may not correlate highly with each other, thereby creating inconsistency in the measurement of a particular trait. Second, test scores may fluctuate over time, thereby creating instability in the measurement process. Finally, observers or raters who measure behavior may disagree among themselves regarding the frequency or occurrence of behavior, thereby introducing error into the assessment process.

Accepting the fact that error exists in all forms of assessment influences practice in two ways. First, it dictates that we be aware of and try to minimize factors that contribute to such errors of measurement. Second, knowing that error is always present makes it essential that we use and interpret assessment data in a cautious and professional manner.

Finally, according to Assumption 5 (good assessment involves gathering information about the environment), the kinds of assessment information that are gathered can directly influence the inferences we make about children's behavior. If we collect information only about the child in question, then we will likely view the problem as a within-child problem. A well-established finding from the field of social psychology indicates that observers of another person's behavior are likely to attribute the causes of that behavior to internal, stable predispositions or traits and minimize environmental or situational causes of that behavior (Jones & Nisbett, 1972). For example, teachers are more likely to attribute a child's aggressive behavior to the internal trait of aggressiveness rather than consider possible situational causes for that behavior (e.g., being provoked, teased, or made fun of).

An alternative assessment practice would be to collect not only teacher rating information but also data on specific environmental factors that may contribute to the child's behavior. For example, we might find that problem behaviors are much more frequent in unstructured settings and activities (e.g., on the playground) than in structured settings (e.g., the classroom). We might also discover that problem behaviors are less likely to occur with preferred peers and more likely to occur in the presence of nonpreferred peers. Finally, we might also learn that these problem behaviors result in peer social attention, which reinforces their continued occurrence. Clearly, by not collecting this type of contextual information, we risk making some faulty assumptions about the cause of behavior problems.

Assessment within a Problem-Solving Model

Good assessment practice takes place within a problem-solving model focused on making screening, classification, progress monitoring, intervention planning, and program evaluation decisions. Problem solving can be defined as the process by which one determines that (1) a significant discrepancy exists between an individual's current level of performance and a desired level of performance and (2) strategies are developed to reduce or eliminate this discrepancy (Gresham, 1991, 2002).

In this model, "problem" is a relative concept because a discrepancy may vary according to the perceptions of different social agents in the child's environment. For instance, parents may not report a discrepancy between how the child is behaving and how they want their child to behave. In contrast, the child's teacher and principal may see a huge discrepancy between current and desired levels of performance in academic, social, personal, and/or behavioral domains.

Once current and desired levels of performance are defined in operational terms, this discrepancy becomes the focus of the problem-solving assessment process. Defining problems in this manner is based on the belief that problems are a result of unsuccessful or discrepant interactions between persons (e.g., child and peers, child and teacher, child and parent, or parent and teacher). As such, the person identified as having the problem, as well as his or her interactions with the environment, must be examined in order to understand and change the problem behavior. Many children with DBDs come to school with a long list of non-school-related risk factors operating in their lives and a learning history that has shaped many of their problems (see Chapter 1). However, the focus of a problem-solving model is to identify and intervene on those variables over which parents, educators, and others have some control.

In this model, problem solving takes place in a four-step process, with specific objectives for each step (Bergan & Kratochwill, 1990). These four steps or phases are (1) *problem identification*, (2) *problem analysis*, (3) *plan implementation*, and (4) *problem evaluation*. In other words, we are attempting to answer the following questions: (1) What is the problem? (2) Why is it occurring? (3) What shall we do to change it? and (4) How will we know it was effective? The first step in this process is to obtain a clear, objective definition of the problem behavior(s). As we see later in this chapter, the screening process uses objective operational definitions of DBDs. Once the problem behavior is clearly defined, the next step is to analyze factors that may be contributing to the acquisition and maintenance of the behavior. After defining specific behaviors and analyzing factors contributing to their occurrence, the next step is to plan and implement an intervention to change the target behaviors. The final step in this problem-solving process is to evaluate the degree to which the implemented intervention was effective in reducing or eliminating the problem behaviors.

Assessment information in each of these four steps is gathered from a variety of sources. Some information is obtained from archival school records, school cumulative folders, and other records. Additional information on the child's developmental history might be gathered from parents. Still other information is gathered from interviews, systematic direct observations, and behavior rating scales, achievement tests, and past evaluations. Table 3.1 shows the objectives for each of the four steps or stages in the problem-solving process.

Subsequent sections of this chapter describe specific problem-solving assessment strategies for making decisions about children and youth who are at risk or are displaying DBDs. We begin with a discussion of risk and protective factors that either contribute to or buffer children from the destructive effects of DBDs. Later sections illustrate procedures for making decisions regarding early screening, classification, and intervention approaches that can be used in progress monitoring and program evaluation.

Identification of Risk and Protective Factors

A number of risk and protective factors operating within family, school, and community contexts have been associated with severe social, emotional, and behavioral excesses and deficits. However, the extent to which these risk and protective factors within these interlocking systems moderate or mediate the development and maintenance of behavioral difficulties is unclear (Crews et al., 2007).

Understanding risk and protective factors in the development of social, emotional, and behavioral difficulties is important for at least three reasons. First, significant numbers of these children and youth experience short-term and long-term negative outcomes and/or fail to achieve positive outcomes (Walker, Ramsey, & Gresham, 2004). Second, current policy imperatives dictate a consideration of risk and protective factors as preventive strategies (Kellam, 2002; Zigler, Taussig, & Black, 1992). Finally, a consideration of risk and protective factors may moderate children's response to intervention (Sugai & Horner, 1999; Walker et al., 1997). Much of the prior meta-analytic risk/protection research has focused on single outcomes or single risk/protective factors; thus, the interrelationships that exist between the entire range of outcomes and contributing factors is not apparent. Research suggests that risk and protective factors can be distinguished and quantified and that risk and protective factors that influence multiple outcomes may exist (Crews et al., 2007).

TABLE 3.1. Objectives of the Problem-Solving Model

Problem identification

- Define behaviors in operational, measurable terms.
- Prioritize behavioral concerns.
- Describe planned methods of assessment.
- Describe events preceding target behavior.
- Describe events following behavior.
- Describe discrepancy between observed and expected performance.
- Set goals for intervention outcomes.

Problem analysis

- Formulate reasonable hypotheses about factors affecting the problem.
- Focus on factors over which we have control.
- Generate solutions based on presumed function of target behavior(s).

Plan implementation

- Define responsibilities of all parties involved.
- Determine need for training intervention implementers.
- Conduct skills training as necessary.
- Assess and monitory treatment integrity.

Problem evaluation

- Evaluate degree to which intervention was implemented.
- Evaluate effectiveness of intervention.
- Evaluate social validity from perspectives of different consumers.

What Are Risk and Protective Factors and How Do They Operate?

Risk factors refer to conditions or characteristics that are associated with poor developmental outcomes or with the failure to achieve positive outcomes (Nash & Bowen, 2002). Many developmental risk factors are not disorder specific, but rather may be related to multiple maladaptive outcomes. Factors such as low socioeconomic status, low academic achievement, and a history of physical and/or emotional abuse all are risk factors in developing DBDs. Given that single risk factors may predict multiple outcomes and that a great deal of overlap occurs between behavioral markers, interventions focusing on reduction of interacting risk factors may have direct effects on multiple outcomes (Coie et al., 1993; Dryfoos, 1990). Risk factors arise in diverse contexts within an ecological model and, as such, interventions addressing risks in a single context are unlikely to be sufficient to eliminate or significantly ameliorate problem behaviors (Rutter, 1982).

Protective factors are variables that reduce the likelihood of maladaptive outcomes given conditions of risk. Positive developmental outcomes are more likely when protective factors are present at multiple system levels (Nash & Bowen, 2002; Kazdin, 1991). Rutter (1985) identified three contexts in which protective factors arise: (1) within-child, (2) family, and (3) community. The within-child context includes characteristics of the individual such as cognitive skills, social-cognitive skills, temperamental characteristics, and social skills. The family context includes the child's interactions with the environment, such as secure attachment to parents. The community context includes bonding or affiliating with prosocial peers or other adults.

The etiology of DBDs is complex and a single risk factor is not likely to be responsible for any given behavior pattern, nor is any single protective factor likely to be sufficient to prevent the development of problematic behavior patterns (Greenberg, Domitovich, & Bumbarger, 2001; Greenberg, Speltz, & DeKylen, 1993). Sameroff and Seifer (1990) concluded that no single factor, whether considered risk or protective, can account for children's emotional or behavioral disorders/adjustment. Moreover, not all children experiencing the same risk factors ever develop emotional and behavioral disorders. Researchers typically find a nonlinear relationship between risk factors and outcomes, suggesting that a single risk factor may have a small effect, but also find that rates of DBDs increase rapidly with the accumulation of additional risk factors (Rutter, 1979; Sameroff, Seifer, Barocas, Zax, & Greenspan, 1987). In addition, risk and protective factors are not equal in importance; accordingly, a primary challenge is to identify and target those risk and protective factors that are of greatest influence when seeking to promote positive outcomes and prevent negative outcomes (Fraser, 1997; Nash & Bowen, 2002).

Meta-Analytic Findings on Risk and Protective Factors

Crews et al. (2007) conducted a literature synthesis of 18 meta-analyses that have investigated risk and protective factors of externalizing behavior problems. This "mega-analysis" was based on 500 primary studies and effect sizes for risk and protective factors were reported in terms of Pearson r in order to have a standard unit of effect size. In this analysis, *risk* described a positive relationship with a negative outcome or a negative relationship with a desirable outcome. *Protection* described either a positive relationship with a desired outcome or a negative relationship with a problematic outcome.

Table 3.2 shows that the risk factors most highly correlated with DBDs are lack of bonding to school (r = .86), having delinquent peers

TABLE 3.2 Risk Factors for Disruptive Behavior Disorders

Risk factor	Median r
Lack of bonding to school	.86
Delinquent peers	.49
Internalizing comorbidity	.47
Prior antisocial behavior	.41
Low academic achievement	.41
Nonsupportive home environment	.41
Corporal punishment by parents	.41
Controversial sociometric status	.41
Violent video game exposure	.29
Rejected sociometric status	.25
Victim of abuse	.14
Substance abuse	.14
Poor social skills	.14
Low socioeconomic status	.12
Criminal commitment	.12
Nonsevere pathology	.10
Neglected sociometric status	.10
Male	.10
Racial minority	.03

(r = .49), and having a comorbid internalizing disorder (e.g., anxiety, depression)(r = .47). Five risk factors showed identical correlations with DBDs (r = .1) and included prior history of antisocial behavior, low academic achievement, nonsupportive home environments, corporal punishment by parents, and controversial sociometric status. Several risk factors showed virtually no relationship with DBDs such as low socioeconomic status, substance abuse, poor social skills, racial minority status, and being male (r = .03 to .14).

Table 3.3 depicts the protective factors associated with DBDs. Age at first juvenile justice commitment (r = .34), adequate academic performance (r = .33), and positive play activities with peers (r = .26) were the three highest protective factors for DBDs. Being popular with peers, having a high IQ, and having high socioeconomic status did not operate as substantial protective factors for this behavior pattern.

The breadth of the contexts in which risk and protective factors arise suggests that interventions targeting factors beyond the individual child may be more effective than focusing solely on building children's

TABLE 3.3. Protective Factors for Disruptive Behavior Disorders

Protective factor	Median r
Age at first commitment	.34
Adequate academic achievement	.33
Play activities	.26
Corporal punishment	.24
Intact family structure	.24
Popular sociometric status	.18
High IQ	.14
Neglected sociometric status	.10
High socioeconomic status	.10

strengths or remediating areas of risk. Several of the identified risk factors are malleable and can be altered, such as lack of bonding to school, internalizing comorbidity, low academic achievement, association with delinquent peers, and nonsupportive home environments. Other risk factors are immutable and thus not amenable to intervention, such as prior antisocial behavior and controversial sociometric status. The three strongest protective factors are reasonable targets for early intervention and include age at first commitment, adequate academic performance, and positive play activities with peers. It is important to note that this analysis identified *moderators* (correlates) of DBDs in terms of risk and protection and it remains for future research to identify *mediators* (causes) of DBDs.

Early Identification and Screening of DBDs

Many fields have well-established practices for early identification of problems that lead to early, more effective treatments. For instance, in medicine routine screening procedures such as Pap tests to detect early stages of cervical cancer or prostate-specific antigen tests to detect prostate cancer have been routine medical practice for years. Unfortunately, similar proactive early identification approaches for DBDs have been the exception rather than the rule. As discussed in the previous section, we know a great deal about risk factors that predict quite accurately which children will develop social and emotional behavioral problems later in life. The technology for making these predictions is gradually becoming

more accurate for children at younger ages, yet the practice of early identification remains static (Severson & Walker, 2002; Walker, Severson &
Seeley, 2010).

Bullis and Walker (1994) have discussed the irony of teachers consistently ranking children with severe behavior disorders as one of their
highest service priorities, even though prevalence studies indicate that
this school population continues to be seriously underidentified (Forness, Kim, & Walker, 2012; Walker, Nishioka, Zeller, Severson, & Feil,
2000). In fact, Kauffman (1999) suggests that the field of education
actually "prevents prevention" of behavior disorders of at-risk children
through well-meaning efforts to protect them from such factors as label-
ing and stigmatization associated with the screening/identification process.

We know that children who have not learned to achieve their social
goals other than though coercive behavioral strategies by about age 8
years of age will likely continue displaying some degree of antisocial
behavior throughout their lives (Bullis & Walker, 1994; Kazdin, 1987;
Loeber & Farrington, 1998). In the absence of early identification, these
problems will morph into more serious and violent behavior patterns.

Technical Considerations
in Early Identification and Screening

Screening instruments and approaches must have established levels of
technical adequacy before they can be used to accurately identify children who are at risk for DBDs. Technical adequacy subsumes the concepts of reliability and validity (predictive accuracy). Reliability refers to
the consistency with which individuals are identified as being either at
risk or not at risk. Three types of reliability are relevant here: *internal
consistency reliability, test–retest reliability,* and *interrater reliability.*
Internal consistency reliability refers to the average interrcorrelations
among items on a screening tool and reflects the extent to which items
"hang" together. Test–retest reliability refers to the degree to which a
screening tool yields comparable scores at two or more points in time (Is
it stable over time?). Interrater reliability refers to the degree to which
two or more raters agree with each other at one point in time (Do they
view the person being rated in the same way?).

The validity of screening approaches is reflected in their accuracy
in identifying or detecting at-risk status. In other words, is the level

of predictive accuracy sufficiently high to justify the use of a screening procedure (Lane et al., 2014). Figure 3.1 shows the dimensions that are germane to assessing predictive accuracy. *Sensitivity* reflects the proportion of persons with a given outcome (e.g., a DBD) who have a particular risk indicator and reflects the correct identification of membership in the at-risk group (i.e., a true positive identification). *Specificity* reflects the proportion of persons without the outcome who do not have the risk indicator (i.e., a true negative identification). Positive predictive power (PPP) is the proportion of individuals classified as at-risk who develop the outcome. Negative predictive power (NPP) is the proportion of persons classified as not at risk who do not develop the outcome.

Two types of errors in predictive accuracy are inherent in the use of behavioral screening measures. As noted earlier, false positive errors involve identifying persons as having a problem when they do not. Thus a person with a risk indicator would be inaccurately identified to have the outcome (DBD) when he or she did not. False positive errors are shown in Cell B of Figure 3.1. False negative errors result from a failure to predict that individuals will have an outcome when in fact they do. In this case, the risk factor is absent, but the outcome is present (DBD). False negative errors are shown in Cell C of Figure 3.1. The *overall accuracy* of a behavioral screening process is the proportion of individuals correctly classified divided by all decisions make (Sensitivity + Specificity/Sensitivity + Specificity + False Positive + False Negative).

A Accurate Prediction (Sensitivity)	B False Positive
C False Negative	D True Negative (Specificity)

Sensitivity: A/A + C
Positive predictive power: A/A + B
Specificity: D/B + D
Negative predictive power: D/C + D
Overall accuracy: A + D/A + B + C + D
Base rate prevalence: A + C/A + B + C + D

FIGURE 3.1. Dimensions of predictive accuracy and inaccuracy.

Screening Tools

Several screening tools have been developed over the past 20 years, and many have been proved useful in correctly identifying at-risk children and youth. These screening tools vary in terms of the dimensions of behavior assessed, age/grade levels of students, and resources needed to implement the screening tool (Lane et al., 2014). In evaluating the utility of screening tools, it is important to pay attention to issues of technical adequacy and feasibility. Screening tools must have empirically established cutoff scores to correctly identify children who have (sensitivity) and who do not have (specificity) an at-risk status while minimizing false positive and false negative error rates. Several screening tools are reviewed in the following sections.

Systematic Screening for Behavior Disorders

The Systematic Screening for Behavior Disorders (SSBD; Walker & Severson, 1990, 2002) is a multiple gating screening device for identifying children having behavior disorders in grades 1–6. It provides a cost-effective mass screening of all students in regular education classrooms on both externalizing and internalizing behavioral dimensions. For the purposes of this book, only externalizing behavior disorders are relevant for students with DBDs. The SSBD is a multiple gating device because it contains a series of linked, sequential assessments known as "gates." It utilizes a combination of teacher nominations (Gate 1), teacher rating scales (Gate 2), and direct observations of classroom and playground behavior (Gate 3) to accomplish the early identification of children who are at risk for DBDs. The SSBD instrument and procedures have long been recognized as a preferred best practice in the universal, proactive, and early screening of students having school-related behavior problems and disorders (Lane, Menzies, Oakes, & Kalberg, 2012).

The SSBD contains three interrelated stages for screening. Gate 1 uses teacher nominations in which teachers are asked to identify three students in their classrooms who match an externalizing behavior profile; that is, problems directed outward by the child toward the external environment. Externalizing behavior problems (sometimes called under-controlled behavior patterns) are viewed as behavioral excesses because they occur too often. Examples include defying the teacher, arguing, aggressing toward others, and noncompliance with teacher directives.

Gate 2 involves teacher ratings of externalizing behavior patterns.

Teachers are asked to rate the three children ranked highest on the externalizing behavioral dimension on the frequency of maladaptive and adaptive forms of behavior. Teachers also rate these children on a Critical Events Index (CEI), or checklist that assesses behavior problems within the past 6 months. Students exceeding normative cutoff points in Gate 2 of the SSBD are then independently assessed in Gate 3 via classroom and playground observations by professional observers.

In Gate 3, a school professional (e.g., school psychologist, guidance counselor, or social worker) assesses students on two measures of school adjustment using direct observation procedures. A duration recording procedure, which estimates the amount of time a target behavior occurs during a specified observation session, is used to measure classroom behavior. The first measure, known as academic engaged time (AET) is recorded during seatwork periods. The second measure, the peer social behavior observation code (PSB), measures the quality, distribution, and level of children's social behavior during recess periods on the playground using a partial interval coding procedure consisting of five categories. Both the AET and PSB coding systems have been positively reviewed in the literature by professionals who have used them in research. Students who exceed normative criteria on these two measures are then considered to pass Gate 3 and are referred for more comprehensive assessments of their behavior.

The SSBD was nationally standardized on 4,500 cases for the Gate 2 measures and approximately 1,300 cases for the Gate 3 measures. These cases were collected from 18 school districts in eight states: Oregon, Washington, Utah, Illinois, Wisconsin, Rhode Island, Kentucky, and Florida. In the second edition of the SSBD, an additional 7,000 cases have been added to the original normative database. The second edition also contains an extensive analysis and description of the empirical knowledge base developed on the instrument by the developers and other researchers. The SSBD has extensive empirical evidence in support of its reliability and validity, which is reported in the SSBD technical manual and in other sources (Severson & Walker, 2002; Walker & Severson, 1990; Walker et al., 1994).

Early Screening Project

The Early Screening Project (ESP) is a downward extension of the SSBD developed for use in preschool and day care settings for children ages 3–5 (Walker, Severson, & Feil, 1995). Like the SSBD, the ESP assesses young children who are at risk for developing externalizing and internalizing behavior problems. For purposes of this book, I focus only on the externalizing domain of the ESP. The ESP was normed on 2,853 children in eight states. The process used by the ESP is the same as in the SSBD except that it incorporates parent ratings of problem behavior at Gate 3 of the screening process. There is strong empirical support for the ESP in terms of its reliability and validity as reported in its technical manual.

The ESP has been shown to be an important component of early intervention programs in which systematic screening occurs on a regular basis (Walker et al., 1998). Use of the ESP in Head Start programs has been particularly beneficial in the early identification process (Del'Homme, Sinclair, & Kasari, 1994; Sinclair, 1993; Sinclair, Del'Homme, & Gonzalez, 1993). The ESP can be used for making screening, classification, and intervention planning decisions and for monitoring progress in evaluating outcomes of interventions for very young preschool children (see Feil et al., 2014; Frey et al., 2014).

Student Risk Screening Scale

The Student Risk Screening Scale (SRSS; Drummond, 1993) has identified a number of behavioral indicators that can predict the development of conduct disorders and later adoption of a delinquent lifestyle (Loeber, 1991; Loeber & LeBlanc, 1990). Parents and teachers are able to accurately rate these behavioral indicators very early in a child's life (preschool). Drummond (1993) has adapted these indicators into a universal, mass screening procedure for use by elementary school teachers in identifying at-risk students. Recently, Lane and colleagues have presented evidence for the reliability and validity of the SRSS at the middle school (Lane, Bruhn, Eisner, & Kalberg, 2010) and high school levels (Lane, Kalberg, Parks, & Carter, 2008; Lane et al., 2013).

The SRSS is a seven-item scale that uses five criteria to guide its development and use:

1. *Brief*: A screening instrument of this type should have no more than 10 items.
2. *Research based*: The items should be those that most powerfully discriminate and predict antisocial behavior patterns.
3. *Easily understood*: The format, scoring, and administration instructions should be as clear and self-explanatory as possible.
4. *Valid*: The instrument should be accurate and valid for the screening and identification of at-risk students.
5. *Powerful*: The instrument should be efficient in identifying those

students who are truly at risk and who could benefit from early intervention programs.

These criteria are carefully reflected in the final form of the SRSS. This instrument has proved to be easy to use, highly effective, and technically sound. It has extensive evidence for reliability and validity and it discriminates at-risk (high sensitivity) from non-at-risk students (high specificity). The seven items on the SRSS are:

1. Stealing
2. Lying, cheating, sneaking
3. Behavior problems
4. Peer rejection
5. Low academic achievement
6. Negative attitude
7. Aggressive behavior

Students are rated on each of the seven items on a 0–3 scale: *0— Never, 1—Occasionally, 2—Sometimes,* and *3—Frequently.* Total scores on the SRSS can range from 0–21. Based on empirical research using the SRSS, Drummond (1993) has established the following risk-score categories for determining at-risk status: High Risk: 9–21, Moderate Risk: 4–8, and Low Risk: 0–3. Thus a child receiving a score of 9–21 should be evaluated more comprehensively for the possible presence of conduct disorder. Children scoring between 4–8 (moderate risk) should be considered to be on the "radar screen" and reevaluated later on with the SRSS to see if their risk status has stayed the same, deteriorated, or improved.

As the profiles in Figure 3.2 show, two students (Frank and Clay) are at high risk for the development of conduct disorder with scores of 16 and 18, respectively. It appears that Frank has more characteristics of a *covert path* of conduct disorder (steals, lies, cheats, sneaks) and Clay appears to have more of an *overt path* of conduct disorder (defies teacher, fights with others, breaks rules). Both Jeff and Seth are at moderate risk for conduct disorder and therefore are on the radar screen for reevaluation using the SRSS at a later time.

BASC-2 Behavioral and Emotional Screening System

The BASC-2 Behavioral and Emotional Screening System (BESS; Kamphaus & Reynolds, 2007) is a mass screening tool developed to assess

Name	Steals	Lies, cheats, sneaks	Behavior problems	Rejected by peers	Low achievement	Negative attitude	Aggressive behavior	Total
Jeff	0	1	3	1	1	1	1	8
Frank	2	2	3	0	3	3	3	16
Jill	1	0	1	0	1	0	0	3
Julie	0	0	0	0	0	0	0	0
Clay	1	2	3	3	3	3	3	18
Seth	0	0	3	1	1	1	0	6
Laura	0	0	0	1	2	0	0	3
Aaron	0	0	1	0	0	1	0	2

0—Never   9–21 High risk
1—Occasionally   4–8 Moderate risk
2—Sometimes   0–3 Low risk
3—Frequently

High-risk students: Frank and Clay
Moderate-risk students: Jeff and Seth

FIGURE 3.2. Student Risk Screening Scale example.

behavioral strengths and concerns for students in preschool through high school. The BESS targets internalizing and externalizing risks, school problems, and adaptive skills. Only the externalizing domain is the focus of this book, since it is most relevant for the development of DBDs. The BESS is a multirater screening tool that uses teacher, parent, and student raters. There are two levels of the teacher and parent versions: preschool (ages 3–5) and grades K–12. Only students in grades 3–12 complete the student self-report form of the BESS.

The BESS is a norm-referenced screening tool that provides percentile ranks and *T* scores with which a child's score are compared to the normative sample. The BESS provides specific cutoff scores for risk classification levels of *normal, elevated,* and *extremely elevated.* The BESS is part of a comprehensive program of behavioral assessment and interventions and can be used to identify at-risk students who might benefit from universal, selected, or intensive interventions targeting DBDs. Its technical manual provides extensive evidence for the reliability and validity of this screening tool. One consideration, however, is that the BESS contains 25–30 items depending on the form used. Screening tools should probably have no more than 10 items; therefore the BESS may be too lengthy for use as a mass screener. The BESS manual states that it will take a teacher 4–6 minutes to rate each student in the classroom. This means that for a classroom of 25 students, it would take 100 to 150 minutes (1.67 to 2.5 hours) to rate each student in the classroom.

Office Discipline Referrals

Office discipline referrals (ODRs) are disciplinary contacts between students and the principal's office that result in written records of the incidents in which the reasons for the referral are noted. Some schools computerize their recording procedures; others use standard referral forms for recording each ODR; still others document the incidents less formally (e.g., via narrative accounts). ODRs can be used as a screening tool to document which students are being referred to the office and to detail the behavioral reasons for these referrals.

ODRs are nearly always initiated by classroom teachers to report behavioral infractions (e.g., teacher defiance, noncompliance, aggression, property destruction, bullying, harassment, or violation of school rules). As a rule, teachers make these sorts of referrals either because they cannot deal with the discipline problem themselves within the classroom context or because they believe the infraction is of such severity that it warrants the involvement of school administrators and/or parents.

ODRs accumulate as part of the normal schooling process and reflect the school's accommodation of students' responses to the routine demands of schooling. They provide a record of the number and types of serious behavioral episodes occurring on a student-by-student basis for each school year. ODRs provide an interesting metric of school adjustment for individual students and also can be aggregated for groups of students within a school population such as by gender and/or by grade level. ODRs can be used by school personnel and researchers to identify behaviorally at-risk students and assess the overall social climate of the school.

In many schools, it is not unusual for most ODRs to be accounted for by less than 10% of the school population. In other words, most students receiving ODRs are "return customers." This finding generally parallels the common one in corrections research showing that approximately 65% of all juvenile crime is accounted for by 6–8% of the juvenile population (Loeber & Farrington, 1998). As a general rule, elementary school students average between 0 and 1 ODRs each school year; the corresponding figure for middle school students is much higher at approximately 3.5 ODRs per student per year. McIntosh, Frank, and Spaulding (2010) analyzed ODRs in 2,500 elementary schools involving more than 990,000 students and found the average ODR rate was 0.59 (SD = 2.24) with a range of 0–154 ODRs. In a longitudinal sample of 40 antisocial boys, studied over a decade, these authors found that many of these students averaged 10 or more ODRs per school year. Furthermore, from grade 4 to 11, this sample of boys had just over 350 arrests—many for serious offenses (Walker et al., 2004). Many experts in law enforcement estimate there is one arrest for every ten arrestable offenses committed.

The typical student with a DBD in the intermediate elementary grades will average 10 or more ODRs per school year (Sugai, Sprague, Horner, & Walker, 2000; Walker et al., 2004). The number for some of these students, however, can range up to 40 or more for the school year. Any student who has 10 or more ODRs per year should be considered to be a *chronic discipline problem* and in need of intervention. Despite substantial differences in recording methods and annual changes in the school population, ODRs show surprising consistency across school years (Walker & McConnell, 1995).

ODRs are an important tool for characterizing the school behavior of students with DBDs and should be incorporated into any comprehensive assessment of them. ODRs represent an unobtrusive, nonreactive measure that is quite inexpensive to collect. Their use extends well beyond that of the individual student with DBDs and, as noted previously, allows school personnel to collect and analyze data that reveal patterns of problem behavior occurring within the school setting. The reader is referred to the excellent work of Rob Horner and his associates on the standardization and Web-based collection and analysis of ODRs (see *www.cacepartnership.org/documents/PBIS/SWIS.ppt*). In summary, the collection of ODRs is an important advance in assessing DBDs in school settings; however, their use has not been without controversy in the professional literature, particularly when used as a program or intervention evaluation tool (see Irvin, Tobin, Sprague, Sugai, & Vincent, 2004; Martella et al., 2010; Nelson, Benner, Reid, Epstein, & Currin, 2002).

Behavior Rating Scales

Behavior rating scales completed by multiple informants (teachers, parents, and children) are useful for identifying children with DBDs.

Unlike the screening tools just described, behavior rating scales offer a much more comprehensive picture of a child's behavior across multiple domains. Behavior rating scales provide norm-referenced assessments concerning an individual with a DBD. These rating scales have large, representative normative data bases and typically are stratified by age/grade and gender. Scores are typically expressed in terms of percentile ranks and T scores and have empirically established cutoff points from which to determine risk status (e.g., 98th percentile).

The most commonly used behavior rating scales are the Achenbach System of Empirically Based Assessment (ASEBA; Achenbach & Rescorla, 2000, 2001), the Behavior Assessment System for Children–2 (Reynolds & Kamphaus, 2004), and the Conners Rating Scales (Conners, 1997). These scales are summarized in Table 3.4.

All the scales contained in Table 3.4 cover the similar age ranges, have equivalent forms across teacher, parent, and child raters, and have developed a similar evidence base for reliability and validity. All these scales provide scores for various types of DBDs such as opposition/defiance and aggression as well as scores for attention/hyperactivity problems that we know exacerbate the developmental course of DBDs.

It should be noted that behavior rating scales are an *indirect* form of assessment because they rely on retrospective ratings of children's behavior. Behavior rating scales measure a child's *typical behavior* rather than his or her actual behavior in a specific situation. One major drawback in the use of behavior rating scales is the low agreement/correlations among multiple raters of the same child (De Los Reyes &

TABLE 3.4. Summary of Selected Broadband Behavior Rating Scales

Scale	Publisher	DBDs assessed
Achenbach System of Empirically Based Assessment	University of Vermont	Aggressive behavior, attention problems, conduct problems, defiance problems, opposition problems, rule-breaking behavior
Behavior Assessment System for Children–2	Pearson Assessments	Aggression, attention problems, covert conduct problems, hyperactivity, learning problems, oppositional behavior
Conners Rating Scales	Multi-Health Systems	Attention problems, hyperactivity, oppositional behavior

Note. Informants for all of the above rating scales are parent, teacher, and child/adolescent.

Kazdin, 2005). As such, there is no "gold standard" informant in rating DBDs.

Systematic Direct Observations

Systematic direct observations (SDOs) are considered by many to be the gold standard in assessment of DBDs because they provide a direct measure of a child's actual behavior in a specific setting. Typically, SDOs are conducted in naturalistic settings such as classrooms or playgrounds using a preestablished observational code. Recall that the SSBD records SDOs in the classroom and the playground using this method. SDOs can be used to measure various *dimensions* of behavior such as frequency, temporality (e.g., duration, latency, interresponse time), intensity/magnitude, or permanent products.

SDOs are based on three core assumptions. One, they are considered to be a sample of an individual's behavior in a specific situation or setting. As such, it is not assumed that the individual's behavior will be generalizable to other settings or situations. Second, they involve the repeated measurement of behavior over time to establish intrasubject variability, which can be used to evaluate a child before, during, and after an intervention. Third, they are considered to provide idiographic data about an individual rather than information about groups of individuals.

Despite several advantages, SDOs have some definite disadvantages as an assessment method for DBDs. First, SDOs are an extremely expensive, labor-intensive form of assessment requiring the use of highly trained observers. Second, there is very little empirical guidance concerning the number or length of observation sessions needed to obtain a representative sample of behavior. Finally, SDOs can be influenced by the *reactivity* of children who know they are being observed, thereby creating an inaccurate measure of the child's behavior.

Direct Behavior Ratings

Direct behavior ratings (DBRs) are hybrid assessment tools combining characteristics of SDOs and behavior rating scales and have been recommended as more practical alternatives to SDOs for progress monitoring purposes (Cook et al., 2014). DBRs are observation tools that meet the following standards: (1) they specify the target behavior(s), (2) they rate behavior(s) at least once per day, (3) they share rating information across individuals (teachers, parents, and students), and (4) they monitor the effects of intervention (Chafouleas, McDougal, Riley-Tilman, Panahon, & Hilt, 2005; Chafouleas, Riley-Tilman, & McDougal, 2002). DBRs are being increasingly used as progress monitoring tools because they are time- and resource-efficient methods for measuring behavior change.

DBRs are flexible because they can be adapted to meet the needs of any measurement situation. They can vary according to the individual, the domain of behavior being assessed, the frequency with which behavior is rated (once or more daily), and/or the rater (teacher, parent, or student). Figure 3.3 provides an example of a DBR to measure a student's DBD pattern.

Functional Behavioral Assessment and DBDs

Functional behavioral assessment (FBA) is being increasingly used by researchers and practitioners to match intervention strategies to behavioral functions in order to enhance the effectiveness of the interventions. Research over the past 30 years in the field of applied behavior analysis indicates that FBA methods contribute to beneficial outcomes for children and youth with challenging behaviors (Martens & Lambert, 2014).

FBA can be defined as a systematic process for identifying events that reliably predict and maintain behavior. It uses a variety of methods for gathering information about antecedents (i.e., events that trigger the occurrence of behavior) and consequences (i.e., events that maintain behavior). Knowledge of the conditions maintaining problem behavior can be used to discontinue or control its sources of reinforcement and teach adaptive, functionally equivalent behaviors as replacements instead (Crone & Horner, 2003; Gresham, Watson, et al., 2001). It should be emphasized that FBA is not a single test or observation but rather involves implementing a collection of assessment methods to determine antecedents, behaviors, and consequences. The major goal of FBA is to identify environmental conditions that are associated with the occurrence and nonoccurrence of problem behaviors.

FBA Defined

The function of behavior refers to the *purpose* that behavior serves for an individual in a setting or situation. Fundamentally, there are only two

Student _____ Teacher _____ School _____
Grade _____ Date _____

Directions: Review each of the items below. For each item, rate the degree to which the student showed the behavior or met the behavior goal. Please rate the student's behavior for **today** only.

1. Frank was noncompliant with teacher instructions during the math lesson.

1	2	3	4	5	6	7	8	9
Never/Seldom				Sometimes			Usually/Always	

2. Frank disrupted the class during individual seatwork activities.

1	2	3	4	5	6	7	8	9
Never/Seldom				Sometimes			Usually/Always	

3. Frank used an inappropriate tone of voice during class.

1	2	3	4	5	6	7	8	9
Never/Seldom				Sometimes			Usually/Always	

4. Frank bothered classmates when they were working on independent assignments.

1	2	3	4	5	6	7	8	9
Never/Seldom				Sometimes			Usually/Always	

FIGURE 3.3. Example of a direct behavior report.

functions of behavior: (1) *positive reinforcement*, which involves anything that brings behavior into contact with a positive stimulus and (2) *negative reinforcement*, in which a behavior or action leads to escape, avoidance, delay, or reduction of an aversive stimulus. In other words, behaviors and actions serving a positive reinforcement function allow the individual to get something preferred and those serving a negative reinforcement function allow the individual to "get out of something" nonpreferred or undesired. For example, if a student engages in disruptive behavior and receives frequent attention for this behavior, this behavior is likely to be positively reinforced, strengthened, and continued. In contrast, if the student engages in disruptive behavior while he or she is supposed to be completing math worksheets, chances are that this behavior is being negatively reinforced by escape from math task demands.

Carr (1994) has further divided the two functions of behavior above into five categories: (1) social attention/communication (positive social reinforcement); (2) access to tangible reinforcement or preferred activities (material or activity reinforcement); (3) escape, avoidance, delay, or reduction of aversive tasks or activities (negative reinforcement); (4) escape or avoidance of other individuals (negative social reinforcement); and (5) internal stimulation (automatic or sensory reinforcement).

FBA Process and Procedures

The FBA process takes place in the following sequences: (1) FBA interviews, which are used to guide direct observations of behavior; (2) observations of behavior, which can be done by teachers, behavior specialists, or school psychologists to allow for confirmation and refinement of hypotheses derived from FBA interviews; (3) formulation of behavioral hypothesis statements concerning the conditions likely to produce problem behavior, providing delineation of problem behaviors, describing consequent events that are likely to maintain the problem behavior; and (4) specification of behavioral interventions based on this information. These interventions might involve such options as changing the conditions that evoke the problem behaviors, teaching new skills (appropriate replacement behaviors), and/or altering consequences that are maintaining the problem behaviors.

FBA methods can be either indirect or direct procedures for behavioral function. Indirect FBA methods are removed in time and place from the actual occurrence of the behavior (Gresham, Watson, et al., 2001). FBA interviews (with teachers, parents, and students), historical/archival records, and behavior rating scales or checklists are the most frequently used indirect FBA methods. Direct FBA methods measure the antecedents, behaviors, and consequences at the time and place of their actual occurrence. SDOs are used to confirm or disconfirm the information produced by indirect FBA methods.

An important class of antecedent events are setting events and establishing or motivating operations. Setting events are antecedents that are removed in time and place from the occurrence of behavior but are functionally related to that behavior (Gresham, Watson, et al., 2001). Setting events can exert potentially powerful influences on behavior. Examples include confrontations on the school bus, physical abuse at home, and negative coercive interactions with parents and siblings. In contrast, establishing or motivation operations are events that temporarily increase the effectiveness of a known reinforcer. For example, food or water deprivation can enhance their appetite and thirst satisfying qualities. In terms of DBDs, sleep deprivation or neglect can each operate as establishing operations for behavior in school.

Behavioral Hypotheses and FBA

Behavioral hypotheses are testable statements regarding the functions of behavior that are based on FBA-derived information. There may be several causal hypotheses for each problem behavior. At a minimum, behavioral hypotheses should include the following: (1) setting events and/or establishing operations, (2) immediate antecedent events, (3) problem behavior(s), and (4) maintaining consequence(s). Behavioral hypotheses are observable, testable, and capable of being accepted or rejected via data collection. The following are examples of testable behavioral hypotheses for a student:

- Frank is more likely to engage in disruptive and noncompliant behaviors when he comes to school without breakfast (establishing operation) and is asked to complete difficult math tasks (immediate antecedent). (Hypothesized function is escape from difficult, nonpreferred tasks.)
- Frank is more likely to engage in disruptive and noncompliant behavior during group instruction activities (immediate antecedent) and when he has had an altercation with peers before school (setting event). (Hypothesized function is peer social attention for disruptive and noncompliant behavior.)
- Frank is more likely to engage in disruptive and noncompliant behaviors when he has not had enough sleep the night before (establishing operation) and is asked to complete tasks within a cooperative learning situation (immediate antecedent). (Hypothesized function is avoidance of nonpreferred activities involving cooperation.)

In summary, there are many reasons for using FBA with students with or at risk for DBDs. It has been shown to be useful in designing interventions for a number of problem behaviors. However, some behaviors exhibited for students with DBDs are simply not amenable to FBA methods. For example, low-frequency but high-intensity behaviors such as physical assaults, fire setting, or sexual assault are virtually impossible to analyze with FBA. Other behaviors that are more covert in nature (e.g., theft, vandalism, cruelty to animals) are very difficult to assess using FBA methods. The reader is referred to the classic text in our field on the use of FBA methods in a range of settings within our field (see O'Neill, Albin, Storey, Horner, & Sprague, 2014).

Chapter Summary Points

- In the assessment of DBDs, five types of decisions can be made: (1) screening decisions, (2) identification and classification decisions, (3) intervention decisions, (4) progress monitoring decisions, and (5) documentation of intervention outcome decisions.

- Screening tools are advantageous because they are brief, inexpensive, and effective in identifying children with DBDs.

- Two types of errors are made in the screening process: (1) *false positive errors* that involve identifying an individual as having a DBD when he or she does not and (2) *false negative errors* that involve failing to identify individuals with a DBD when they in fact have one.

- Classification decisions are based on comprehensive and expensive assessments of DBDs and typically use broadband norm-referenced rating scales.

- Progress monitoring decisions are used to determine whether an intervention is producing desired results and typically uses direct observations, work samples, and direct behavior ratings.

- Intervention decisions are based on assessment information that has *treatment validity* (i.e., the degree to which assessment information contributes to beneficial treatment outcomes).

- Program evaluation decisions are based on data concerning the effectiveness of intervention programs and are important in deciding to continue, modify, or discontinue an intervention program.

- Assessment practices are based on five assumptions: (1) individual differences among children and adolescent are *relative* rather than *absolute*, (2) assessments are samples of behavior, (3) the primary reason for assessment is to improve interventions, (4) all types of assessment contain error, and (5) good assessment involves gathering information about the environment.

- Problem solving assessment is based on (1) determining whether there is a significant discrepancy between current levels of performance and desired levels of performance and (2) strategies designed to eliminate this discrepancy.

- Problem solving assessment occurs in four stages: (1) *problem identification* (What is the problem?), (2) *problem analysis* (Why is it occurring?), (3) *plan implementation* (What should be do to change it?), and (4) *problem evaluation* (How will we know it was effective?).

- *Risk factors* are factors or variables associated with poor developmental outcomes and may be related to multiple maladaptive outcomes.

- *Protective factors* are factors or variables that reduce the likelihood of maladaptive outcomes that operate at multiple system levels (within-child, family, and community).

- Children who do not achieve their social goals other than through coercive behavior by about 8 years of age will likely continue displaying a degree of antisocial behavior throughout their lives.

- The *sensitivity* of a screening process reflects the proportion of persons with a given outcome (e.g., having a DBD) and reflects a *true positive* identification.

- The *specificity* of a screening process reflects the proportion of persons without a given outcome (e.g., not having a DBD) and reflects a *true negative* identification.

- Three commonly used screening tools that have abundant data concerning their reliability and validity are: (1) Systematic Screening for Behavior Disorders, (2) Early Screening Project, and (3) Student Risk Screening Scale.

- Screening tools should meet the following criteria: (1) brief (no more than 10 items), (2) research based, (3) easily understood, (4) valid, and (5) powerful.

- Office discipline referrals can be used as a screening tool and important metric to assess the number and types of behavioral episodes in schools.

- Broadband behavior rating scales are completed by multiple informants (teachers, parents, and children) and provide norm-referenced scores to determine which students have DBDs.

- Systematic direct observations are used to make progress monitoring decisions and compare an individual's baseline level of performance to his or her intervention level of performance.

- Direct behavior ratings are hybrid assessment tools combining characteristics of direct observations and behavior rating scales that are more cost effective and less labor intensive than direct observations.

- Functional behavioral assessment is a process of identifying events that reliably predict and maintain behavior.

- Behavior function consists of two functions: (1) *positive reinforcement* (anything that brings behavior into contact with a positive stimulus) and (2) *negative reinforcement* (a behavior that leads to escape, avoidance, delay, or reduction of an aversive stimulus).

- Behavioral hypotheses are testable statements regarding the functions of behavior.

- Behavioral hypotheses should include: (1) setting events and/or establishing operations, (2) immediate antecedent events, (3) problem behavior(s), and (4) maintaining consequences.

Issues and Guidelines
in Implementing Interventions

This chapter provides a context for understanding and applying the material presented in the remainder of this book. I focus on the social ecology and culture of schools as they relate to interventions for students with DBDs. This chapter describes procedural guidelines and key concepts governing the implementation of evidence-based intervention programs.

This information will be useful in making it more likely that best-practice interventions for children with DBDs can be delivered in a manner that will have a better chance of improving the adjustment problems of these children and youth. This chapter focuses on school-based interventions; however, these children and youth often require interventions that address issues and needs extending beyond the school setting. Chapters 6 and 7 describe these evidence-based interventions that take place in non-school settings.

It is important to understand that schools provide a vital setting and a potent context for intervening with students with DBDs. As mentioned in Chapter 1, this population of students constitute approximately 9–10% of a given school population. Unfortunately, schools often do not have the knowledge, motivation, or resources to help these children. Moreover, these students typically do not qualify for special education and related services under the category of emotional disturbance. As such, schools often resort to reactive, punitive practices to deal with these students' problem behaviors, including suspension, expulsions, reprimands, "talk" therapies, and other ineffective non-evidence-based strategies.

Schools provide a critical setting for intervening with students with DBDs, but are complex and fragile organizations. Trying to infuse effective evidence-based interventions into a school culture requires sensitivity, tact, and careful attention to details. The goals of this chapter are twofold: (1) to document the external factors affecting the DBD pattern that constrains schools' ability to effectively address these behaviors and (2) to describe specific techniques to facilitate the identification and implementation of best-practice interventions for reducing and replacing the DBD pattern.

School Responsibilities in Dealing with DBDs

Schools are the ultimate vehicle for accessing children who need services, supports, and interventions that affect their physical and mental health such as medical and sensory screenings as well as various interventions. In fact, all states have compulsory school attendance laws that require parents to send their children to school up until a certain age (e.g., 16 years). As such, schools are the ideal setting to deliver mental health and other interventions because they provide a "captive audience" for those providing these services. Many schools provide instruction in bullying prevention, sex education, drug awareness, wellness, and health promotion as well as basic parenting skills as part of their curricula. Historically, schools provided one of the only safe places for at-risk children and youth; however, that safety has been seriously compromised in many parts of our country. Currently, we are reducing our investment in public schools but, paradoxically, we are asking schools to revise their curricula in order to attain higher academic performance standards.

Differences among first-grade children in beginning reading literacy provide a good example of how many at-risk children from impoverished backgrounds are severely disadvantaged as they begin their school careers. An investigation by Juel (1988) showed that if a child was a good reader in grade 1, the probability of staying a good reader in grade 4 was .87. However, if a child was a poor reader in grade 1, the probability of continuing to be a poor reader in grade 4 was equally likely at .88. In short, the good news is if you start to school ready to learn and are a good reader, you will remain so; the bad news is that, if you start to school not ready to learn and you are a poor reader, you will remain so. These findings speak to the critical importance of school readiness skills and the early literacy development for all children.

There is an interesting parallel between reading success or failure in grade 1 and emerging patterns of disruptive behavior. If challenging forms of behavior are not addressed effectively at the point of school entry, the behavior will likely worsen as these students progress through school. Kazdin (1987) showed in a comprehensive review of the literature that if children's antisocial behavior problems are not remediated by the end of grade 3, they were highly likely to continue this behavior pattern through adolescence and adulthood.

It has been estimated that 20–40% of the school-age population is at risk of school failure and school dropout due to long-term exposure to societal conditions of risk (Lyon, 2002). Many of these children will also follow a trajectory leading to antisocial behavior and, ultimately, conduct disorder, delinquency, and criminality. Schools must be broadly supported and encouraged to develop partnerships with families and social service agencies that can address those critical, unmet needs of children that affect their education and quality of life. School districts, private foundations, and consortia of social service agencies across the country are developing school-linked models of *wraparound services* and supports targeted to families and at-risk children.

Eber and colleagues (Eber, Malloy, Rose, & Flamini, 2014) describe the history, theory base, and evidence associated with wraparound services for at-risk children and youth. These wraparound services indicate that schools, mental health agencies, and juvenile justice systems struggle to meet their responsibilities for supporting at-risk children and youth. The U.S. Surgeon General, for example, argued that approximately one in every five children between the ages of 9 and 17 has a diagnosable mental health or addictive disorder, but special education only identifies 1–2% of students as emotionally disturbed (U.S. Department of Health and Human Services, 1999). It is important that federal, state, and local governments invest aggressively in school-linked wraparound services if we are to have any chance of dealing effectively with the problems of at-risk children and youth. Schools can play a critical role in this process if they are supported in the process.

Considerations in Using Psychotropic Medications

Our society has become increasingly "drug obsessed" and is being constantly exposed to advertising campaigns from drug manufacturers that promote prescription and nonprescription drugs to treat a variety of ailments. The use of psychotropic medications for disorders such as ADHD and other related conditions of childhood and adolescence has increased exponentially in the last 20 years. There is an ongoing debate about the benefits and drawbacks of psychotropic medications for numerous disorders of childhood and adolescence (see Jensen & Cooper, 2002).

A working group of psychologists from the American Psychological Association reviewed the empirical literature on the use of psychoactive medications with children and adolescents (American Psychological Association, 2004). The bottom-line conclusion of this working group was that there is more use of psychotropic medication with children and adolescents than there is research data to support its use. The Department of Children and Families from the state of Connecticut concluded that there is a lack of scientific evidence for pediatric psychopharmacology and expressed concerns about the use of selective serotonin reuptake inhibitors (SSRIs; e.g., Prozac, Paxil, Celexa) for the treatment of depression. The U.S. Food and Drug Administration (FDA) in 2004 looked at published and unpublished data on trials of SSRI antidepressant medications involving 4,400 children and adolescents and found that 4% of those taking antidepressants thought about or tried suicide compared to 2% of those receiving placebos (sugar pill).

It is fair to note that most psychotropic medications to treat children and adolescents are safe and effective. However, many medications have not been studied or approved for use with children. Physicians often prescribe a medication to help a patient even though the medicine has not been approved for a specific mental disorder or age. Examples of this can be found with various ADHD medications. Concerta, Ritalin, and Vyvanse have been approved by the FDA for children ages 6 and older, yet some physicians may prescribe these medications for children younger than 6.

What does this have to do with children and youth with DBDs? Increasing numbers of children with DBDs are labeled as having ADHD, and attempts to control their behavior often rely on a prescribed drug regimen of stimulant medication. It may well be the case that this drug regimen will have little or no effect on the child's main behavior problems (e.g., noncompliance, aggression, and defiance). Psychotropic medications can be a useful adjunct for some behavior problems but should not be the sole or even the major component of a comprehensive intervention for DBDs.

Importance of Evidence-Based Interventions

The effectiveness of school-based interventions for DBPs is a source of continuing debate among professionals and laypersons. These interventions have been variously described as a "magic bullet" that works every time, lasts indefinitely, and is easy to implement. Such interventions for DBPs do not exist. Instead, these students require powerful, multicomponent, multisetting interventions implemented over a relatively long period of time.

Frequently, interventions implemented in schools are not empirically based, and the most effective interventions are typically not those used most frequently by schools. Instead, interventions are selected that allow the implementer to address the problem and that appeal to him or her. When dealing with DBDs, we do not have the luxury of selecting interventions on this basis. Although no current intervention approach can claim to be a "cure" for a behavior pattern, some practices are clearly more effective than others.

Recall from Chapter 2 the discussion of what constitutes *evidence* and basing intervention actions on how we define it. Some professionals accept what they consider evidence only if it fits into preexisting belief systems and may reject any evidence that does not conform to these beliefs. For example, many teachers believe that the use of rewards to increase desirable behaviors is a form of bribery that should not be used in their classrooms. They maintain this belief in spite of evidence to the contrary.

Strategies for teaching beginning reading provide another good example. It seems prudent to use a teaching method that produces the lowest rate of reading failure among students. Based on years of accumulated empirical research, this strategy should involve instruction in phonics and phonemic awareness (National Reading Panel, 2000). In spite of this accumulated evidence, many schools continue to invest in less effective approaches to teaching beginning reading (e.g., whole word approaches). The social and human costs of this failure are reflected in the 4 out of 10 beginning readers who need structured assistance to master the complexities of reading (Lyon, 2002). This is analogous to an oncologist who uses a treatment regimen that (1) he was trained in, (2) is easier to implement, and (3) he simply likes better. This treatment regimen may have a 20% mortality rate when an alternative regimen may have a 5% mortality rate. Such a practice by medical personnel would not be tolerated given the stakes, yet many educators use a similar logic in dealing the DBDs.

Multi-Tiered Intervention Approaches: Response to Intervention

The U.S. Public Health Service developed a valuable schema for classifying different types of prevention outcomes. Instead of viewing prevention as a means to an end, this classification conceptualized intervention as a tool or instrument for achieving prevention outcomes. This schema has three levels of prevention: *primary prevention, secondary prevention,* and *tertiary prevention.* Primary prevention refers to intervention efforts designed to keep problems from emerging—that is, to *prevent harm.* Secondary prevention refers to interventions whose purpose is to *reverse harm* of children and youth who already exhibit signs of behavior problems. Tertiary prevention refers to interventions for the most severely involved at-risk children and whose purpose is to *reduce harm.*

This three-level schema served as the foundational basis of what is known today as *response to intervention* (RTI; Gresham, 2002; Jimmerson, Burns, & VanDerHeyden, 2007). RTI is based on the notion of determining whether an adequate or inadequate change in behavior has been achieved via an intervention. In an RTI approach, decisions regarding changing or intensifying an intervention are made based on how well or poorly a student responds to an evidence-based intervention that is implemented with integrity. RTI is used to select, change, or titrate interventions based on how the child responds to it. RTI assumes that if a child shows an inadequate response to the best intervention available and feasible in a given setting, then that child can and should be eligible for additional assistance, including more intense interventions, special assistance, and special education and related services. RTI is not used exclusively to make special education entitlement decisions, although it may be used for that purpose.

Several important points should be noted in considering a RTI approach. First, intervention *intensity* is increased only after data suggest that an individual shows an inadequate response to the intervention. Second, treatment decisions are based on objective data that are collected continuously over a period of time (i.e., data-based decision making). Third, the data that are collected are well-established indicators of behavioral functioning (generalized outcome measures [GOMs]). Finally, decisions about treatment intensity are based on the collection of more data as the individual moves through each stage of treatment intensification.

Several factors are related to a behavior's response to intervention. Ones that seem most relevant for school-based interventions are: (1) severity of behavior, (2) chronicity of behavior, (3) generalizability of behavior change, (4) treatment strength, (5) treatment integrity, and (6) treatment effectiveness. Each of these factors is discussed in the following sections.

Severity

Behavioral severity can be defined using objective dimensions such as frequency/rate, duration, intensity, and permanent products (Cooper et al., 2007). Behavioral severity that is operationalized by higher frequencies, durations, and/or intensities is more resistant to intervention than behaviors having lower levels of these dimensions (Gresham, 1991; Nevin, 1988). These behaviors are not only *more resistant* to interventions, but also tend to produce high rates of positive reinforcement (via social attention or access to tangible reinforcers) and/or negative reinforcement (e.g., escape or avoidance of task demands). The net result is that these behaviors continue and even escalate despite interventions designed to reduce them. Using an analogy to physics, the "force" (strength of intervention) is insufficient to change the "momentum" (behavioral severity) of the behavior.

Many children and youth with DBDs exhibit rather severe behavior patterns that are highly resistant to change. Recall from Chapter 1 that many children with this behavior pattern have had these behaviors shaped and reinforced from a very early age. This was termed the *coercive family process* in which the child's behavior gets both negatively reinforced by the removal of demands or directives and positively reinforced by getting his or her way. The parent's behavior is negatively reinforced by the termination of the child's aversive behavior pattern. This process is repeated literally thousands of times during the child's life, which makes this behavior pattern highly resistant to change. Based on this learning history, interventions must have sufficient "force" (strength) to change this resistant behavior pattern.

Chronicity

The chronicity of behavior is an important aspect of behavior change. The term implies a condition that is constant, continuing, and long term. Another definition of *chronic* is habits that resist all efforts to eradicate them, or deep-seated aversion to change. This use of the term is directly related to the concept of response to intervention. The RTI approach embraces this second meaning of the term chronic (resistance to change). One distinguishing feature of DBDs is that it is a pattern of behavior that continues despite interventions designed to change it (Gresham, 1991, 2005). In addision, another use of the term is the recurrence of behavior problems once they have been changed by an intervention. This use of *chronic* represents a problem in *maintenance* of behavior change over time.

Generalizability of Behavior Change

Generalization and maintenance of behavior change is directly related to RTI. If a behavior pattern is severe (in terms of frequency, intensity, and/ or duration) and chronic (it has been resistant to change), it will tend to show less generalization across different nonintervention conditions and will show less maintenance over time when the intervention procedures are withdrawn (Horner & Billingsley, 1988; Nevin, 1988). Students who demonstrate severe behavior patterns over an extended period of time are quick to discriminate intervention from nonintervention conditions, particularly when intervention conditions are vastly different from non-intervention conditions. For instance, when students are exposed to a highly structured point system that uses a response cost component for inappropriate behaviors and a reinforcement component for appropri-ate behaviors, they will readily discriminate when the program is not in effect. Since discrimination is the polar opposite of generalization, behavior under these conditions is likely to deteriorate to baseline levels of performance when one returns abruptly to preintervention conditions (e.g., withdrawal of the point system).

Students with DBDs often show excellent initial behavior change, particularly in terms of behavioral excesses, but fail to show generaliza-tion and maintenance of behavior changes. A reason for this lack of gen-eralization and maintenance is that interventions often exclusively target decreasing inappropriate behavioral excesses at the expense of targeting the establishment of appropriate or prosocial behaviors. The process of replacement behavior training in this regard is described extensively in Chapter 9. Recent advances in positive behavior support in which entire schools recognize and abide by a common set of behavioral expectations for students should enhance generalization and maintenance of interven-tion effects (Sugai, Horner, & Gresham, 2002).

Treatment Strength

The strength of a treatment reflects the ability of a given treatment to change behavior in the desired direction. Strong treatments produce greater amounts of behavior change than weak treatments. Treatment strength is not absolute, but rather situationally, behaviorally, and individually specific (Gresham, 1991). Some treatments are strong in some situations or settings, but not others (e.g., home vs. school). Some treatments are strong for changing some behaviors, but not other behavior (e.g., work completion vs. physical aggression). Some treatments are strong for some individuals, but not other individuals (e.g., students with DBDs vs. students without DBDs). In short, treatment strength is determined by the interaction of situational, behavioral, and individual factors.

In behavioral interventions, treatment strength is not always clearly quantifiable a priori as it is in other fields. For example, a 500-milligram antibiotic is twice as strong as a 250-milligram antibiotic in treatment of many bacterial infections. In contrast, four points awarded in a reward system for appropriate behavior is not necessarily twice as strong as two points awarded. The fundamental difference between a specification of treatment strength in medical and behavioral treatments is that the former specifies treatment strength a priori (e.g., dosage of a drug) and the latter specifies treatment strength a posteriori (e.g., magnitude of behavior change). Treatment strength in a RTI model is indexed by treatment outcome or magnitude of behavior change produced by the treatment.

Treatment Integrity

Treatment integrity refers to the accuracy with which interventions are implemented as planned, intended, or programmed (Peterson, Homer, & Wonderlich, 1982). Historically, treatment integrity has been conceptualized as involving three dimensions: (1) treatment adherence, or the degree to which a treatment is implemented as intended or planned; (2) interventionist competence, or the interventionist's skill and experience in implementing a particular treatment; and (3) treatment differentiation, or the extent to which differ on critical dimensions (Nezu & Nezu, 2008). Conceptually, treatment adherence represents a quantitative dimension of treatment integrity because it can be measured or quantified by the number of critical treatment components that are implemented. Therapist competence can be conceptualized as more of a qualitative dimension of treatment integrity because it reflects how well treatment procedures are implemented or delivered. Finally, treatment differentiation represents theoretical distinctions among different aspects of various treatments.

In adopting an RTI approach, one must be able to demonstrate that measurable changes in behavior (i.e., the dependent variable) can be attributed to systematic and measurable changes in the environment (i.e., the independent variable). Without objective and documented specification that the intervention was implemented as planned or intended, one cannot conclude whether inadequate response to an intervention was due to an ineffective or weak intervention or due to a poorly implemented, but potentially effective, intervention. In an RTI approach, the systematic and frequent measurement of treatment integrity is an essential aspect of service delivery.

Despite the importance of treatment integrity in RTI models, one should be aware that there is not a one-to-one correspondence between the level of treatment integrity and the level of outcome produced by any given treatment. Some treatments may be implemented with less than perfect integrity, yet may produce substantial and beneficial outcomes. Other treatments may be implemented with perfect integrity, yet may produce few or no beneficial outcomes. As such, the integrity of treatments is probably moderated by the relative strength of those treatments (Yeaton & Sechrest, 1981). That is, strong treatments are more resistant than weak treatments to lapses in treatment integrity.

As I described above, treatment strength in educational and psychological interventions cannot be known a priori. We can only gauge the strength of a treatment by the level of outcomes it produces. Some aspects of treatment strength such as the amount of treatment, the duration of treatment, and the intensity of treatment may all be related to treatment strength. However, long and intense delivery of weak treatments may not produce significant changes in behavior, whereas relatively short and less intense delivery of strong treatments may produce dramatic changes in behavior.

One common assumption is that interventions must have perfect integrity in order to be maximally effective. This assumption presumes a perfect linear relationship between treatment integrity and treatment outcome. This assumption, however, is not based on empirical data, and there is little published research showing a one-to-one correspondence between level of integrity and level of treatment outcome. In fact, my colleagues and I found only a .58 correlation between level of treatment integrity and outcome level in our review of 158 school-based intervention studies (Gresham, Gansle, Noell, Cohen, & Rosenblum, 1993).

There may be a ceiling effect above which treatment integrity improvement may not be effective or cost beneficial. The problem the field faces is that we do not know what level of integrity is necessary with what treatments to produce beneficial treatment outcomes. We also do not know at this time how far one might drift away from a treatment protocol and still have positive outcomes.

What are the implications of this dilemma for delivering interventions to students with DBDs? Some problems might be effectively resolved with an intervention implemented with 75% integrity, whereas other problems might require interventions implemented with close to 100% integrity. Currently, the best advice is to assess and monitor treatment integrity levels and assess and monitor treatment outcomes. If an evidence-based treatment is implemented with 70% integrity but is not producing adequate outcomes, then the procedures should be implemented to increase the level of treatment integrity. On the other hand, if a treatment is implemented with 60% integrity but is producing beneficial outcomes, then increasing treatment integrity may not be cost beneficial.

Treatment Effectiveness

The conceptualization of DBDs within the context of an RTI approach requires that if a school-based intervention is implemented with integrity but does not show beneficial outcomes, then decisions must be made about increasing the strength of the intervention or changing the intervention all together. In short, if a behavior pattern continues at an unacceptable level, then changes in the intervention are warranted. In an RTI approach, how does one know whether a given treatment was effective in changing a pattern of behavior? What standards or criteria might one use to make this decision? Two general approaches have been proposed to quantify whether treatments are effective: (1) visual inspection of data and (2) various effect size estimates.

Visual inspection of graphed data is the standard method used by behavior analysts to determine whether an intervention produced a substantial change in behavior from baseline to intervention phases. Visual analysis involves consideration of four fundamental aspects of the graphed data: (1) variability, (2) level, (3) trend, and (4) immediacy of change. *Variability* refers to the extent to which multiple measures of a behavior produce different outcomes. Data showing a high degree of variability within a condition indicate that there is little control over the behavior of interest. Data showing little variability within a condition indicates that there is a great deal of control over the target behavior. Generally speaking, the greater the variability within a condition, the more data points one needs to establish a predictable pattern of behavior.

Level refers to the average degree of behavior change produced by an intervention. Level can be quantified by using either the mean (arithmetic average) or the median (middle data point). For example, if a student's median level of disruptive classroom behavior was 10 during baseline and 2 during intervention, then that intervention produced a median change of 8, or 80% reduction in disruptive behavior.

Trend reflects the overall direction and magnitude of change from one phase to another. Trend can be either positive (increasing behavior), negative (decreasing behavior), or zero (no behavior change). The direction and degree of trend in graphed data is represented by a trend line of progress. Trend lines can be calculated mathematically by a formula known as the ordinary least squares regression equation.

Immediacy of effect refers to the time it takes for an intervention to produce a detectable change in behavior. Some interventions produce effects during the first several days or sessions of an intervention, whereas others may take somewhat longer. In general, interventions producing immediate effects are stronger than those interventions producing delayed effects.

Unlike traditional statistical analysis, visual inspection relies on the "interocular" test of significance. The logic of visual inspection is quite simple: If a meaningful effect was produced by the treatment, it should be obvious or noticeable by simply viewing graphed data. Potential drawbacks of relying exclusively on visual inspection include: (1) absence of standards or benchmarks for deciding whether behavior change is clinically or educationally significant, (2) potential for unacceptably high Type I error rates, and (3) difficulty in interpreting autocorrelated time series data (Gresham, 2005).

Various effect size estimates have been proposed to quantify the effectiveness of interventions using single-case experimental designs. One metric is *percent nonoverlapping data points* (PND) that is computed by calculating the percentage of nonoverlapping data points between baseline and intervention phases (Mastropieri & Scruggs, 1985–1986). If the goal is to decrease problem behavior, one computes PND by counting the number of intervention data points exceeding the *highest* baseline data point and dividing by the total number of data points in the intervention phase. For example, if 9 of 10 intervention data points exceed the highest baseline data point, the PND would be 90%. Alternatively, if the goal is to increase desirable behavior, then one calculates PND by counting the number of intervention data points that are below the *lowest* baseline data point and dividing by the total number intervention data points.

PND provides a quantitative index to document the effects of an intervention that is easy to calculate. There are several drawbacks using this method. One, PND often does not reflect the magnitude of effect of an intervention. That is, one can have 100% nonoverlapping data points in the intervention phase yet have an extremely weak treatment effect. Two, unusual baseline trends (high and low data points) can skew the interpretation of PND. Three, PND is greatly affected by floor and ceiling effects. Four, aberrant or outlier data points can make interpretation of PND difficult (see Strain, Kohler, & Gresham, 1998, for a discussion). Five, there are no well-established empirical guidelines for what constitutes a large, medium, or small effect using the PND metric.

An alternative to PND is calculation of percentage of all nonoverlapping data (PAND; Parker, Hagan-Burke, & Vannest, 2007). Similar to PND, PAND reflects the data nonoverlap between phases of a single-case experimental design but differs in several key respects. First, PAND uses *all data* in baseline and treatment phases and thus avoids the criticism of PND not considering all data and including unreliable or skewed data. Second, PAND is easily translated into a *phi coefficient* which is a Pearson *r* for a 2 × 2 contingency table. As such, PAND has a known sampling distribution that makes the calculation of *p* values and estimation of statistical power possible. Third, PAND can be transformed to Cohen's *d* and thus can be interpreted as a standardized mean difference effect size.

Perhaps the easiest and most relevant index to quantify the magnitude of behavior change in single-case designs is to calculate the percentage of behavior change from baseline to intervention levels of performance. This index, *percent exceeding the median* (PEM) is calculated by taking the median data point in baseline and comparing that value to the median data point in the intervention phases. The median is used rather than the mean because it is less susceptible to outlier effects. For example, if a student's baseline was eight occurrences of a behavior and the median number of behavioral occurrences in intervention was two, the PEM reduction in behavior would be 75% ([8–2]÷8 = 75%).

The PEM metric is not unlike methods used by physicians to quantify weight loss or reductions in blood cholesterol levels. The difference, however, is that there are well-established medical benchmarks for ideal weights and cholesterol levels, but not for problem behaviors or social skill levels. Also, PEM only reflects change in the *level* of a target behavior from baseline to intervention phases and not changes in *trend*.

Effect size estimates in single case designs can also utilize a modification of the standardized mean difference metric known as Cohen's *d* that is used frequently in meta-analytic research. Busk and Serlin (1992) proposed two methods for calculating effect sizes using Cohen's *d*. The first method makes no assumptions about the distribution of data points in baseline and intervention phases. It is calculated by subtracting the intervention mean from the baseline mean and dividing by the standard deviation of the baseline mean. For example, if the intervention mean is 3, the baseline mean is 12, and the standard deviation is –2, then Cohen's *d* would be –4.5 ([12–3] ÷ –2 = –4.5). The second approach makes an assumption about the homogeneity of variance in the data points and uses the *pooled standard deviation* calculated from baseline and intervention data points in the denominator. A drawback of using Cohen's *d* is that it often yields unrealistically large effect sizes that cannot be interpreted in the same way as effect sizes calculated using group experimental design data.

Importance of Social Validity in DBDs

Social validity deals with three fundamental questions faced by those who implement interventions for children and youth with DBDs: What should we change? How should we change it? How will we know it was effective? There are sometimes disagreements among professionals as well as treatment consumers (parents vs. teachers) on these three fundamental questions. Wolf (1978) is credited with originating the notion of *social validity* within the field of applied behavior analysis. In Wolf's view, social validity refers to establishing the *social significance* of the goals of an intervention (What should we change?), the *social acceptability* of intervention procedures to attain those goals (How should we change it?), and the *social importance* of the effects produced by the intervention (How will we know it was effective?).

For all intents and purposes, social validation is a means of assessing and analyzing consumer behavior. Schwartz and Baer (1991) indicated that the most important element in studying consumer behavior is the decision-making process. In the study of consumer behavior, this decision-making process consists of four steps: (1) recognizing the problem, (2) evaluating alternative solutions to the problem, (3) "buying" the product or service, and (4) evaluating the decision. This decision-making process parallels the problem-solving model of behavioral consultation (Bergan & Kratochwill, 1990) that involves the four steps of *problem identification, problem analysis, plan implementation,* and *problem evaluation.* Each of these dimensions of social validation are discussed in the following sections.

Social Significance of Goals

Deciding the goals to be accomplished in interventions for children and youth with DBDs is the most vital aspect of the intervention process. One of the most important aspects of the behavior consultation process is the adequacy of problem identification (Bergan & Kratochwill, 1990; Martens, DiGennaro Reed, & Magnuson, 2014). An adequate definition of behavior, however, does not necessarily establish its social significance. It may even be easier to identify and define simplistic, trivial behaviors than complex, socially significant behaviors. The social significance of behavior can be established in relation to how consumers value certain behaviors. In other words, do consumers consider the behavior to be socially significant rather than trivial or insignificant?

Social significance can be assessed using questionnaires that sample consumer opinions. These assessments are designed to reflect opinions of relevant communities of consumers and to use this information to select or change program goals or consumer opinions (Schwartz & Baer, 1991). Social invalidity is not necessarily the inverse of social validity. Instead, social invalidity is represented by consumers who disapprove of or complain about some aspect of an intervention program and who do something about that disapproval. For example, some conservative politicians and groups might express their disapproval of the Common Core State Standards by writing editorials, letters, calling school board members, and taking out ads in newspapers.

Hawkins (1991) argues that the term *social validity* is misleading because what is really being measured in social validation is consumer satisfaction. Basically, consumer satisfaction is obtained by asking for a second opinion from another source. If the second opinion agrees with another professional's opinion, then the goal of an intervention is considered "socially validated." If the second opinion disagrees with that of a professional, then the goals are viewed as socially invalid or socially insignificant. It may well be the case that the second opinions obtained from consumers are less informed than those of professionals. Disagreements between professionals and treatment consumers merely reflect the absence of interobserver agreement and not necessarily the invalidity of goals, procedures, or outcomes. For example, many cardiac patients would probably prefer medication to a triple-bypass surgery, although the former treatment may not solve the patient's problem in terms of a medically important outcome (preventing death).

Hawkins (1991) made a strong case for using the concept of *habilitative validity* instead of social validity. Goals, procedures, and outcomes in interventions should promote behaviors that allow for successful functioning or adaptation to school, home, and community settings. Habilitative validity can be defined as the degree to which the goals, procedures, and/or outcomes of an invention maximize overall benefits and minimize overall costs to that individual and to others (Hawkins, 1991). Gresham and Noell (1993) used a similar heuristic in their model of consultation based on the notion of functional outcome analysis. In this model, the goals of interventions are considered socially valid if the benefits of an intervention (both objective and subjective) outweigh the costs.

Establishing the social significance of target behaviors is an exercise in identifying *functional behaviors*. The questions asked in the process are: Is this a functional target behavior to change? Will changing this behavior result in short-term and long-term benefits for the individual? Is the cost of changing the behavior less than the benefits produced by the change (a positive cost–benefit ratio)? Consumers may not always be in the best position to judge the habilitative validity or functional utility of target behaviors.

Cooper et al. (2007) provided a useful series of questions that can be used to prioritize target behaviors for intervention. In this approach, a pool of potentially eligible target behaviors are identified and decisions are made about the relative priority of each behavior. The outcome of this process is that often a group of highly related target behaviors are identified. Behaviors that are highly related are considered to be part of the same response class and by changing one or two behaviors in this response class, the other behaviors in the response class should change in the same direction (Evans, Meyer, Kurkjian, & Kishi, 1988). The following questions can be used to prioritize and establish the social significance of target behaviors:

- Does this behavior present danger to the client or to others? These behaviors should receive first priority in the intervention process.
- How many opportunities will the person have to exhibit this new behavior, or how often does this problem behavior occur?
- How chronic is the problem behavior? A chronic or long-standing

behavior problem should take priority over a sporadically occurring behavior.

- Will changing the behavior produce higher rates of reinforcement
  for the person? Behaviors that produce higher levels of reinforcement for the individual should take priority over behaviors that
  result in little reinforcement.
- What will be the relative importance of this target behavior to
  future skill development and adaptive functioning? Behaviors
  that have habilitative validity should take priority over behaviors
  with little or no habilitative validity.
- Will modifying this behavior reduce or eliminate negative attention from others? Some problem behaviors elicit negative attention or criticism from others. If this is the case, these behaviors
  should take priority over behaviors that do not elicit such negative attention.
- How amenable is the target behavior to change? Some behaviors
  are easier to change than others because some behaviors are more
  resistant to change. It may be prudent to change behaviors that
  are relatively easier to change in the beginning of an intervention
  and then move on to changing more difficult behaviors later.
- What is the cost–benefit ratio of changing this behavior? As mentioned earlier, behaviors that have a positive cost–benefit ratio
  should receive priority in behavior change programs. Remember,
  "costs" are not limited to monetary costs, but also include time
  and effort of persons involved in the intervention.

Social Acceptability of Procedures

Not all interventions for treating DBDs are necessarily acceptable
to consumers. This is particularly true of interventions developed via
the behavioral consultation process with teachers and parents. Kazdin
(1981) first defined treatment acceptability as a judgment of whether a
treatment is fair in relation to a problem, is reasonable and nonintrusive,
and is consistent with what a treatment should be. Elliott (1988) suggested that *acceptability* is the initial issue in treatment selection and
use. If a treatment is considered acceptable, then the probability of using
it is high relative to treatments judged to be less acceptable. Use and
effectiveness of treatments are moderated by the integrity with which
they are implemented. The major reason for the ineffectiveness of many
treatments developed in behavioral consultation for DBDs is the lack of
treatment integrity (Gresham, 2014).

Most of the early research on treatment acceptability was conducted in analogue settings using hypothetical behavior problems and treatments. The typical paradigm involved presentation of a written problem and treatment vignettes and subsequently asking participants to rate the acceptability of different treatments. This literature base told us that complex treatments were less acceptable than simpler treatments, positive treatments were more acceptable than punishment-based treatments, all treatments become more acceptable as problem severity increased, and more knowledgeable treatment consumers of behavioral principles found treatments more acceptable than less knowledgeable consumers (Elliott, 1988).

This literature, while informative with respect to pretreatment acceptability, may not correspond to what consumers might tell us about the acceptability of treatments after they have tried them. The pretreatment acceptability paradigm is similar to judging the sales and consumption of products based on verbal descriptions and ratings rather than actual sales or consumption of products.

A more direct measure of acceptability would use the concepts of *integrity* and *use* as direct behavioral markers of acceptability. If a treatment is not implemented as planned, then some aspects of the treatment may be unacceptable. Similarly, if a treatment is not used, for whatever reason, it can be considered unacceptable. In this revised conceptualization, integrity and use are behavioral markers for treatment acceptability (see Gresham & Lopez, 1996, for an extensive discussion).

Consumer satisfaction with intervention procedures may not reflect the most effective treatment procedures or what is in the best interests of children and youth. Some consumers (e.g., parents and teachers) may reject legitimate interventions simply because they lack the skills for their implementation, because they are philosophically opposed to them, or because they may have motives other than the implementation of interventions. The net effect of any of these reasons is that children and youth may not receive the best practices of evidence-based interventions.

Social Importance of Effects

The social importance of the effects produced by an intervention establishes the clinical or practical significance of behavior change. That is, does the quality or quantity of behavior change make a difference in an individual's everyday functioning? Does the change have "habilitative validity"? Is the behavior now in a functional range? All of these questions capture the essence of what is meant by establishing the social importance of intervention effects.

Social importance can be established at several levels: the level of proximal effects, of intermediate effects, and of distal effects (Fawcett, 1991). Proximal effects represent changes in target behaviors as a function of an intervention (e.g., decreases in problem behaviors or increases in social skills). Intermediate effects represent concomitant changes in collateral behaviors and outcomes as a function of changes in target behaviors (e.g., changes in teacher and parent behavior ratings or higher academic achievement). Distal effects represent long-term changes in behavior or outcomes as a function of proximal and intermediate effects (e.g., increased friendships, improved peer acceptance, or reductions in school disciplinary referrals).

One reason that many practitioners may fail to utilize the research literature in guiding their practice is that this literature typically is not presented in a readily consumable form. Conventional methods for reporting research outcomes have relied primarily on parametric statistics ($p < .05$). Although parametric statistics have contributed to our understanding of intervention effects, these methods do not present research outcomes in a readily understandable and usable form.

There is often no relationship between statistical significance and practical significance, particularly when statistical significance is a function of large sample sizes rather than strong effects of an intervention (Baer, 1977; Jacobson, Follette, & Revenstorf, 1984). Traditional statistical analyses were not designed for and therefore cannot address the issue of what constitutes socially important effects. Most behavior problems vary on a continuum of functioning involving a range of differences in behavioral functioning. Some approaches to social validation contend that an intervention produced a socially important effect if the problem is successfully resolved. This approach, however, leads to thinking about outcomes in terms of false dichotomies (problem present vs. problem absent).

One means of establishing the social importance of intervention effects is to conceptualize behavioral functioning as belonging to either a *functional* or *dysfunctional* distribution. This could be accomplished by using norm-referenced behavior rating scales or social skills measures that have an adequate normative database. Thus if teacher and parent ratings of problem behaviors moved from the 95th percentile to the 50th percentile, then the behavior could be considered as having moved from a dysfunctional to a functional distribution. This approach is problematic because it requires a normative database for both functional and dysfunctional populations. Many behaviors targeted for intervention do not have a normative database and fewer still have separate norms for functional and dysfunctional populations.

More practical approaches to establishing the social importance of effects were first proposed by Kazdin (1977), who recommended three general approaches to social validation: social comparisons, subjective evaluations, and combined social validation procedures. *Social comparisons* involve comparing an individual's behavior after an intervention with the behavior of relevant peers. Social comparisons, however, may not necessarily reflect changes in behavior that have habilitative validity. It is possible to produce changes in behavior that is comparable to a child's peers, yet the behavior may not have habilitative validity. Social importance might be evaluated by specifying different levels of performance. For example, one could specify *ideal* (best performance available), *normative* (typical or commonly occurring performance), or *deficient* (poorest performance available). Interventions that move an individual from a deficient level of performance to normative or ideal levels of performance could be considered socially important (Fawcett, 1991). This procedure is not unlike *goal attainment scaling* that has been used in the mental health literature for a number of years.

Subjective evaluations represent another approach to establishing the social importance of intervention effects. These evaluations consist of having treatment consumers rate the qualitative aspects of an individual's behavior. These global evaluations of behavior assess how well the child is functioning and provide an overall assessment of performance. Subjective evaluations can be used not only for assessing the quality of behavior change, but to assess consumer satisfaction with treatment procedures and interventionist's behavior.

Combined social validation procedures take advantage of social comparisons and subjective evaluations in assessing the social importance of intervention effects. The practical importance of an intervention could be bolstered if we could demonstrate that: (1) the child's behavior moved into the same normative range than nonreferred peers and (2) treatment consumers felt that the intervention produced socially important changes in behavior. This combined approach to social validation captures not only how much a behavior changed (a quantitative criterion), but also how consumers of an intervention view this change (a qualitative criterion).

The ultimate goal in intervention for students with DBDs is to change their standing on *measures of social impact*. A social impact measure is characterized by changes that are recognized by most people as being critically important in everyday life (Kazdin, 2003a). Treatments that produce reliable effects may be quite different in their impact on a child's functioning in everyday life. One way of thinking about social impact is in terms of the following outcomes: *true positives, false positives, true negatives,* and *false negatives.* A true positive reflects an individual who is correctly identified as having made a socially important change on a proximal measure and who shows a corresponding change on a social impact measure. A false positive is an individual who shows a socially important change on a proximal measure but does not show a change on a social impact measure. A true negative is an individual who does not show a socially important change on a proximal measure or a change on a social impact measure. A false negative is an individual who does not show a change on a proximal measure but who does show a change on a social impact measure.

Social impact measures represent socially valued intervention goals because social systems such as schools and mental health agencies utilize them to index the success or failure of interventions. Examples of social impact measures include: school dropout, arrest rates, days missed from school, and school suspensions/expulsions. These measures might be considered criterion measures against which behavior changes can be socially validated.

The drawback of relying exclusively on social impact measures is that they are not particularly sensitive in detecting short-term intervention effects. Many treatment consumers consider these social impact measures to be the bottom line in gauging successful intervention outcomes, however exclusive reliance on these measures may overlook a great deal of behavior change (Kazdin, 2003b). As such, exclusive use of social impact measures may result in unacceptably high Type II error rates (i.e., concluding that an intervention was ineffective when, in fact, it was effective).

It is often the case that rather large and sustained changes in behavior are required before these changes are reflected on social impact measures. Sechrest, McKnight, and McKnight (1996) suggested using the psychophysical method of *just noticeable differences* (JND) to index intervention outcomes. The JND approach answers the question: How much of a difference in behavior is required before is it "noticed" by significant others or reflected on social impact measures? In the case of a student with a DBD, how much of a decrease in aggressive/noncompliant behavior is required before it is reflected in a decrease and subsequent elimination of office discipline referrals?

Chapter Summary Points

- Most students with DBDs do not qualify for special education under the category of emotional disturbance and schools often resort to reactive, punitive, intervention practices (e.g., suspensions, expulsions, reprimands, and other weak, non-evidence-based strategies) in dealing with this population.

- Schools are ideal settings to deliver mental health services because they provide a "captive audience" for professionals providing these services.

- If children's conduct problems are not remediated by age 8 (end of third grade), they are highly likely to continue this behavior pattern through adolescence and adulthood.

- School districts, private foundations, and consortia of social service agencies are developing school-linked models of wraparound services and supports targeted to families and at-risk children.

- Approximately one in every five children between the ages of 9 and 17 has a diagnosable mental health or addictive disorder, but special education only identifies 1–2% of these students as emotionally disturbed.

- Most psychotropic mediations used with children to treat a variety of behavior problems lack sound scientific research supporting its use. Psychotropic medications can be a useful adjunct for some behavior problems, but should not be the sole or even the major component of a comprehensive intervention for DBDs.

- Multi-tiered interventions for children and youth with DBDs can be viewed as consisting of three levels of prevention: primary, secondary, and tertiary.

- These three levels of prevention served as the foundational basis of what is known today as response to intervention.

- Several factors are related to a behavior's response to intervention and include: severity of behavior, chronicity of behavior, generalizability of behavior change, treatment strength, treatment integrity, and treatment effectiveness.

- The more severe a behavior problem is, the more resistant it will be to change.

- Long-standing or chronic behavior problems are more resistant to change than less chronic behavior problems.

- Students with DBDs often show excellent initial behavior change, but fail to show generalization and maintenance of these behavior changes.

- The strength of treatments is not absolute, but rather is situationally, behaviorally, and individually specific.

- Treatment integrity is conceptualized as involving three dimensions: treatment adherence, interventionist competence, and treatment differentiation.

- Treatment effectiveness is evaluated using two general approaches: visual inspection of graphed data and various effect size estimates.

- Social validation occurs on three levels: establishing the social significance of behavioral goals, evaluating the social acceptability of intervention efforts, and gauging the social importance of intervention effects.

- Social validation may be accomplished using social comparisons, subjective evaluations, and combined social validation procedures.

Evidence-Based School Interventions

A Multi-Tiered Approach

Not too long ago, school-based consultants and teachers relied on interventions based on familiarity and relative ease of implementation rather than on scientific evidence. Over the past decade, this practice has changed dramatically. In this time, school personnel have increasingly relied on evidence-based practices to assist students in overcoming their learning and behavioral problems. Recall from Chapter 2, *evidence-based practices* are those practices based on rigorous, systematic, and objective evidence using well-established research methodologies. Multiple types of research evidence can be used to support evidence-based practices. These include: observations of disruptive behavior problems to formulate hypotheses about these behaviors; qualitative research to capture the real-world experiences of children with DBDs; single-case experimental designs that are used to draw causal inferences about the effectiveness of interventions for individuals; randomized controlled trials or efficacy studies that are used to draw casual inferences about groups; mediator and moderator studies used to identify correlates of intervention outcomes; and meta-analyses of the research literature to provide a quantitative index concerning the effectiveness of multiple studies.

It cannot be overemphasized that schools are vital settings for intervening with students having DBDs. Schools are unique because they are the one place where teachers and students spend a significant amount of time together in both structured and unstructured contexts, thereby creating numerous intervention-related opportunities. Many school administrators often view students' behavioral problems as stemming from factors outside the school and therefore do not view schools as proactive agents in the process of prevention and/or behavior change (Shinn & Walker, 2010). In fact, schools often utilize interventions that are either patently ineffective or, in some cases, downright harmful (Dishion & Andrews, 1995).

Developing and implementing behavioral interventions in the school requires knowledge, skill, sensitivity, and tact, particularly for interventions delivered within a consultation model of service delivery (see Erchul & Sheridan, 2014). To build effective behavioral interventions requires attention to establishing effective systems of schoolwide positive behavioral interventions and supports that I describe in Chapter 8. We know, however, that not all children will respond adequately primary prevention or Tier 1 interventions and will require more intensive Tier 2 (selected) or Tier 3 (intensive) interventions. Based on the best available evidence, we know that about 15% of students will require Tier 2 selected interventions and about 5% will require Tier 3 intensive interventions (Walker & Shinn, 2010).

It is important to note that the above percentages are useful only as a heuristic or a guide to thinking about a problem. This heuristic represented by multiple tiers of intervention and their respective percentages provides a conceptual roadmap for allocating resources, defining populations, and differentiating among interventions. The following things are true about multi-tiered interventions:

- No single tier solves all problems.
- A well-designed multi-tiered system will have hierarchical tiers of increasing intensity.
- Effective interventions at lower-level tier reduce the need for interventions at subsequent tiers (Walker et al., 1996).

Conceptualization of School-Based Behavioral Interventions

Behavioral interventions, as the term is used in this chapter, can be conceptualized using four broad theoretical categories: (1) applied behavior analysis, (2) social learning theory, (3) cognitive behavioral theory, and (4) neobehavioristic S-R theory. Applied behavior analysis (ABA) derives directly from Skinner's (1953) operant conditioning work and is based on the three-term contingency that describes the functional relationship between antecedents, behaviors, and consequences. ABA uses functional behavioral assessment methods to target antecedent and consequent events in order to design function-based interventions to change socially significant behaviors (Baer, Wolf, & Risley, 1968; Gresham, Watson, et al., 2001). The goal of ABA-based interventions is to determine the *function* (reason or purpose) that a problem behavior serves for an individual in a specific situation so that more socially appropriate replacement behaviors can be facilitated (see Chapter 9). Most school-based interventions for problem behaviors are based on ABA techniques (Cooper et al., 2007).

Social learning theory emanates largely from the work of Bandura (1977, 1986) and utilizes the concept of vicarious reinforcement and the role of cognitive mediational processes in determining which environmental events are attended to, retained, and subsequently performed when an individual is exposed to modeling stimuli. Several factors influence the efficacy of learning via modeling such as model-observer similarity, narrated modeling, and reinforced modeling (Bandura, 1977).

Cognitive-behavioral theory (CBT) assumes that an individual's behavior in response to environmental events is mediated by their cognitions or thoughts. The goal of CBT is to change maladaptive cognitions that then lead to changes in behavior. Techniques such as self-instruction, self-evaluation, correction of maladaptive self-talk, and problem solving are commonly used to treat problem behaviors.

Finally, neobehavioristic S-R models are based on features of classical (respondent) conditioning and avoidance learning in which maladaptive responses are conditioned to stimuli in the environment (conditioned stimuli paired with unconditioned stimuli to elicit conditioned responses). Procedures such as systematic desensitization and exposure-based treatments (flooding) for treatment of anxiety disorders and obsessive–compulsive disorders are based on the S-R model of learning.

Clearly, behavioral interventions encompass a diverse array of theoretical orientations leading to a number of different intervention strategies. Each of the above behavioral intervention models makes different assumptions about the causes and maintenance of problem behaviors. Some behavioral interventions in schools may require intervention strategies using only one model, whereas other behavioral difficulties may require strategies from all four theoretical models. For example, an intervention for disruptive behavior in the classroom may only involve the use of differential reinforcement of incompatible behaviors (DRI) delivered by the teacher. Other behavioral difficulties such as an individual having a comorbid DBD, depression, and obsessive–compulsive disorder may require a combination of differential reinforcement, modeling of appropriate behaviors, CBT, and exposure-based strategies.

Matching Intensity of Intervention to Problem Severity

Perhaps the most important concept in delivering school-based behavioral interventions is the notion of matching the intensity of the intervention to the intensity and severity of the problem behavior. I discussed the U.S. Public Health Service model of primary, secondary, and tertiary prevention strategies in Chapter 4. This prevention model has subsequently been recast into various types of interventions that differ in terms of the nature, comprehensiveness, and intensity of the intervention as well as the degree of unresponsiveness of individuals to a given type of intervention. This model of intervention serves as the basis of *response to intervention*, or RTI, and is composed of three levels of intervention intensity: universal, selected, and targeted/intensive interventions (Gresham, 2002, 2007).

Universal, or Tier 1, strategies are discussed extensively in Chapter 8. These interventions are delivered to all students and are delivered in the same manner and under the same conditions. These interventions are implemented classwide, schoolwide, or districtwide; are implemented either daily or weekly; and each student receives an identical "dosage level" of the intervention. Some examples of these universal interventions are school vaccinations, schoolwide discipline plans, districtwide bully prevention programs, and social skills training curricula in the regular classroom.

Selected, or Tier 2, interventions focus on the inadequate responders to the universal, or Tier 1, intervention. These students are at risk for more severe problem behaviors and will require more intensive, individualized interventions. Many of these students may respond to relatively simple, individually focused behavioral interventions such as behavioral contracts, self-management strategies, and token systems (Walker et al., 2004). Various reductive strategies such as response cost, time out, and differential reinforcement represent effective, evidence-based selected interventions for problem behaviors in the classroom (Cooper et al., 2007).

The goal of selected interventions is to manipulate antecedent and consequent events that might set the occasion for problem behavior to occur and to provide students with effective social-behavioral repertoires that will make them more responsive to universal interventions. These interventions are typically not based on an analysis of behavioral function (functional behavioral assessment) and therefore can be characterized more accurately as *behavior modification* rather than behavior analytic. These interventions utilize procedures such as reinforcement and reductive strategies that overpower whatever function is maintaining problem behavior.

The most intense level of intervention focuses on students who are the most recalcitrant to change and who exhibit chronic behavioral difficulties. It is estimated that this group of students constitutes about 1–5% of any given school population, that they are responsible for 40–50% of behavioral disruptions in schools, and they drain 50–60% of school building and classroom resources (Colvin, Kame'enui, & Sugai, 1993; Sugai et al., 2002). These students do not respond adequately to universal or selected interventions and often require intense, individualized, and comprehensive systems of intervention care such as mental health, juvenile justice, and social services (Eber et al., 2014). The goal of interventions for this group of students is to decrease the frequency and intensity of their problem behaviors and to teach positive replacement behaviors that will successfully compete with their problem behaviors. Unlike selected interventions, these interventions are based on a functional behavioral assessment to determine the consequent events maintaining problem behaviors. The role of functional behavioral assessment in designing behavioral interventions is discussed in a subsequent section of this chapter.

RTI as a Basis for Selecting Interventions

In any intervention, one must have a basis for deciding whether to maintain, modify, intensify, or withdraw an intervention; the RTI model can be used to make this decision. RTI is defined as the change in behavior as a function of intervention (Gresham, 1991, 2002). It uses a student's lack of response to an evidence-based intervention that is implemented with integrity as *the* basis for intensifying, modifying, or changing an intervention. RTI is based on the notion of discrepancy between pre- and postintervention levels of performance and is consistent with a problem-solving model of intervention in which problems are defined as a discrepancy between current and desired levels of performance (Bergan & Kratochwill, 1990; Martens et al., 2014). Any intervention that does not produce a discrepancy between preintervention and postintervention levels of performance should be modified or intensified in an RTI problem-solving model.

Consider a student who exhibits relatively high rates of disruptive and noncompliant behavior in a classroom. The teacher has an established system of classroom rules and procedures that are posted and reviewed in class. The entire school also operates using a schoolwide positive behavior support (SWPBS) model. These are the universal interventions in place that are effective with the majority of students in the class, but are clearly ineffective with this particular student. The teacher consults with the school psychologist, who conducts systematic behavioral observations of the student in the classroom over several days to obtain baseline levels of performance. Based on this observational assessment, along with teacher interviews, the use of differential reinforcement of incompatible behavior (DRI) may be recommended to reduce rates of disruptive, noncompliant behavior (a selected, or Tier 2, intervention).

Subsequently, an observation of the student and teacher is conducted in the classroom to ensure that the intervention is being implemented as intended and to assess rates of disruptive/noncompliant behavior in the classroom to determine the student's response to the DRI intervention. If the student either does not respond to this intervention or responds at an unacceptable level, a more intensive Tier 3 intervention based on a functional behavioral assessment might be implemented to more accurately determine the function of the noncompliant/disruptive behaviors.

Using an RTI approach for making decisions regarding the modification of interventions has several advantages. The most compelling reason for using this approach is that it provides immediate assistance to students who are having difficulties with behavioral challenges. In an RTI approach, there is no need to wait for a student's difficulties to become more severe before effective intervention services are delivered.

Universal screening can be combined with RTI, thereby allowing for proactive identification of at-risk children and establishing baseline data against which to compare the effects of the intervention. Chapter 3 described various evidence-based screening tools that can be used for the early identification of disruptive behavior problems. An excellent and validated example of proactive, universal screening is the Systematic Screening for Behavior Disorders (SSBD; Walker & Severson, 1990). The SSBD consists of a three-stage multiple gating process in which students are screened for externalizing and internalizing behavior problems. The SSBD is norm referenced, has excellent psychometric properties, and is used in a number of states to screen for behavioral difficulties (Walker et al., 2004).

Another advantage of using an RTI approach is that it incorporates assessment procedures that have *treatment validity*, which refers to the degree to which an assessment procedure informs or contributes to beneficial outcomes for individuals (Hayes et al., 1987). Treatment validity contains the idea of incremental validity because it requires assessments to improve prediction above and beyond existing assessment procedures (Gresham, 2004). It also includes principles of utility and cost–benefit analysis as well the notion of evidential bases for test use and interpretation (Messick, 1995). Assessment procedures having treatment validity must meet several technical requirements: (1) the ability to track or model behavior over time, (2) the availability of evidence-based interventions or treatment protocols, (3) ability to inform behavioral decisions, and (4) sensitivity in detecting intervention effects (Gresham, 2002).

Some critics of using an RTI approach might argue that medical diagnoses are not ruled in or out based on how a patient responds to more intensive treatment efforts. This is partially true; however, medical diagnoses often have direct treatment implications (e.g., cancer, diabetes, high cholesterol) and the causes of many medical problems are well known. Moreover, the intensity of medical treatments is often matched to the severity of the medical diagnosis and the progression of the disease (e.g., Stage I vs. State III cancers). Increases in the "dose" of treatment and where it is delivered (outpatient setting vs. hospital setting) are calibrated to the degree of unresponsiveness to that treatment. The fundamental point here is that not all students will require the most intense form of behavioral intervention and the strength, intensity, and duration of treatment should be increased in direct proportion to the student's unresponsiveness to that treatment (Gresham, 1991, 2002).

Types of RTI Used in Schools

There are two basic approaches to delivering interventions within an RTI model: (1) problem-solving RTI and (2) standard-protocol approaches (Gresham, 2007). These two approaches are described in the following sections. Some RTI models combine the two approaches, particularly within a multi-tiered model of service delivery, and may be particularly useful in school settings. These models are best described as multi-tiered RTI approaches to intervention (Barnett, Daly, Jones, & Lentz, 2004).

Problem-Solving RTI

Problem solving can be traced back to the behavioral consultation model first described by Bergan (1977) and later revised and updated by Bergan and Kratochwill (1990). Behavioral consultation takes place in a sequence of four phases: (1) problem identification, (2) problem analysis, (3) plan implementation, and (4) problem evaluation. The goal in behavioral consultation is to define the problem in clear, unambiguous, and operational terms (problem identification), to identify the environmental conditions related to the referral problem (problem analysis), to design and implement an intervention plan with integrity (plan implementation), and to evaluate the effectiveness of the intervention (problem evaluation). Behavioral consultation addresses four fundamental questions: (1) What is the problem?, (2) Why is the problem occurring?, (3) What should be done about it?, and (4) Did it work? These problem-solving steps are described in the following section.

Problems are defined in a problem-solving approach as a discrepancy between current and desired levels of performance; that is, the larger the discrepancy, the larger the problem. For example, if the baseline frequency of noncompliant behavior is 10 episodes per school day and the teacher can tolerate only 2 episodes per school day, the discrepancy is 8 episodes per day. As such, an intervention will have to create an 80% reduction in noncompliant behavior to be considered effective by the teacher. This same type of logic can be applied to any type of referral problem as the first step in a problem-solving approach.

Most types of DBDs result from motivational or so-called *performance deficits*, meaning that the child knows how to perform a more appropriate behavior, but does not do so. Reasons for not performing the behavior may be due to the lack of reinforcement to perform the appropriate behavior (recall the matching law) or the lack of opportunities to perform the behavior. In this case, remedial interventions would involve increasing the rate of reinforcement for appropriate behavior, decreasing the rate of reinforcement for inappropriate behavior, and providing multiple opportunities to perform the appropriate behavior.

The final stage of a problem-solving model involves determining whether the intervention was effective in changing behavior. This process involves *data-based decision making* in which the effectiveness of an intervention is determined empirically by direct measurement of intervention outcomes. RTI models insist on direct measurement of behavior and the environment as the core foci of a comprehensive assessment. RTI is concerned primarily with the assessment of measurable and changeable aspects of the environment and its relationship to the occurrence of problem behavior.

Standard-Protocol RTI Approaches

A second RTI approach is the use of validated treatment protocols that can be implemented with students having DBDs. These protocols are manualized and can be implemented with integrity by most professionals in schools. Standard protocols are described in Chapters 6 (home interventions) and 7 (multicomponent interventions). Manualized treatments have the following characteristics: (1) a clear description of procedures, strategies, and activities that should be implemented and those that should be avoided; (2) specification of the length, duration, and intensity of intervention services; and (3) definition of the target population (Perepletchikova, 2014).

Manualized treatments have several advantages. One, manuals reduce the variability in treatment implementation thereby increasing treatment integrity. Two, manuals can specify the theoretical basis for a given treatment, specify interventionist's behaviors, describe the sequence of intervention components to be implemented, and specify procedures for dealing with deviations from a treatment protocol. Three, manualized treatments can specify built-in flexibility procedures in the implementation of a treatment.

The primary advantage of a standard-protocol approach compared to a problem-solving approach is that it can be used to ensure the integrity of an intervention. It should be noted that most behavioral interventions implemented in schools do not use or even have a manual to guide implementation (Gresham, 2007). This is not to say that school-based interventions cannot be manualized, but we currently do not have an adequate library of manualized school-based behavioral interventions.

Evidence-Based School Interventions

The Behavior Education Program

The Behavior Education Program (BEP) is a school-based program targeting students who are at risk for developing serious or chronic behavior problems (Crone, Horner, & Hawken, 2004). Students who fail to respond adequately to Tier 1 universal interventions and who receive several office discipline referrals (ODRs) per year may benefit from a Tier 2 intervention like the BEP. The BEP is based on a *Check-In/Check-Out* system providing students with immediate feedback on their behavior using a Daily Progress Report (DPR) and contingent adult positive attention. In the BEP, behavioral expectations are clearly defined and students receive immediate and delayed reinforcement for meeting these expectations. School and home communication is established by sending a copy of the DPR home to parents (i.e., a daily behavioral report card) to be brought back to school signed by the parent or guardian the next day. A crucial feature of the BEP is the use of data to evaluate the effectiveness of the program in changing the student's behavior. Points recorded on the DPR are summarized and graphed, and these data are reviewed every 2 *weeks* to decide whether to continue, change, or fade the program.

The BEP is based on several core features of positive behavior support as follows:

- Clearly defined behavioral expectations.
- Instruction of teaching appropriate social skills.
- Increased positive reinforcement for following behavioral expectations.
- Contingent consequences for problem behavior.
- Increased positive contact with an adult in the school.
- Improved opportunities for self-management.
- Increased home–school collaboration.

Features of the BEP

The BEP is continuously available, can be implemented within 3–5 days of identifying a problem, and requires no more than 5–10 minutes per teacher per day. All teachers and staff at a school can implement the BEP, and it has relatively low time demands. The program is a Tier 2, or selected, intervention, and therefore does not require a functional behavioral assessment that is typical of Tier 3 intensive behavioral interventions. Based on an RTI model, it is estimated that approximately 15–20% of students in a school will need a Tier 2 behavioral intervention such as the BEP. For example, in a school with 600 students, about 90–120 students will need a Tier 2 intervention because they typically not respond adequately to a Tier 1 universal intervention.

The BEP has several advantages over other types of Tier 2 interventions. First, based on the size of a school, up to 30 students can be supported by the BEP at one time. Second, the BEP has a built-in progress monitoring system in which students obtain feedback on their behavioral performances via the DPR. Third, the program is easily generalizable to other students in the school and therefore does not require extensive training.

The daily cycle of the BEP consists of the following:

- The student arrives at school and checks in with an adult or BEP coordinator at the school.
- After check-in, the student receives his or her DPR.
- The student carries the DPR throughout the day and hands it to the teacher or supervisor at the start of the school day (elementary school) or class period (middle school and high school).
- The student receives the DPR after each class period and receives feedback from the teacher or supervisor related to expected social behaviors.
- At the end of the day the student returns the DPR to the BEP coordinator, determines whether point goals were met, and carries a copy of the DPR home.
- Family members receive the DPR, deliver recognition for success, and sign the form. The student returns the signed DPR the next day to the BEP coordinator.

Which Students Should Receive the BEP?

The BEP is designed for students who are at risk for developing serious and chronic behavior problems. Most of these students exhibit relatively low-intensity problem behaviors such as being tardy to class, coming to school unprepared, talking out in class, and minor disruptions in the classroom. This disruptive behavior interferes with academic instruction, with the student's learning, and with the learning of others in the classroom. The BEP is based on frequent positive social interactions between students and teachers and utilizes frequent progress monitoring of behavior at school and home. Students who are not reinforced by adult attention or who even may find it aversive are not good candidates for the BEP (Crone et al., 2010).

The BEP is not an adequate intervention for students who engage in serious or violent behaviors. These students will require more intensive interventions typically based on a functional behavioral assessment. Also, the types of behaviors addressed by the BEP will be different in elementary school versus middle or high school. In elementary school, students may have difficulty in taking turns, remaining seated in class, refusing to share materials, or completing tasks independently. In middle or high school, students may use inappropriate language, be frequently tardy to class, become defiant to adults, and refuse to complete assigned work. Table 5.1 summarizes the characteristics of appropriate and inappropriate candidates for the BEP.

Research on the BEP with elementary school students has shown it to be effective in reducing problem behaviors. Filter et al. (2007) and Hawken, MacLeod, and Rawlings (2007) demonstrated that the BEP was effective in reducing office discipline referrals (ODRs) by 67% and 75%, respectively. Other studies have shown similar effects in elementary schools (Crone et al., 2004; Fairbanks, Sugai, Guardino, & Lathrop, 2007; McCurdy, Kunsch, & Reibstein, 2007) and middle schools (Hawken, 2006; March & Horner, 2002). Overall, the effects of the BEP on problem behavior can be summarized as follows:

- Typical schools are able to implement the BEP successfully.
- Use of the BEP is functionally related to reduced levels of problem behavior, and for some students, increased levels of academic achievement.
- The BEP is likely to be effective with 60–75% of at-risk students.
- Students who do not find adult attention rewarding are least likely to respond successfully to the BEP.
- If a student is not successful on the BEP, conducing a functional behavioral assessment and using this information to adapt the BEP support can be effective in improving behavioral outcomes (Crone et al., 2010).

First Steps to Success

First Steps to Success (FSS) is a coordinated school and home intervention program designed to prevent the development of antisocial behavior among at-risk children in kindergarten through third grade. FSS consists of three interrelated modules that can be implemented separately or collectively. These modules were designed to be applied in concert with each other in order to provide a comprehensive screening and home–school intervention package coordinated with a single linked process. These modules consist of (1) universal screening and early detection of behaviorally at-risk students in grades K–2, (2) implementation of a school intervention component that teaches an adaptive pattern of behavior for school success and development of friendships, and (3) parent instruction in how to teach and reward school success at home. The FSS program provides a comprehensive and highly effective approach to

TABLE 5.1. Appropriate and Inappropriate Students for the BEP

Appropriate students for the BEP	Inappropriate students for the BEP
Engage in problem behavior throughout the day in multiple settings.	Engage in problem behaviors in one class or only in unstructured settings (lunchroom, playground, bus area).
Engage in mild acting-out behaviors such as talking out, off-task, out-of-seat.	Engage in serious or violent behaviors such as extreme noncompliance, aggression, injury to others.
Problem behaviors are not related to trying to escape difficult academic tasks.	Problem behaviors typically occur when the student is trying to escape a difficult task or academic subject.
Problem behaviors are maintained by adult attention and/or the student finds adult attention reinforcing.	Problem behaviors are maintained by escape or avoidance of academic tasks and/or the student does not find adult attention reinforcing.

the prevention of antisocial behavior patterns among young children. The program is designed to detect at-risk children when they begin their formal school careers and to work cooperatively with them and their parents, teachers, and peers intensely over a 3-month period to ensure that they get off to the best start possible early in their school careers. A behavioral coach coordinates the FSS program; this individual may be an early interventionist, school counselor, school psychologist, or behavioral specialist.

Universal Screening and Early Detection

The screening component of the FSS is proactive, involves multiple gates or screens, and is designed to give every child an equal chance to access the intervention based on their behavioral characteristics. Classrooms of students in kindergarten and the primary grades are systematically screened to detect behaviorally at-risk children who show signs of emerging antisocial behavior using the SSBD (Walker & Severson, 1990). Four screening options are provided ranging from inexpensive (teacher nominations) to more expensive (a three-stage multiple gating procedure using teacher nominations and rank ordering, teacher ratings on measures of adaptive and maladaptive behavior and critical behavioral events, and direct observations recorded in classroom and playground settings). The total cost of the FSS, including the coach's time and required materials, is approximately $400 per case. The coach invests about 40–50 hours of time over the 3-month implementation period for the program.

School Intervention

The Contingencies for Learning Academic and Social Skills (CLASS) program for acting-out children makes up the school intervention component of the FSS program. CLASS requires 30 school days for implementation. It is intended as a behavior management program that overlays the curricular content and instructional routines of regular education settings.

CLASS is divided into two major phases: consultant and teacher. The consultant phase lasts five program days and is characterized by proximal and intense monitoring of the target student's classroom behavior. Red and green signaling cards are used to this purpose during two 20–30-minute periods daily. Points and praise for following classroom rules and remaining academically engaged are awarded frequently during these periods (every 1–2 minutes). The red side of the card is used to signal inappropriate behavior or lack of academic engagement. If the red side is showing when it is time to award a point, then the point goes on the red rather than the green side, thereby serving as a response cost contingency (i.e., loss of points). The student must earn at least 80% of the available points in order to earn access to a group activity reward that immediately follows the period. If the target student meets the reward criteria for both daily sessions, then a special privilege or reward is prearranged with the student's parents. The student takes the card home, shows it to his or her parents, and returns the card to school the next day.

The teacher phase of the CLASS program lasts from day 6 to day 30 and is divided into reward and maintenance phases. The reward phase (program days 6–20) involves the continued use of home and school rewards and the awarding of points. The maintenance phase (program days 21–30) relies only on teacher and parent praise to maintain the behavioral gains achieved in the previous phase. Brief time-out procedures are implemented to deal with teacher defiance, fighting, property destruction, and severe tantrums.

On program day 6, the regular teacher assumes primary control of the CLASS program's daily procedures with the support and assistance of the behavioral coach. By this time, the monitoring, point awarding, and praising requirements CLASS have been reduced to levels at which the teacher can manage the program as part of his or her regular teaching duties. The teacher phase begins with the intermittent use of the red and green point cards for monitoring and awarding points but this is completely faded out by day 15 of the program. The magnitude of available rewards at both home and school increases as the program progresses, as does the length of the intervals required to earn them. For instance, during days 16–20, the student must work five full school days in order to meet the reward criterion.

Family Support and Parent Training

The third component of the FSS program is called Homebase. Homebase is a parent skill-building program based on more than 30 years of research of research and clinical trials at the Oregon Social Learning Center that conducts research on deviant families (i.e., those families that produce antisocial, delinquent children). This research is reviewed in Chapters 1 and 6 of this volume (see Patterson, 2002). Homebase is a child-focused program for improving adjustment to kindergarten. The program consists of six sessions in the home and a midweek telephone call to discuss parent and child performances of the previous lesson content. Homebase is implemented over consecutive weeks to maximize parents' mastery of the material and corresponding parenting skills. Its lessons are designed to complement the CLASS program and are organized around key elements of good school adjustment (e.g., following rules, being ready for school, cooperating, accepting limits, and getting along with others).

Each in-home meeting follows a standard format. A behavioral coach presents the skill and provides a rationale for its importance. Next, the parent and behavioral coach complete a current skill-level assessment for the child. Some lessons are enhanced using videotape examples shown during the home visit. Activity cards and other instructional materials for the week's lesson are presented and reviewed with the parents. A daily time is chosen for practicing the skill. Barriers to practicing the exercises are discussed and strategies for implementation are developed that are fine-tuned to parents' preferences and skill levels.

After 6 weeks of skill development, groups of parents may meet monthly to share their successes and discuss strategies for responding to difficulties they encounter during the daily practice sessions geared toward managing their child's behavior problems at home. Groups also discuss their successes and difficulties in collaborating with the school intervention components.

Outcomes of the FSS Program

Twenty-one studies have been conducted that investigated the effectiveness of the FSS program. Two of these studies were randomized controlled trials (RCTs) that met the What Works Clearinghouse evidence standards without reservation and three studies met these standards using the single-case design standards. Walker et al. (1998) randomly assigned 46 kindergartners to the FSS program or to a wait-list control condition. Students were described as exhibiting antisocial behaviors including victimizing others, severe tantrums, and aggression. Results from this study showed that children in the FSS program showed large increases academic engaged time ($d = 0.97$) and adaptive behavior ($d = 1.17$) and large decreases in aggressive behavior ($d = 0.99$) and maladaptive behavior ($d = 0.93$) with an overall effect size of $d = 1.02$.

Walker et al. (2009) randomly assigned 198 students in grades 1–3 to the FSS program or to a control condition. The FSS program showed large increases in teacher rated social skill ($d = 0.78$) and adaptive behavior ($d = 0.72$) and moderate decreases in teacher and parent ratings problem behavior ($d = 0.50$) and teacher ratings of maladaptive behavior ($d = 0.50$). Overall, the FSS program is an effective, evidence-based treatment for preventing serious and chronic antisocial behavior patterns. It appears to produce the strongest effects on teacher ratings of prosocial behavior and academic engaged time.

Intensive School-Based Interventions

Depending on the school, it is estimated that Tier 3 (intensive) interventions will be needed to address the behavioral needs of about 5–10% of a school population. These students do not respond adequately to Tier 1 (universal) or Tier 2 (selected) interventions. Tier 3 behavioral interventions can be characterized as individualized, assessment-based, and consisting of intense, durable procedures. A key feature of most Tier 3 interventions is that they are based on a *functional behavioral assessment* (FBA). I described FBA procedures in Chapter 3 of this volume and will revisit that topic briefly in the following section.

Functional Behavioral Assessment

FBA derives from operant learning theory that is grounded in a philosophy of science known as functionalism. Functionalism rejects an understanding of behavior based on topography (form or structure) because behavioral topographies are merely descriptive and, as such, explain nothing about the controlling functions of behavior (Skinner, 1953). The topography of behavior is simply what the behavior looks like. For example, children with oppositional defiant disorder exhibit behaviors such as noncompliance, arguing, annoying others, loss of temper, and blaming others for their mistakes. Each of these behaviors have different topographies (i.e., they look different to an observer).

A good example of a structural or descriptive account of behavior can be found in clinical classification systems such as the fifth edition of the *Diagnostic and Statistical Manual of Mental Disorders* (DSM-5; American Psychiatric Association, 2013). The DSM-5 provides a topographical rather than a functional account of behavior. The emphasis in DSM-5 is on "What?" (topography) rather than "What for?" (function) of behavior. There is nothing particularly wrong with a structural or descriptive account of behavior except that it provides no information regarding important, identifiable, and controllable environmental events surrounding those behaviors. For example, a diagnosis of conduct disorder in DSM-5 requires the presence of at least 3 of 15 symptoms (behaviors) such as bullying others, fighting, lying, stealing, truancy, and so forth. A mere description of these behaviors does not yield the most important information for treatment planning: the function served by these behaviors. Some behaviors may be maintained by social attention, others by access to tangible reinforcers (e.g., money or someone's possessions), and still others might be maintained by escape or avoidance of aversive events. To effectively treat these behaviors requires identification of the function served by these behaviors.

TYPES OF FBAs

There are two basic types of FBAs: *descriptive FBA* and *experimental FBA*. A descriptive FBA uses systematic direct observations of antecedents, behaviors, and consequences in a naturalistic environment (e.g., classrooms) to determine the occurrence of behavior as a function of antecedents and maintaining consequences. As described in Chapter 3, an antecedent–behavior–consequence, or ABC, recording chart is used for this purpose. Invariably, certain behaviors only occur in the presence of some antecedents and not others and certain behaviors are maintained by some consequences but not others. Knowing when behaviors occur and which consequences follow them can be useful in designing effective interventions. It should be noted, however, that a descriptive assessment is *correlational* and not causative in that it identifies antecedents and consequences that are correlated with the occurrence of behavior.

Another type of FBA, known as experimental functional analysis, involves a more rigorous experimental methodology that allows for stronger statements regarding behavioral function. Iwata, Dorsey, Slifer, Bauman, and Richman (1982/1994) pioneered this methodology in their long-term study of self-injurious behavior in individuals with developmental disabilities. Experimental functional analysis involves exposing an individual to each of the possible maintaining conditions in a tightly controlled experimental design such as a multi-element or reversal design. Typically, an individual is exposed to four possible maintaining contingencies in a controlled analogue situation (social attention, access to tangibles, escape from aversive stimuli, and automatic reinforcement plus a control condition (e.g., free play). Using a multi-element design, these conditions are counterbalanced and rapidly alternated. Rates of target behavior under each of the conditions are graphed and compared to the condition producing dramatically higher rates of responding.

Although the methodology developed by Iwata et al. (1982/1994) for studying self-injurious behavior has undergone a number of iterations, the essentials remain basically the same. By controlling the delivery and rate of reinforcement and the influences of extra-experimental variables, one can make stronger statements regarding behavioral function and can design functionally specific interventions. Despite the methodological rigor of experimental functional analysis, there are limitations regarding the external validity of the findings and the amount of time and expertise required to conduct a valid functional analysis.

SUMMARY OF FBA

Many school-based interventions for DBDs may be ineffective because these interventions are selected and implemented without an adequate assessment and consideration of behavioral function. At least four problems can arise when interventions are selected without considering behavioral function: (1) the intervention may strengthen a problem behavior via positive reinforcement, (2) the intervention may strengthen a problem behavior via negative reinforcement, (3) the intervention may be functionally irrelevant to a problem behavior, and (4) the intervention may not provide alternative sources of reinforcement for more desirable behaviors.

A key question when using FBA is whether interventions matched to the operant function of behavior are more effective than non-FBA-based interventions. That is, does FBA have treatment validity?

Prescribed interventions without FBA data can be effective under three conditions: (1) when assessment costs exceed treatment costs, (2) when consequences of delaying treatment are minimal, and (3) there is no link between behavioral function and treatment selection. A good example of this from the applied behavior analysis literature is illustrated in a study by Lalli et al. (1999). These researchers showed that all five participants who clearly had escape-motivated disruptive behavior (maintained by negative reinforcement) responded better to a positive reinforcement intervention (edibles) than a negative reinforcement treatment (30-second escape from tasks).

It should also be noted that not all behaviors exhibited by children and youth with DBDs are amenable to an FBA. Many behaviors exhibited by children and youth with DBDs occur at such low frequencies that it is nearly impossible to observe and determine baseline levels of performance. For example, behaviors such as fire setting, bringing a weapon to school, and abusing animals are examples of these high-intensity but low-frequency behaviors. Other behaviors exhibited by these children are not amenable to a FBA because they are virtually unobservable by others. For example, behaviors such as breaking into someone's home or car, stealing, and lying are difficult to detect and thus are not amenable to an FBA.

In an insightful article critiquing the use of functional behavioral assessments in schools, Walker and Sprague (1999) suggested that there are two models or approaches to the assessment of behavior problems. One, the longitudinal or risk factor exposure model, grew out of research on the development of antisocial behavior patterns and seeks to identify molar variables operating across multiple settings that put students at risk for long-term negative outcomes (e.g., delinquency, school dropout, arrests). The second, called the functional assessment model, seeks to identify microvariables operating in specific situations that are sensitive to environmental contingencies. Both models are useful, but answer quite different questions.

Walker and Sprague (1999) suggest the following: If one's goal is to understand and manage problem behavior in a specific setting, then functional assessment is a useful procedure. However, if one's goal is to understand the variables that account for risk across multiple settings and predict a student's future, then one need to know something about the student's genetic–behavioral history (risk factors). This is the goal of longitudinal research and is not of pressing concern to school study teams or special education placement committees.

ARE FBA-BASED INTERVENTIONS MORE EFFECTIVE?

A fundamental question to be answered is whether FBA-based interventions are more effective than interventions not based on an FBA. In other words, do the benefits of produced by an FBA outweigh the costs of conducting it? Gage, Lewis, and Stichter (2012) conducted a meta-analysis of 69 studies that used FBA to design an intervention for children and adolescents with emotional and behavioral disorders. These studies used either a descriptive or experimental FBA to design the interventions. Gage et al. calculated several indices of effect size in the meta-analysis. First, the percent of nonoverlapping data (PND) was calculated for each study. PND was calculated by computing the percentage of data points in the treatment phase that exceeded the most extreme baseline data point in the intended treatment direction. The average PND from baseline to intervention was 73.25%. Second, the authors conducted a hierarchical linear model (HLM) analysis of the data. The HLM analysis showed that FBA-based interventions produced an average level change or mean shift of −32.46% that can be interpreted as the percentage of change from baseline to intervention. This indicates that FBA-based interventions reduce the percentage of the dependent variable by 70.5% from baseline to intervention.

The HLM analysis also showed a significant effect for slope or rate of change from baseline to intervention. The mean rate of change from baseline to intervention was −0.52, indicating a negative or decreasing slope, thus demonstrating a declining trend. The HLM analysis also revealed a great deal of variability in baseline and intervention levels and trends across studies. Overall, this meta-analysis suggests that FBA-based interventions for students with DBDs are effective in reducing problem behaviors. However, since no non-FBA-based interventions were included in this study, no statements could be made about the relative effectiveness of FBA-based and non-FBA-based interventions.

Some Effective Tier 3 Interventions

I will describe two major categories of effective, evidence-based Tier 3 interventions for reducing problem behaviors associated with DBDs. These categories are: (1) punishment-based procedures and (2) reductive non-punishment-based procedures. The discussion of these procedures will necessarily be relatively brief given space considerations, but I will refer the reader to more extensive discussions of these procedures in the text.

Punishment-Based Procedures

Punishment teaches each of us not to repeat behaviors that are painful or harmful. Punishment is equally important to learning as reinforcement because, like reinforcement, punishment creates certain consequences. Accidentally putting your hand on a hot stove is punishing and teaches you to be more careful around hot stoves. Punishment, like reinforcement, has survival value for all of us. Punishment, as the term is used in operant learning, is different from everyday vernacular uses of the term punishment. Our legal system "punishes" offenders by sending them to jail, fining them, and, in the most extreme cases, by capital punishment. This use of the term implies some sort of retribution for an individual. In operant learning, punishment refers to consequences of a *behavior* that affect its future probability of occurrence.

Punishment can be defined as a stimulus that follows a behavior that *decreases* the future probability of that behavior. Recall that reinforcement is a stimulus that follows a behavior that *increases* the future probability of behavior. Thus punishment and reinforcement are mirror images of one another. Punishment consists of two fundamental types: positive punishment and negative punishment. Positive punishment refers to the *presentation* of a stimulus following a behavior that decreases the future probability of that behavior. Putting your hand on the hot stove is an example of positive punishment. Negative punishment can be defined as removal or termination a stimulus that decreases the future probability of that behavior. Receiving a speeding ticket from the police is an example of negative punishment (contingent loss of money via a fine).

It should be noted that the terms positive and negative punishment, like positive and negative reinforcement, do not imply the desirability of behavior change. Positive and negative simply describe whether a stimulus is presented or removed (similar to the mathematical operations of addition and subtraction). Unfortunately, positive punishment and negative reinforcement are frequently confused because both procedures involve a form of aversive control of behavior (Cooper et al., 2007). Remember, positive punishment refers to the presentation of a stimulus that reduces the future frequency of behavior and negative reinforcement refers to the removal of a stimulus that increases the future frequency of behavior.

There are several factors that influence the effectiveness of punishment as an intervention procedure. One, punishment is much more effective if it is delivered immediately after a behavior rather than being delayed. Two, punishment is more effective if it is of relative high intensity or magnitude. Three, the schedule of punishment dramatically affects the future probability of a behavior. For example, a punisher delivered on a continuous schedule of punishment is more effective in suppressing behavior than a punisher delivered on an intermittent schedule.

EXAMPLES OF POSITIVE PUNISHMENT PROCEDURES

Two types of punishment procedures have been used to reduce behaviors characteristic of DBDs. *Verbal reprimands* delivered by teachers and/or parents are one such procedure. Verbal reprimands are perhaps the most common attempted punishment procedure by teachers and parents. A teacher who uses a high frequency of verbal reprimands will probably not see a huge reduction in problem behaviors. Cooper et al. (2007) recommend that the teacher would be better off issuing one strong verbal reprimand such as BE QUIET! If reprimands are issued repeatedly, students often habituate to the reprimand and do not attend to it. It also should be noted that verbal reprimands can function as a reinforcer instead of a punisher, particularly for students whose problem behaviors are maintained by social attention. Before using verbal reprimands as an attempted punisher, it would be wise to conduct an FBA to determine the function of the problem behavior.

Another positive punishment procedure is *overcorrection* that requires the student to engage in effortful behavior that is directly related to the problem behavior. Overcorrection consists to two types: restitution and positive practice. In *restitutional overcorrection,* the student is required to return the environment to its original state or condition and to improve the environment to a better state than it was prior to the misbehavior. For example, a student who has a tantrum in which he turns over desks in the classroom and kicks the trashcan might be required to put the desks back where they belong, pick up the spilled trash, and then clean the entire classroom. This form of overcorrection is based on the notion of high response effort that is aversive to most individuals.

A variation of overcorrection is known as *simple correction*, in which the student is required to restore the environment to its previous state, but not to make the environment better than it was prior to the misbehavior. Breaking in the lunch line, littering at school, and breaking another student's possessions may be best handled by simple correction. Simple correction is perhaps most appropriate for behaviors that are not severe, do not occur frequently, and are not deliberate (Azrin & Besalel, 1999).

Yet another type of correction procedure is known as *precorrection*. In precorrection, the student is told the situations and contexts in which he or she is having behavioral difficulties. For example, some students may have difficulty in transitioning between activities in the classroom by exhibiting unruly inappropriate behaviors. Precorrection typically involves the following seven steps:

- The teacher identifies the contexts and behaviors of concern.
- The teacher specifies expected appropriate behaviors to perform instead.
- The teacher modifies the context or situation in which problem behaviors are occurring.
- The teacher conducts behavioral rehearsals with the student.
- The teacher provides strong reinforcement of performance of expected behaviors.
- The teacher prompts expected behaviors before performance.
- The teacher monitors the precorrection plan.

Precorrection is a relatively simple, effective procedure for preventing the occurrence of problem behaviors. Many students with DBDs exhibit problem behaviors in some contexts and not others. Precorrection attempts to identify the contexts in which problem behaviors are exhibited and tries to modify that context and teach expected behaviors to take the place of problem behaviors. Many students may simply need to be reminded of their problem contexts and how to avoid these contexts, thereby preventing the occurrence of problem behavior.

Another type of overcorrection is known as *positive practice overcorrection,* in which the student is required to repeatedly perform a correct form of a behavior or a behavior that is incompatible with that behavior (Cooper et al., 2007). For example, is a student says negative or hurtful things to another student, he might then be required to say nice things about that student and all the students in the class. Positive practice overcorrection has been effectively used to reduce rates of disruptive behavior in the classroom, to reduce aggressive behavior, and to decrease oral reading errors (Cooper et al., 2007).

EXAMPLES OF NEGATIVE PUNISHMENT PROCEDURES

There are two commonly used negative punishment procedures: (1) time out and (2) response cost. *Time out* (technically, time out from positive reinforcement) is the withdrawal of the possibility or opportunity to

earn positive reinforcement or the loss of the access to positive reinforcers for a specified period of time contingent upon a behavior (Cooper et
al., 2007). Time out reduces the future probability of behavior based on
the removal of access to positive reinforcement and therefore is a negative punishment procedure. Three important considerations are vital to
the definition of time out: (1) the difference between the time-in and
time-out environments, (2) the contingent loss of access to the positive
reinforcement for period of time, and (3) the decrease in the future frequency of behavior subsequent to time out.

Cooper et al. (2007) indicate that time out can be considered from
procedural, conceptual, and functional perspectives. In terms of procedure, time out is that period when an individual is removed from a positively reinforcing environment or loses access to reinforcers in that environment for a period of time. Conceptually, the difference between the
time-in and time-out environments is of central importance. The more
reinforcing the time-in environment is, the most effective time out will
be in decreasing behavior and vice versa. Functionally, time out involves
reducing the frequency of an undesirable behavior. If a student's problem
behavior is maintained by escape or avoidance (negative reinforcement
function), then time out will lead to *increases* rather than decreases in
the problem behavior. In this case, time out must be considered a reinforcer rather than a punisher.

Two fundamental types of time out are typically used: (1) nonexclusion time out and (2) exclusion time out. In nonexclusion time out, the
child is not completely removed from the time-in setting but remains in
that setting during the time-out procedure. There are three variations of
the nonexclusion time out procedure: (1) planning ignoring, (2) contingent observation, and (3) a time-out ribbon. In planned ignoring, social
reinforcers such as attention, physical contact, or verbal interaction are
withheld for a brief period of time contingent on the occurrence of a
problem behavior. *Planned ignoring* assumes that the problem behavior
is functionally maintained by social attention and that its removal will
reduce the frequency of a problem behavior. The advantage of planned
ignoring is that it is easy to implement, nonintrusive, and convenient.

Contingent observation involves removing the individual to another
physical location within the classroom where he or she can observe the
other class members engaging in classroom activities. During contingent
observation, the individual loses access to positive reinforcement for a
period of time. At the end of the contingent observation period, the child
rejoins the group and can access ongoing positive reinforcement that is
available in the time-in environment.

A *time-out ribbon* is a colored band or badge usually placed on the child's wrist and serves as a discriminative stimulus for the receipt of positive reinforcement. When the band on the child's wrist, he or she is able to earn positive reinforcers. Contingent on misbehavior, the time-out ribbon is removed and all types of social interaction with the child ceases for a short period of time. Like all other forms of time out, the ribbon signals to the child that he or she has lost all access to positive reinforcement for a period of time.

Exclusion time out involves removing an individual from the physical environment to another location contingent on the occurrence of problem behavior. Exclusion can involve sending the child to a time-out room, using a partition in the classroom (e.g., cubicle or screen), or sending the child to hallway time out. There are advantages and disadvantages of each these time-out procedures. The advantage of a time-out room is that one can control access to all forms of positive reinforcement. The primary disadvantage of this procedure is that many students become highly resistant to going to the time-out room and display high-intensity emotional outbursts. The chief advantage of partition time out is that it allows the student to remain in the classroom to hear ongoing academic instruction. The disadvantage of partition time out is that the student may still access positive reinforcement from other students via social attention (laughing, sighing, and so forth). Although hallway time out is easy to implement, it is not recommended because it is impossible to control the student's access to multiple forms of reinforcement while in the hallway.

The primary advantages of time out for reducing problem behaviors is that it is relatively easy to implement, acceptable to most teachers (appropriate, fair, and effective), and it leads to relatively rapid decreases of problem behavior. To be most effective, several steps should be taken while implementing time out. One, it is important to enrich the availability of reinforcement in the time-in environment. One way of doing this is to give the entire class access to free time or other preferred activities while the offending student is in time out. Two, it is important to specify what behaviors that will lead to time out. Three, it is important to specify the duration of time out. As a rule of thumb, the duration of time out should be relatively short (e.g., 2–5 minutes). Four, one should consider using non-punishment-based procedures first (e.g., differential reinforcement or extinction) before using time out.

A final negative punishment procedure is response cost. In *response cost,* a specified amount of a positive reinforcer is lost contingent on the occurrence of problem behavior. Examples of response cost include losing minutes of recess, loss of points in a token economy intervention, loss of time available to engage in preferred activities (lost computer time), or other "fines" for misbehavior. Response cost is highly acceptable to teachers, convenient, and leads to moderate to rapid decreases in problem behavior. To be maximally effective, response cost should be combined with positive reinforcement. For example, a student may earn points for appropriate behavior in the classroom, but may lose a specified number of those points contingent on the occurrence of problem behavior.

REDUCTIVE NON-PUNISHMENT-BASED PROCEDURES

There are two basic procedures for decreasing the frequency of behavior using non-punishment-based procedures: (1) extinction and (2) differential reinforcement. *Extinction* refers to a gradual decrease in behavior when reinforcement for a previously reinforced behavior is discontinued or withheld. A student who constantly interrupts the teacher in class to get attention (positive reinforcement) creates problems in the learning of others. In this case, the teacher might ignore these interruptions (withholding reinforcement) and the behavior should gradually decrease over time. Extinction consists of two basic types: (1) extinction of behavior maintained by positive reinforcement and (2) extinction of behavior maintained by negative reinforcement.

Extinction

Extinction of behavior maintained by positive reinforcement occurs when a positive reinforcer for a previously reinforced behavior is withheld. This procedure will only work if the positive reinforcer if it is withheld *every time* the behavior occurs. If the reinforcer is withheld every nine times a problem behavior occurs but is not withheld on the tenth time it occurs, the behavior will not extinguish because the behavior in this case is being maintained by a *partial* or *intermittent* schedule of reinforcement. A good example of this is a child who whines to his mom that he wants candy (which is conveniently placed at the cash register in the store). The mom says "No" nine times they go to the store but says "Yes" on the tenth time. The behavior of whining for candy will not extinguish and will, in fact, *increase* and become more *intense* over time. Unlike the effects of punishment, extinction produces a *gradual* (rather than an immediate) decrease in behavior over time. The problem with using extinction in classrooms to decrease behavior maintained by social attention is that the behavior may disrupt ongoing academic instruction and learning in the classroom.

Extinction of behavior maintained by negative reinforcement involves behavior that does *not* produce removal of an aversive stimulus. In other words, the individual cannot escape the aversive situation. This form of extinction is known as *escape extinction*. For example, a child exhibits high rates of disruptive behavior when the teacher instructs him to complete math worksheets in the classroom. A functional behavioral assessment determined that this behavior was being maintained by escape from math task demands (negative reinforcement). The teacher decided to use escape extinction to decrease the disruptive behavior; that is, the disruptive behavior would no longer lead to escape from task demands. This procedure should produce a gradual decrease and elimination of disruptive behavior during math worksheet activities.

When using extinction, one should consider the following three concepts: (1) extinction burst, (2) spontaneous recovery, and (3) schedule of reinforcement. An *extinction burst* refers to an immediate increase in a behavior following the removal of a positive or negative reinforcer. Going back to the previous example of the student who interrupts the teacher to gain social attention, the immediate effect of the teacher ignoring the behavior will be a temporary *increase* in interrupting behavior. If the teacher continues to ignore the behavior, it will decrease over time. Similarly, the student's disruptive behavior during math worksheet activity should temporarily increase during the escape extinction process, but should eventually decrease over time. Extinction bursts are quite common, and one must be prepared for dealing with these temporary increases in problem behaviors when using extinction.

Spontaneous recovery refers to an increase in the frequency of a behavior that has been reduced or eliminated by the extinction process. Spontaneous recovery occurs even though the behavior does not produce reinforcement. Cooper et al. (2007) suggest that spontaneous recovery is temporary, and those using extinction should be prepared for this occurrence.

Finally, the *schedule of reinforcement* determines how quickly a behavior will extinguish. Behavior maintained on a continuous schedule of reinforcement (i.e., the behavior is reinforced every time it occurs) will extinguish more rapidly than behavior maintained on intermittent schedules of reinforcement. The "thinner" (less reinforcement) the schedule of reinforcement for a behavior, the *more resistant* that behavior will be to extinction. For instance, a behavior that is reinforced, on average, every 10 times it occurs will be more resistant to extinction than a behavior that is reinforced every five times it occurs. Many problem behaviors are highly resistant to extinction because they are maintained on relatively thin intermittent or partial schedules of reinforcement. In these cases extinction is probably not the intervention of choice, and one might consider alternative reductive strategies (e.g., response cost or time out).

Differential Reinforcement

Differential reinforcement involves the reinforcement of one response class and withholding reinforcement for another response class (Cooper et al., 2007). Differential reinforcement has two components: (1) delivering reinforcement contingent on a behavior other than a problem behavior and (2) withholding reinforcement for the problem behavior. In other words, differential reinforcement involves the dual processes of positive reinforcement and extinction. There are four basic forms of differential reinforcement: (1) differential reinforcement of incompatible behavior, (2) differential reinforcement of alternative behavior, (3) differential reinforcement of other behavior, and (4) differential reinforcement of low rates of behavior.

In differential reinforcement of incompatible behavior (DRI), a behavior that is incompatible with the problem behavior is reinforced and reinforcement for the problem behavior is withheld. For example, staying seated in the classroom is incompatible with being out of one's seat (i.e., the two cannot occur at the same time). A DRI intervention would provide reinforcement to in-seat behavior and would withhold reinforcement for out-of-seat behavior. There are numerous appropriate behaviors incompatible with disruptive, oppositional behaviors that could be increased using DRI. For example, saying "Yes sir" or "OK" is incompatible with talking back, following directions is incompatible with noncompliance, being in one's seat when class begins is incompatible with being tardy, and being on task is incompatible with being off task.

Differential reinforcement of alternative behavior (DRA) is identical to DRI, *except* the alternative behavior is not incompatible with the problem behavior. Alternative behavior can be any behavior that is performed instead of the target problem behavior.

Differential reinforcement of other behavior (DRO) refers to the delivery of a reinforcer whenever the problem behavior has not occurred during a specified time period. In other words, DRO involves the reinforcement of *not responding* or engaging in a behavior for a period of time. DRO typically involves a time schedule of reinforcement for the nonoccurrence of a problem behavior. For example, suppose you have a target problem behavior of verbal outbursts in the classroom. A DRO 2-minute schedule of reinforcement would provide reinforcement for the first occurrence of *any behavior* except the target problem behavior after 2 minutes had elapsed. This is known as fixed-interval DRO and is relatively easy to implement in a classroom. Generally speaking, the higher the frequency of a problem behavior, the shorter the DRO schedule of reinforcement should be. For example, behaviors occurring at very high rates should have much shorter DRO schedules (e.g., DRO 30 seconds) than behavior occurring at much lower rates (e.g., DRO 5 minutes).

Differential reinforcement of low rates of behavior (DRL) is a schedule of reinforcement in which a behavior is reinforced if it is separated from the previous behavior by a minimum interresponse time (i.e., time elapsing between occurrences of a behavior) or is contingent on the number of behaviors in a time period that does not exceed a predetermined criterion (Cooper et al., 2007). DRL is designed to reduce, but not completely eliminate, the overall frequency of behavior. There are two types of DRL: (1) full-session DRL and (2) spaced-responding DRL. In full-session DRL, reinforcement is delivered if the frequency of a target behavior in a specified period does not exceed a certain criterion. For example, in a full-session DRL 3 schedule, reinforcement is delivered if the frequency of behavior during a session is three or fewer occurrences. Full-session DRL is an effective, efficient, and easy way of reducing the overall frequency of behavior.

In spaced-responding DRL, a reinforcer is delivered following the occurrence of a behavior that is separated by a minimum amount of time elapsing between occurrences of a behavior. For example, suppose a teacher wished to decrease, but not eliminate, the frequency of question-asking in the classroom. In a spaced-responding DRL, the teacher would only answer a question if 5 minutes had elapsed since the student asked the last question. This intervention would decrease but not totally eliminate question asking.

Chapter Summary Points

- Schools are vital settings for intervening with students having DBDs because they are the one place that teachers and students spend a significant amount of time together in both structured and unstructured contexts.
- Developing and implementing behavioral interventions in schools requires knowledge, sensitivity, and tact, particularly for interventions delivered within a consultation model of service delivery.

- About 15% of students will require Tier 2 interventions and about 5% of students will require Tier 3 interventions.

- We know that no single tier of intervention can solve all problems, a well-designed multi-tiered system will have hierarchical tiers of increasing intensity, and effective interventions at lower tiers reduce the need to intervene at subsequent tiers.

- Behavioral interventions in schools can be conceptualized using four broad theoretical categories: (1) applied behavior analysis, (2) social learning theory, (3) cognitive-behavioral theory, and (4) S-R learning theory based on respondent conditioning.

- The most important concept in delivering school-based interventions is that the intervention intensity should be matched to the intensity of the problem behavior.

- Students requiring Tier 3 interventions are responsible for 40–50% of behavioral disruptions in schools, and drain 50–60% of a school's resources in dealing with their problem behaviors.

- Unlike Tier 2 interventions, Tier 3 interventions typically will require an FBA to design the intervention.

- A useful way of thinking about interventions for students with DBDs is the notion of RTI.

- In an RTI approach, a student's lack of response to an evidence-based intervention implemented with integrity is the basis for intensifying, modifying, or changing an intervention.

- There are two basic models or approaches in an RTI approach: (1) problem-solving RTI and (2) standard-protocol RTI.

- Problem-solving RTI is based on the behavioral consultation model and proceeds in four distinct phases: (1) problem identification, (2) problem analysis, (3) plan implementation, and (4) problem evaluation.

- Standard-protocol RTI is based on manualized scripted treatments that specify the procedures and strategies to be used in implementing the intervention.

- The BEP is a validated Tier 2 intervention based on a Check-In/Check-Out procedure.

- The BEP is designed for students who are at risk for developing more serious and chronic behavior problems. It is not an appropriate intervention for students who engage in serious or violent behaviors.

- The FSS program is a coordinated Tier 2 school- and home-based program designed to prevent the development of antisocial behavior among at-risk children in kindergarten through third grade.

- FSS consists of three components: (1) universal screening and early detection, (2) school intervention based on the CLASS program, and (3) a home-based intervention using parent training.

- Tier 3 interventions are based on an FBA to design the intervention.
- There are two basic types of FBA: (1) descriptive FBA and (2) experimental FBA or functional analysis.
- Not all behaviors exhibited by children and youth with DBDs are amenable to FBA because they either occur at very low frequencies (e.g., fire setting or bringing weapons to school) or they are covert and are therefore unobservable.
- A meta-analysis of the FBA literature showed that FBA-based interventions showed a 70.5% reduction in problem behaviors and a significant declining trend from baseline to intervention phases of the studies.
- Punishment-based procedures consist of two basic types (1) positive punishment procedures (verbal reprimands and overcorrection) and (2) negative punishment procedures (time out and response cost).
- Reductive non-punishment-based procedures consist of two types: (1) extinction and (2) differential reinforcement.

Evidence-Based Home Interventions

From the moment of birth, infants shape the behavior of their parents through their behavior. By crying, fussing, and having tantrums, infants with virtually no language skills can control their social environments and have their immediate needs met by caregivers. An infant's behavior reliably produces certain caregiver reactions and therefore establishes a *contingency*. A contingency expresses the relationship between an individual's behavior and certain proximal or distal environmental events (Patterson, 2002). For example, in the course of development, the infant learns that crying reliably produces attention from a caregiver. The caregiver tries a number of actions to stop the infant's crying, but the crying does not stop until the caregiver displays the "correct" action. This cycle occurs literally thousands of times in the course of normal child development and shapes both parent and child behavior.

The above scenario is both a normal and expected part of child development. Once a child develops language, he or she can communicate needs and desires verbally and does not have to rely on crying or tantrums. However, children with DBDs such as noncompliant or oppositional behavior or who display antisocial behavior patterns learn to control their social environments in quite a different, less desirable way.

Earlier in this book, I described the concept of *coercion* as the key mechanism by which children with DBDs learn to control their social environment(s). Longitudinal research has shown that these children often exist in dysfunctional family contexts and display relatively low levels of aversive behaviors at a young age, such as noncompliance, whining, and defiance (Snyder & Stoolmiller, 2002). If their problems are not systematically addressed, however, many of these children will bring this behavior pattern to school and continue it within elementary school, middle school, and beyond. For some of them, this behavior pattern will become elaborated and increasingly destructive in the absence of effective intervention. As the child matures, his or her behavioral repertoire may comprise very serious acts such as bullying, high-level aggression, assault, defiance, delinquency, and self-destructive behavior (Patterson, Reid, & Dishion, 1992; Walker et al., 2004). Thus it is imperative to recognize that what may appear to be low-level problems early in a child's life (e.g. noncompliance with adult directives) may be a harbinger of severe problems later on. Well-implemented parenting programs, such as those described here, can prevent the elaboration and transformation of these problems into something far more serious.

Many psychodynamic theories of child development argue that to understand the development of oppositional/defiant or antisocial behavior patterns, one must analyze internal characteristics or traits. The empirical literature on the DBD student population does not support this view. Reid et al. (2002) argue convincingly that to change oppositional/defiant and antisocial behavior, *we must change the environmental conditions that support it*. The primary social environment in which these children develop is the home for at least 5 years before school entry. The home environment provides a setting in which coercive interactions serve as the vehicle by which these problem behaviors are learned and maintained.

This chapter describes evidence-based strategies and proven interventions for changing DBDs within the home context. Before describing these intervention strategies, I provide a description of the mechanisms responsible for the development of this behavior pattern.

Understanding DBD Developmental Mechanisms

It is quite evident that DBDs stem from cumulative daily social interactions among persons in the home environment (Patterson & Bank, 1989). *Coercion* is the key mechanism in the development of this behavior pattern in which children with DBDs live in a highly contentious and hostile home environment wherein pain and coercion are the fundamental strategies for controlling the behavior of others. Coercion, which functions as a powerful controlling mechanism in the short term, can and often does produce long-term negative consequences for children and youth with DBDs (e.g., social isolation and rejection, impaired peer and teacher relationships, school failure).

In Chapter 1, I described the role of this coercive family process in the development of DBDs. We mentioned that typically developing children usually learn through a process of positive reinforcement and respond well to social praise, rewards, and encouragement. Children with DBDs, however, learn primarily through the process of *negative reinforcement* in that they learn to escape, avoid, delay, or reduce aversive demands placed on them by parents. A negative reinforcement contingency is one in which the occurrence of behavior leads to the removal, termination, reduction, or postponement of an aversive stimulus (i.e., condition or event), causing an increase in future occurrences of that behavior.

The coercive process that explains the development of DBDs can be characterized as a five-step interaction between parent (or other family members) and the child: (1) the child uses coercive tactics to achieve a social goal (e.g., control, dominance, escape or avoidance); (2) the parent reacts negatively to the child's aversive behavior; (3) the child escalates the level of aversiveness and/or intensity using coercive tactics; (4) the parent "gives in" and allows the child to have his or her way in order to reduce the aversiveness and eliminate the coercion; and (5) the child then reduces the level of his or her aversiveness and terminates the coercion. In this sequence of events, both the parent and the child are powerfully reinforced: the parent by termination of the child's aversive behavior and the child by getting his or her way or by achieving the sought-after goal. Thus it is easy to see how this unfortunate behavior pattern is powerfully sustained over time and often generalizes across settings.

The mechanisms by which children develop DBDs are now extensively researched and well documented as a result of the work of such investigators as Patterson (1982). This development has important implications for designing interventions to reduce this behavior pattern. Coercion becomes a typical part of a child's interactions within the home setting and, as such, the child's behavior problems produce a high rate of reinforcement. This, in turn, increases the likelihood that the child will continue to use coercive behavioral tactics to control the social environment. The longer the child displays DBDs, the more opportunities he or she has to enter into coercive processes with diverse sets of individuals within other contexts (e.g., teachers, peers, and others in the larger social environment). If this behavior pattern persists across settings, it will become more and more resistant to change, thus making any attempted intervention less likely to succeed. An effective intervention in this instance must, at a minimum, teach the child that one's social goals can be met without resorting to coercion. However, doing so is no easy task!

This chapter focuses on evidence-based *home interventions* for children with DBDs. I also describe *adjunctive interventions* such as social problem solving and anger control training. The home-based interventions and strategies described here primarily focus on the age range of 3 to 7 because (1) this is the age range that has been subjected to the most stringent empirical research involving DBDs and (2) it is a critical developmental period in which behavior patterns are established that will determine the direction and life course of most children. Parental influence is likely at its peak during this formative period. Whether or not a child acquires a disruptive behavior pattern or instead enters school ready to learn can often be traced to family circumstances and risk factors experienced within this developmental period. We strongly believe that the most effective way to address the child's behavior problems is to work directly within natural home and school settings, in a collaborative fashion, to deliver the most powerful and effective intervention(s) possible.

Overview of Parent Training

As described in Chapter 1, there are a number of individual and family risk factors that tend to place a child on the path to disruptive behavior problems. Recall that one of the most salient risk factors in this regard is the age at which children start this pernicious pattern of behavior. Being an *early starter* for defiant/oppositional and antisocial behavior problems is the single most important risk factor for this behavior pattern (Loeber & Keenan, 1994). Early starters or what have been called "life-course-persistent" conduct problems are characterized by an early onset, typically in the preschool years, that continues throughout childhood and into adolescence and young adulthood in the absence of intervention (Moffitt, 1993).

Child temperamental characteristics such as irritability, fussiness, and emotional volatility predispose many children to the development of DBDs. All too often, parents are unskilled in dealing with these behavioral tendencies and the interaction of a child's difficult temperament with unskilled parenting can form a toxic mix. In addition, deficits in children's *social-cognitive skills* may put them at greater risk for developing DBDs. Crick and Dodge (1994), for example, have shown that children with DBDs demonstrate serious deficiencies in social information processing. That is, they tend to develop hostile attributional biases about the intentions of others rather than more neutral ones. As a result, they make numerous errors in the interpretation of social cues within the social environment. Furthermore, youth with DBDs tend not to develop appropriate solutions to challenging social situations and instead are likely to default to coercion, aggression, or noncompliance. This is usually their only choice in pursuing their social goals and solving their social-behavioral challenges. Typically, if a coercive strategy doesn't work initially, these youth tend to reapply it but with more intensity rather than consider a different strategy. This is a major reason for teaching students problem-solving skills and the ability to generate and select more than one alternative in responding to situations.

Parenting practices play a crucial role in the development of DBDs for young children. Disciplinary practices that are unpredictable, explosive, inflexible and/or harsh or punitive, weak parent involvement in the child's life, and poor supervision are all characteristics of an incompetent parenting style (Chamberlain & Patterson, 1995). Unfortunately, they provide a fertile breeding ground for DBDs and the emergence of antisocial behavior patterns. Given these kinds of parenting practices, the focus of home-based interventions for children and youth with DBDs must be on altering this style of discipline and promoting positive, effective parenting strategies.

Development of Parent Training Programs

Parent training has strongly evolved in research and practice over the past 40 years and has been used to improve multiple types of child problems and conditions including autism spectrum disorder, ADHD, anxiety disorders, sleep problems, and feeding difficulties (McMahon & Forehand, 2003). Although parent training can be used from preschool to adolescence, as I have noted, it has been used most often with preadolescent children from preschool through elementary school.

Parent training has several important advantages over traditional psychotherapeutic interventions in which a therapist often works in an office setting divorced from target problem behavior settings. Parent training approaches teach parents to manage the behavior of their children in the naturalistic ecologies of the home, school, and community settings. Typically, children being treated in office settings do not generalize any achieved therapeutic effects back to home, school, and community environments. Prior to school entry, children spend the majority of their time with parents and siblings. As such, the home is the logical choice for being the primary setting in which treatment should take place prior to beginning school.

Although there are a number of parent training programs available (see review by Eyberg et al., 2008), most of the evidence-based parent training programs have been substantially influenced by the important work of Hanf (1969, 1970) with families. Eyberg et al. (2008), in an excellent review of the parent training literature, have recommended three such programs as being probably efficacious interventions for children having DBDs: (1) *Helping the Noncompliant Child* (McMahon & Forehand, 2003), the *Incredible Years Parent Training* (Webster-Stratton & Hammond, 1997; Webster-Stratton, Reid, & Hammond, 2001), and *parent–child interaction therapy* (Schulmann, Foote, Eyberg, Boggs, & Angina, 1998). These programs are described in more detail later in this chapter. Four other evidence-based parent training programs have been developed: *Parent Management Training* (Patterson, Chamberlain, & Reid, 1982), *multisystemic therapy* (Henggeler, Melton, & Smith, 1992), *Multidimensional Treatment Foster Care* (Chamberlain & Reid, 1998), and *Parent Management Training* (Kazdin, 2005). These programs are also described briefly later in this chapter.

Theoretical Basis for Parent Training Programs

More than any other group of family-focused researchers over the past four decades, Gerald R. Patterson, John B. Reid, and their colleagues at the Oregon Social Learning Center (OSLC) have made perhaps the most meaningful contributions to our understanding of deviant family processes. It is worth noting that they have based development of their home intervention approaches and parent training models on the outcomes of their seminal research. The OSLC scientists and therapists have achieved international recognition for their outstanding research that has significantly advanced our ability to understand and foster changes in the family ecologies and parenting practices that consistently produce disruptive and antisocial children (Patterson, 1982; Patterson et al., 1992; Reid et al., 2002). Before beginning the task of intervening in the home setting to address DBDs, the reader is strongly advised to review this impressive body of work (See the Oregon model of Parent Management Training and supporting research at *oslc.org*.)

Evidence-based parent training programs, as a rule, consist of intervention procedures derived primarily from a combination of applied behavior analysis and core principles of social learning theory and research outcomes. This knowledge base enables parents to implement proven practices in order to change their child's behavior in desired directions. Kazdin (2005) has described four distinguishing but interrelated components of parent training as follows: (1) a conceptual framework regarding how to change children's social behavior; (2) a set of principles and techniques that flow from this framework; (3) development of specific skills in parenting through modeling, coaching, role play, behavioral rehearsal, and performance feedback; and (4) the integration of assessment and evaluation outcomes in treatment planning and decision making. Each of these components is described following.

First, Kazdin's conceptual framework of child behavior change is based on learning theory. Specifically, evidence-based parent training programs are, as a rule, based primarily on the principles of *operant learning*. Operant learning is the foundation for applied behavior analysis, which uses the three-term contingency as a primary basis for understanding and changing behavior. The three-term contingency consists of identifying and changing the *antecedents and consequences* of problem behaviors. Known as an ABC approach, this contingency seeks to identify environmental events that consistently precede problem behavior (antecedents) and environment events that consistently follow behavior (consequences).

Second, parent training is based on two important principles derived from the operant learning paradigm: *positive reinforcement* and *negative reinforcement*. Numerous intervention strategies are derived from the principle of reinforcement and are used in parent management training along with other strategies such as reductive techniques (time out, response cost, extinction). However, positive and negative reinforcement are the foundational approaches used in parent training.

Third, specific behavior management skills are taught to parents or caregivers using principles of coaching (Tell), modeling (Show), behavioral rehearsal (Do), and role playing (Practice)—all supported by performance feedback from experts. This type of parent training does not simply rely on counseling parents about how to manage their child's behavior but rather teaches them how to directly apply proven parenting strategies within the home setting to change their child's problem behavior.

Fourth, parent training incorporates assessment and evaluation in the planning and treatment process. Central to this approach is the concept of systematic *progress monitoring* to directly assess whether the treatment is producing the desired results. A fundamental part of decision making in treatment is obtaining information about how parents and children are progressing in the parent training program. The evaluation of treatment integrity is crucial in determining whether a treatment is being implemented as planned or intended (Gresham, 2014).

Outcomes of Systematic Parent Training

Parent training is one of several evidence-based treatments for childhood DBDs. Other treatments include problem-solving skills training (Kazdin, Siegel, & Bass, 1992) and anger control training (Lochman, Coie, Underwood, & Terry, 1993). Kazdin (2005) indicates, however, that no other treatment for children and adolescents has been as well investigated as systematic parent training. Parent training has been the focus of numerous well-controlled empirical studies, reviews, and meta-analyses. It remains the treatment of choice for DBDs (McMahon & Forehand, 2003; Kazdin, 2005; Weisz, 2004).

Although most children will improve as a result of parent training, it is not universally effective. Patterson (1974) noted that about 22% of families in his parent training program did not show significant improvement. Others have reported that almost one-third of treated families did not have sustained improvement 1 year after treatment (Webster-Stratton, Hollinsworth, & Kolpacoff, 1989). Forehand and colleagues reviewed 22 parent training studies and found that the overall dropout rate averaged 28% (Forehand, Middlebrook, Rogers, & Steffe, 1983).

Research has shown that specific child and family characteristics moderate or limit the effectiveness of parent training interventions (Reid et al., 2002). The severity of a child's conduct behavior problem(s) appears to be the strongest variable affecting poor parent training outcomes (McMahon & Forehand, 2003). A child's gender does not appear to moderate treatment outcomes, but the research clearly points to parent training as being more effective with younger children (preadolescents) than older children (McMahon, 1999).

Fundamental Principles Underlying Parent Training

As I noted earlier, parent training is based on principles derived from social learning theory and primarily emphasizes operant learning principles. The most fundamental principle of operant learning is referred to as *contingencies of reinforcement.* Contingencies of reinforcement involve the three-term contingency described earlier: antecedents (events occurring prior to behavior), target behavior (the focus of change), and consequences (events following behavior that either strengthen or weaken it). Behavior change interventions, based on the three-term contingency, involve understanding the influences of antecedents and consequences and how they can be used to increase and maintain behavior. A behavior that occurs more frequently under some antecedent conditions is called a *discriminated operant.* Discriminated operants occur at a higher frequency in the presence of a particular stimulus than in the absence of that stimulus; thus the behavior is said to be under *stimulus control.* Answering the telephone when it rings brings the behavior of answering the telephone under stimulus control, and answering the telephone does not occur in the absence of the telephone ringing.

The three-term contingency is considered the basic unit of analysis in the study of operant behavior (Cooper et al., 2007). Although the term *contingency* has several meanings, the most common use of the term refers to the *dependency* of a particular consequence on the occurrence of behavior. When a reinforcer or punisher is said to be *contingent* on a particular behavior, the behavior must obviously occur in order for the consequence to be delivered. If the teacher says to the student, "Name a type of fish," and the student responds, "Shark," and the teacher, in turn, responds with, "Good job," then this describes the straightforward contingent relationship between the antecedent, the behavior, and the consequence.

Antecedents of Behavior

STIMULUS CONTROL

Reinforcement of behavior increases the future frequency of that behavior and influences the stimuli or behavioral events/conditions that immediately precede it. The stimuli that precede the behavior are known as *antecedent stimuli* and acquire an evocative effect on a behavior. For example, loud talking and active behavior may be appropriate on the playground, but not in the classroom. In this case, the playground functions as an antecedent stimulus for loud talking and high activity levels, and the classroom functions as an antecedent stimulus for their absence. Thus the playground is said to be a *discriminative stimulus*, or S^D, for loud talking/high-rate activity and the classroom is said to be a *nondiscriminative stimulus*, or SΔ, for loud talking/high-rate activity. When a behavior is reinforced in the presence of a discriminative stimulus, that behavior comes under the control of that stimulus. Stimulus control occurs when the rate, frequency, duration, or amplitude of a behavior is altered in the presence of a discriminative stimulus (Dinsmoor, 1995).

Stimulus control plays a basic role in everyday behavioral operations such as language systems, problem solving, and social interactions. Behaviors might be considered appropriate in one situation or context, but not in others. Some behaviors that parents and teachers might consider inappropriate are not necessarily behavior problems per se. The problem is that the behavior is performed at a time and place considered inappropriate by social agents in the environment. This illustrates a problem in the *stimulus control* of behavior. Interventions for these types of problems necessarily involve teaching the individual to *discriminate* the times and places in which the behavior is appropriate and inappropriate.

Antecedent stimuli that have a history of prompting a behavior that has been reinforced in their presence are likely to lead to increases in that behavior in the presence of similar stimuli. This tendency is known as *stimulus generalization*. Noncompliant behavior might be reinforced in the presence of a mother in the home, which may generalize to noncompliance in the presence of a father, and siblings in the home or a teacher at school. In contrast, *stimulus discrimination* refers to a situation in which different stimuli do not evoke a behavior (i.e., the behavior is under stimulus control). Using the above example, a child may learn to display high rates of noncompliant behavior withthe mother, but not with the father. In this case, the mother is a discriminative stimulus for noncompliance and the father is a nondiscriminative stimulus for noncompliance.

The development of stimulus control is accomplished by a procedure known as *stimulus discrimination training*. This procedure requires one behavior and at least two antecedent stimulus conditions. Behaviors are reinforced in the presence of one stimulus condition, the S^D, but not in the presence of the other stimulus, the SΔ. Over time, behavior will become more frequent in the presence of the S^D and less frequent in the presence of the SΔ. Many of the home-based interventions described in this book are based on this fundamental principle of the stimulus control of behavior.

SETTING EVENTS

Setting events are antecedent stimuli that also influence the occurrence of behavior. Unlike discriminative stimuli, setting events are *temporally* and *physically remote* from the occurrence of behavior. Whereas discriminative stimuli immediately precede behavior, setting events occur at a different time and place from the occurrence of behavior. For example, a boy having a fight on the school bus on the way to school may increase the occurrence of noncompliance or defiance later in the school day. Setting events might be considered events that set the stage for the occurrence of behavior. Because setting events are temporally and physically remote to behavior, they are difficult to control because of their unobservability.

A particularly effective behavioral intervention strategy, based on the manipulation of setting events for appropriate behavior, is known as *precorrection*. Precorrection is an instructional prompt presented before an individual enters a setting that may lead to problem behavior or a setting previously associated with problem behavior. It includes verbal prompts such as rule reminders or descriptions of the desired behavior or nonverbal prompts such as gestures or demonstrations of the appropriate behavior (Colvin & Sugai, 1989).

Precorrection also involves communicating behavioral goals and expectations for appropriate behavior before inappropriate behavior can occur and can therefore be considered a setting event for appropriate behavior in a given environment. Chapter 5 described how precorrection can be effectively used in schools to manage student behavior.

As I have emphasized in this book, children with DBDs very often come from coercive, contentious home environments in which there are frequent arguments and coercive interactions characterized by extreme hostility. These interactions often operate as powerful setting events for different problem behaviors occurring in school. As such, one goal of parent training is to reduce the occurrence of these setting events at home so they do not lead to problem behaviors in other settings and situations. For example, having an argument with a parent before school about being late might serve as a setting event for disruptive behavior problems in the classroom later that day. In turn, the school's attempts to discipline the child (e.g., being sent to the office) may serve as a setting event for additional problem behaviors with parents when the child gets home from school that day. An important goal of parent training programs is to reliably identify these setting events that lead to or "set off" problem behaviors and thereby prevent their occurrence.

ESTABLISHING OPERATIONS

An establishing operation (EO) refers to any environmental event that alters the effectiveness of a reinforcer and changes the frequency of all behavior that has been previously strengthened by it. For example, not having access to water for a period of time on a hot day will increase the effectiveness of water as a reinforcer and lead to other behaviors that result in accessing water (i.e., careful planning). Michael (2007) has identified nine establishing operations that increase the effectiveness of a reinforcer.

EOs accomplish their influence on behavior by altering an individual's motivational state. EOs are based on temporary states of deprivation and satiation. In the latter case, eating Halloween candy immediately after Halloween is most likely to be less reinforcing than eating the candy early in October, since one's appetite becomes temporarily sated with the immediate prior ingestion of candy. EOs may result from conditions of abuse and neglect in which either physically painful stimuli are inflicted on a child or a child's basic needs (e.g., food, water, sleep) are not met. This can have a profound impact on a child's behavior in other environments such as school.

Typical EOs for children with DBDs might include sleep deprivation, emotional trauma, physical punishment, abuse, and neglect. All of these EOs might alter the motivational state of a child and lead to increases in oppositional/defiant and antisocial behavior patterns.

PROMPTS

Prompts are antecedent events that cue the performance of certain behaviors. Prompts can be differentiated from setting events, which are broader, contextual influences on behavior that are temporally and proximally remote. Prompts can be distinguished from discriminative stimuli because they do not bring a behavior under stimulus control through the establishment of an S^D. Prompts include reminders to engage in a behavior (e.g., "Do your homework"), cue or reminders (creation of "to-do" lists), gestures (e.g., stop, sit down), and modeling (e.g., showing how a behavior is done). Prompts are antecedent events that help initiate a desired behavior, which, in turn, can be reinforced when it occurs.

Kazdin (2005) indicates that prompts play a substantial role in developing adaptive behavior. Individuals who are not engaging in a desired or expected behavior can be given prompts to show the individual what to do, how to do it, and when to do it. Often a specific behavior will not occur without a direct prompt. If a behavior does not occur, it obviously cannot be reinforced and thereby strengthened. Prompts are not elaborate explanations for why a behavior should be performed; rather, they are short, specific statements that direct or encourage a behavior (e.g.,

"Pick up your toys," "Remember you have homework due tomorrow," or "Make your bed").

Prompts are especially important in increasing behavior that occurs infrequently. Early on, numerous prompts may be required to increase the target behavior to a desired frequency. Later, these prompts can be withdrawn, or *faded*. Fading refers to the gradual removal of a prompt. It is important to remember that fading is the *gradual removal* of a prompt, but not a complete elimination of it. Prompts that are faded too quickly will lead to the behavior being performed less frequently and ultimately not at all.

An excellent example of the use of prompts in the treatment of non-compliance can be found in the parent training program called *Helping the Noncompliant Child* (McMahon & Forehand, 2003). These authors describe what they have named the *clear instruction sequence*. It begins with a parent giving an explicit instruction to the child. If the child complies with the initial instruction or with a subsequent prompt or warning, then the parent communicates approval or provides positive attention and the sequence is ended. Clear instructions are called *alpha commands* and are presented in unambiguous and behaviorally specific terms. Examples of clear instructions are statements like "Turn off the TV," or "Come to dinner now." Use of the clear instruction sequence in the management of childhood noncompliance is described in more detail later in this chapter.

The Organization of Interrelated Forms of Behavior

The field of applied behavior analysis has contributed greatly to our understanding of the relationships between antecedent events (discriminative stimuli, setting events, establishing operations, prompts) and consequences (punishment, positive and negative reinforcement). However, in the view of many, the field of applied behavior analysis focuses too heavily on rather narrow, discrete behaviors that may have high face validity but low social validity (Wolf, 1978) in terms of their ultimate impact and social significance. Targeting isolated behaviors is valuable at some level, but may not address the bigger picture in terms of what to change via an intervention that will make a difference in an individual's functioning within society.

What is often missing in this conceptual framework is an understanding of how multiple behaviors may be organized or interrelated. A clearer understanding of the principles of behavior organization would put the field in a better position to design and implement interventions that will produce not only short-term but also long-term positive outcomes.

There are various ways in which behavior patterns can be organized into meaningful, coherent units. One of the most common ways in which behavior is organized is the *response class*. A response class consists of two fundamental types: (1) *topographical response class* and (2) *functional response class*. A topographical response class organizes behavior based on how it looks via its form. The DSM-5 (American Psychiatric Association, 2013) provides a good example of the classification of behavior based on a topographical response class. For example, the diagnostic criteria for oppositional defiant disorder (e.g., noncompliance, defiance, arguing, and annoying others) are all behaviors based on behavioral or response topographies (form). A functional response class organizes behavior based on the *function* it serves rather than how it looks (its form). For example, noncompliance, defiance, and arguing with adults may all be maintained by serving a negative reinforcement function because each one results in the removal of task demands, thereby increasing its frequency in the future. Most parent training programs focus on the functions that maintain problem behaviors and attempt to change their consequences.

In identifying behaviors belonging to a functional response class, one conducts a *functional behavioral assessment* (see subsequent discussion of consequences). In this process, one systematically identifies the antecedents and consequences surrounding the occurrence of a problem behavior. Once these are identified, one can design and implement interventions based on this information. Topographical response classes have no inherent treatment validity, whereas functional response classes do.

Another way in which behaviors might be organized is that of a *response chain*. A response chain is an organizing principle in which one behavior immediately follows another. The first behavior in a behavioral chain sets the occasion (signals) for the performance of the next behavior in a behavioral chain, thereby functioning as a discriminative stimulus (see earlier discussion). Many patterns of behavior consist of tasks or routines in which a series of behaviors are learned and performed in a sequence. With DBDs, the first behavior in a chain might be agitation (based on some environmental event) that is subsequently followed by crying, task refusal, name calling, and ultimately throwing task materials.

Conceptualizing this behavior pattern as a behavioral chain can lead to effective prevention of more intense responses occurring later in the chain. For example, temporarily removing task demands and directives when a child is agitated may prevent the occurrence of the rest of the behavioral chain. Parents are taught in most parent training programs to recognize problem behaviors occurring early in a behavior chain and intervene (via ignoring or leaving the room) before the behavior escalates out of control. A common mistake that parents make in this regard is to escalate this response chain by attempting to impose their authority over the child. This often leads to the behavior spiraling out of control.

The Role of Behavioral Consequences

It is a truism that behavior is a function of its consequences. In the realm of operant learning, behavior can be increased or decreased by manipulating the consequences that follow the behavior and are contingent upon it. Behavior is increased by the contingent delivery of *reinforcement* and behavior is decreased by the contingent delivery of *punishment*. Reinforcement consists of two fundamental types: (1) positive reinforcement and (2) negative reinforcement. Punishment also consists of two fundamental types (1) positive punishment and (2) negative punishment. These concepts are discussed in the following sections and throughout this book because they are vital to the design of interventions to change DBDs.

POSITIVE REINFORCEMENT

Positive reinforcement is the contingent delivery of a reinforcing stimulus immediately following a focus behavior that increases the future likelihood of that behavior. The stimulus is presented as a consequence and can consist of virtually anything in the environment. There are differing types of reinforcers or rewarding events. Positive reinforcers can be either primary (e.g., food or water) or secondary or conditioned (e.g., praise, money, points, preferred activities). Primary or unconditioned reinforcers do not have to be learned and fulfill some biological need for an individual (food, water, comfort, warmth). Conditioned or secondary reinforcers are learned and achieve their rewarding properties by being paired repeatedly with a primary reinforcer.

Positive reinforcers are typically classified into categories such as: (1) edible reinforcers (food, candy, snacks), (2) sensory reinforcers (tactile stimulation, lights, music), (3) tangible reinforcers (stickers, trinkets, toys), (4) activity reinforcers (using high-probability behaviors as a reinforcer for lower probability behaviors), and (5) social reinforcers (attention, praise, approval). It should be noted that not all of the above types of reinforcers will be effective with all individuals. The reinforcing value of a reinforcing stimulus depends on such things as individual differences in learning histories, access to a given reinforcer in a given time frame, and the delay between the behavior's occurrence and delivery of the reinforcer.

The identification of positive reinforcers for individuals typically uses *preference assessments* in which the person is asked what kinds of things he or she finds reinforcing. This can take a variety of forms such as asking open-ended questions ("What do you like to do in free time?"), multiple choice ("Which of the following would you do a lot of hard work to get?"), or rank ordering ("Rank order the following from most to least preferred"). Other assessment methods might include asking significant others (parents and/or teachers), observations (recording the amount of time a person spends in given activities), or trial-based methods in which stimuli are presented to the person to determine their preference for that individual.

Most parent training programs rely on positive reinforcement strategies in the form of differential attention, privileges, and token or point systems to increase appropriate behavior. McMahon and Forehand's (2003) parent training program consists of two phases: (1) teaching the skills of differential attention and (2) teaching the skills of compliance training. In the first phase, parents learn that their child probably engages in a fair amount of positive behaviors that go unrecognized by the parent. Attention can be either positive (praise) or negative (criticism or scolding). Many behaviors that a child might display result in negative attention, which (at least from the child's perspective) is better than no attention at all. Based on the matching law described earlier, problem behaviors reinforced more frequently via negative adult attention will occur more often than appropriate behaviors reinforced with positive adult attention.

SCHEDULES OF REINFORCEMENT

It is well established that the *schedule of reinforcement* has a profound effect on the frequency of behavior. A schedule of reinforcement is a rule that describes a contingency of reinforcement which importantly determines the conditions under which behaviors will produce reinforcement (Cooper et al., 2007). Reinforcement schedules can be continuous schedules in which reinforcement is delivered after each occurrence of a target behavior or intermittent schedules of reinforcement in which reinforcement only occurs after some, but not all, occurrences of the behavior.

Schedules of reinforcement can be either *ratio schedules* or *interval schedules*. Ratio schedules require a certain number of responses before one response produces a reinforcer. If the ratio requirement for a behavior is six correct responses, then only the sixth correct response will produce reinforcement. Interval schedules require an elapse of time before a response produces reinforcement. If the interval requirement is 3 minutes, then reinforcement is provided contingent on the first response after 3 minutes have elapsed.

Schedules of reinforcement can also be either *fixed schedules* or *variable schedules*. A fixed schedule provides reinforcement if it meets a ratio or time requirement, whereas a variable schedule provides reinforcement for the response ratio or time requirement that changes over time. Based on the concepts of ratio and interval schedules and fixed and variable schedules, there are four basic types of reinforcement schedules.

In a fixed-ratio schedule of reinforcement, reinforcement is contingent on a number of responses to produce the reinforcer. For example, in a fixed-ratio 15 schedule (FR 15), a response is reinforced every 15 times it occurs. In a variable-ratio schedule of reinforcement, a behavior is reinforced based on a variable number of responses to produce the reinforcer. For instance, a variable-ratio 5 (VR 5) schedule of reinforcement will deliver reinforcement, on average, every five times a behavior occurs. In a fixed-interval schedule of reinforcement, a behavior will be reinforced after a fixed amount of time elapses. For example, a fixed-interval 2-minute schedule (FI 2 minutes) will provide reinforcement for each response after 2 minutes have elapsed. In a variable-interval schedule of reinforcement, a response will be reinforced after variable durations of time have elapsed. For instance, a variable-interval 10-minute schedule (VI 10 minutes) will produce reinforcement, on average, after 10 minutes have elapsed.

These four types of reinforcement schedules produce different rates of behavior. A fixed-ratio schedule will produce high rates of responding, whereas a variable-ratio schedule will also produce rapid, high rates of responding (depending on the amount of reinforcement provided). Fixed-interval schedules of reinforcement produce initially slow but gradually accelerating rates of responding from the beginning to the end of the interval. After the reinforcement is delivered, there is a postreinforcement pause in responding until the next interval begins. A variable-interval schedule of reinforcement will produce low to moderate response rates with the larger average interval producing the lowest rates of behavior (e.g., VI 5 minutes vs. VI 20 minutes).

What do these rather esoteric-sounding schedules of reinforcement have to do with the acquisition and maintenance of DBDs? They actually contribute greatly to our understanding of the conditions under which problem behaviors are occurring. In real life, a single behavior is not typically maintained by a single type of schedule of reinforcement (e.g., fixed ratio or variable interval). It is best to think about behaviors as involving a "choice" between displaying one behavior versus another at any given time. This "choice" is dictated by the schedule of reinforcement for one behavior versus all other behaviors that might be "chosen" at that time.

Thus it is more realistic to think about *concurrent schedules of reinforcement* operating simultaneously rather than any one type of schedule as described above. A concurrent schedule is reinforcement of two or more behaviors according to two or more schedules of reinforcement available at the same time (i.e., concurrently). For example, suppose defiant behavior is reinforced, on average, every five times it occurs (VR 5) and suppose compliant behavior is reinforced, on average, every 15 times it occurs (VR 15). Based on what we know about concurrent schedules of reinforcement, defiant behavior will occur three times as often as compliant behavior (15÷5 = 3). This is a result of the matching law described earlier in this book. A common mistake made by parents of defiant/noncompliant and antisocial children is the reinforcement of problem behaviors at high rates with negative attention and the failure to reinforce desired behaviors just as frequently, or more so, when they occur.

NEGATIVE REINFORCEMENT

Negative reinforcement refers to the occurrence of a response that produces the removal, termination, reduction, or postponement of an aversive event or condition (i.e., negative stimulus) that leads to an increase in the future occurrence of that response. Earlier in this chapter we noted that the development of DBDs is primarily due to process of negative reinforcement in which a child engages in a coercive behavior pattern that leads to the withdrawal or termination of adult commands or directives to change behavior. Whereas both positive and negative reinforcement lead to an increase in future occurrences of behavior, they do so in quite a different manner (Iwata & Smith, 2007). You will recall that positive reinforcement involves the *presentation* of a stimulus contingent on the occurrence of behavior that increases the future occurrence of that behavior. Negative reinforcement involves the contingent *removal* or *termination* of an aversive stimulus that increases the future occurrence of the behavior that causes it to be removed (Cooper et al., 2007).

It is important to note that negative reinforcement is sometimes confused with punishment. Many equate negative reinforcement with punishment because both involve aversive stimuli. However, the terms positive and negative do not connote "good" and "bad," but rather the presentation (positive) or removal (negative) of a stimulus. Aversive stimuli can function as negative reinforcers in one situation and as punishers in another situation. The key in making this distinction is the effect the aversive stimulus has on the future occurrence of behavior. Negative reinforcement always increases the future occurrence of the focus behavior, and punishment always decreases the future occurrence of the focus behavior.

Negative reinforcement often involves an *escape contingency*, in which a response terminates or leads to an "escape from" an ongoing aversive stimulus. For example, a child given a written math assignment that is beyond his or her skill level may engage in disruptive behavior to avoid or escape the math assignment. Disruptive behavior in this case will be negatively reinforced if it leads to delay or termination of the math assignment.

Many situations such as the above avoid–escape contingency occur in everyday life; however, it is fair to say that most behavior maintained by negative reinforcement can be characterized as an *avoidance contingency* (Cooper et al., 2007). An avoidance contingency is one in which a response prevents or postpones the presentation of an aversive stimulus. For example, a child given a command by his parents to complete a homework assignment might engage in any behavior that leads to avoiding or postponing completion of homework. If this occurs, then any behavior leading to this avoidance or postponement will be negatively reinforced and will, if successful, lead to an increase in the future occurrence of these behaviors. This type of arrangement has been called *discriminated avoidance* because a response in the presence of one stimulus ("Do your homework") is discriminated from the absence of that stimulus. Thus the command of "Do your homework" serves as a discriminative stimulus (S^D) for any behavior that leads to avoidance or postponement of that stimulus.

PUNISHMENT

Punishment is one of the foundational principles of operant learning. However, it is often misunderstood and misapplied in everyday life

(Vollmer, 2002). Part of this misunderstanding and misapplication stems from confusing punishment within an operant learning context with everyday and legal interpretations of this concept. Everyday connotations of punishment involve the delivery of physical pain, loss of privileges, or fines for the purposes of teaching a person a "lesson" so as to reduce the likelihood of the behavior's future occurrence. In the legal system, punishment involves sanctions such as community service, home confinement, being sent to jail, or fining a person for speeding such that lawbreakers atone for and "repay" their debt to society (Cooper et al., 2007).

Legal conceptions of punishment have very little to do with punishment as a fundamental principle of behavior. Punishment refers to the presentation or removal of a stimulus that leads to a *decrease* in the future occurrence of a behavior. Like reinforcement, punishment can be either *positive* or *negative* punishment. Positive punishment occurs when the presentation of a stimulus immediately following a behavior leads to a decrease in that behavior. For example, if a child engages in disruptive classroom behavior and the teacher points her finger at the child and says "No, stop that," and the child stops engaging in the behavior, then the behavior is said to be punished (i.e., the teacher's reprimand leads to a decrease in that behavior). The above example is positive punishment because a stimulus was *presented* that led to a decrease in the behavior.

Negative punishment involves the termination or decrease in the magnitude of a stimulus following a behavior that leads to a decrease in the behavior. In other words, negative punishment involves the contingent removal of a specified amount of a positive reinforcer that ordinarily leads to a decrease in the future probability of behavior. Common behavior change strategies based on negative punishment include the contingent loss of reinforcers immediately following undesirable behavior (i.e., response cost) or the removal of the opportunity to acquire rewards for a period (i.e., time out from positive reinforcement). Many evidence-based home interventions for DBDs involve the contingent use of response cost (i.e., fines) and time out.

Several factors influence the effectiveness of punishment in decreasing behavior, including: (1) immediacy, (2) intensity or magnitude, (3) schedule, (4) rate of reinforcement for a target behavior, and (5) availability of reinforcement for alternative forms of behavior. Punishment will be maximally effective in reducing problem behavior if it is delivered *immediately* or as soon as possible after the occurrence of a target behavior. The longer the time delay between the occurrence of behavior and the delivery of a punisher, the less effective it will be. For example, a mother saying to a child who has misbehaved, "Wait until you father comes home," to control the misbehavior will be sorely disappointed in the effectiveness of this strategy in changing behavior. The *intensity* or *magnitude* of a punishing stimulus also has a substantial effect in reducing behavior. The more intense the magnitude of the punishing stimulus, the greater the behavioral reduction.

Like schedules of reinforcement discussed earlier, the *schedule of punishment* has a dramatic effect on the frequency of behavior. The more frequently a behavior is punished, as in a continuous punishment schedule (FR 1, in which every response is punished), the more behavioral reduction will occur. Intermittent punishment schedules (e.g., variable-ratio or variable-interval schedules) can be effective under some circumstances. The effectiveness of punishment is moderated by the frequency of reinforcement for the target behavior. Thus if the target behavior is frequently reinforced, then punishment will be less effective. Punishment will be maximally effective in reducing the target behavior if reinforcement maintaining the target behavior is substantially reduced or eliminated. Finally, punishment will be more effective in reducing behavior if an alternative behavior is reinforced more frequently. This phenomenon is simply a restatement of the matching law. That is, response rate matches reinforcement rate so that an alternative behavior that is reinforced more frequently will occur more often and the problem behavior will be reinforced less frequently.

EXTINCTION

Extinction is a procedure that involves the discontinuation of reinforcement for a target behavior that results in a *decrease* in that behavior. Like punishment, extinction decreases the future probability of behavior but does so by withholding reinforcement for a previously reinforced behavior. For example, if a student disrupts the classroom by making noises and getting out of his seat, the teacher may choose to ignore this behavior and its frequency, in time, should decrease. However, if the disruption interferes substantially with the teaching–learning process, more direct and immediate reductive procedures are called for.

Extinction consists of two fundamental types: (1) extinction of behavior maintained by positive reinforcement and (2) extinction of behavior maintained by negative reinforcement. In the former, behaviors that are maintained by positive reinforcement are placed on extinction when those behaviors no longer result in positive reinforcement. For example, suppose a young child throws temper tantrums when she does not get her way. Previously, the parent attending to the tantrum and trying to console the child positively reinforced these tantrums. Subsequently, the parent simply leaves the room where the tantrum occurred, thereby placing tantrumming on extinction and decreasing its frequency.

Behaviors maintained by negative reinforcement are placed on extinction when these behaviors no longer produce a removal of the aversive stimulus, meaning that the person cannot avoid or escape from the aversive situation (Cooper et al., 2007). This procedure is known as *escape extinction*. For instance, a child in a reading tutoring session with a paraprofessional starts engaging in disruptive and inattentive behavior to escape the task demands of the reading instruction session. If these behaviors do not lead to avoidance or escape, then the disruptive and inattentive behaviors will be placed on extinction via the process of escape extinction.

Extinction results in a gradual reduction in behavior over time and can produce emotional behavior in the form of frustration. Extinction is often difficult for parents and teachers to apply because the initial effect of behavior undergoing extinction is an immediate increase in the behavior being extinguished. This is known as an *extinction burst*. Extinction bursts, in the long run, are actually a good thing because they indicate that the reinforcer maintaining the problem behavior has been successfully identified and therefore extinction should be an effective intervention over time. The key in using extinction is to "hold your own" and not succumb to the temptation of providing reinforcement, in the form of negative attention, for the problem behavior when emotional bursts become more intense.

It should be noted that behavior reinforced on intermittent schedules of reinforcement (FR, VR, FI, VI) are more resistant to extinction than behaviors reinforced on continuous schedules. Generally speaking, the more frequently a behavior is reinforced the more easily it is extinguished. Thus behaviors reinforced on relatively *thin schedules of reinforcement* (e.g., VR 20 or VI 15 minutes) will be more resistant to extinction than behaviors reinforced on thicker schedules of reinforcement.

One caveat about the use of extinction has to do with the occurrence of extreme, harmful forms of behavior. Behaviors such as severe physical aggression against others should not be placed on extinction because of the harmful effects of these behaviors. In such cases, other procedures like differential reinforcement and/or mild punishment would be considered more appropriate strategies.

Evidence-Based Home Treatments for DBDs

The basic goals of most home-based intervention programs are twofold: (1) to change the parents' behavior and (2) to change how the parents and the child interact with one another. The fundamental strategy is to teach parents effective behavior change strategies based primarily, but not exclusively, on principles of operant learning. Parents learn the concepts described earlier in this chapter such as antecedent events (discriminative stimuli, setting events, establishing operations), concepts of positive and negative reinforcement/punishment and the use of extinction procedures as in ignoring mildly noxious child behavior (i.e., sometimes referred to as "nattering"). Parents are taught to operationally define the target behaviors they want to change, develop skills in observing and recording target behaviors, to implement behavior change procedures based on principles discussed earlier in this chapter, and to monitor progress in the intervention program. Progress monitoring is a key component in all home-based intervention programs. Kazdin (2005) describes four ways in which progress is monitored in most home-based intervention programs: (1) review of the program at the beginning of the treatment session; (2) role plays to assess what the parent can do in the session and does do at home; (3) telephone calls, text messages, or e-mails during the week to determine how the program is working; and (4) contact sessions in which both the parent and child are seen together to reenact interactions that occur in the home.

Participants and Roles

Parent training programs involve a therapist, a parent or parents, and sometimes the child in some, but not all, treatment sessions. The therapist is responsible for the parent training program and functions as a coach or trainer in leading the training sessions (Kazdin, 2005). Typically, the mother comes to the parent training sessions, but both mothers and fathers may choose to attend some sessions. Some research suggests that maintenance of treatment gains is greater when both parents are involved in the treatment sessions. Although there are a number of differences between single-parent, blended, and two-parent families, the research suggests that parent training with single-parent families is often very effective (Kazdin, 2005).

It is extremely desirable, when feasible, to have the child's teacher involved in the parent training program so their role can be integrated into a comprehensive home- and school-based intervention program (see

Chapter 7 for a discussion of this topic). It is most effective when the therapist or parent trainer-coordinator is in frequent contact with the child's teacher either by telephone, text messaging, or e-mail to determine how the child is behaving in school. School–home notes are particularly effective when the child's teacher gives daily feedback to parents on how the child has behaved in school that day (Kelley, 1990).

Kazdin (2005) cogently points out that parents often see the child's behavior problems as residing within the child. As such, some parents may think that the focus of treatment should be on the child and not parent–child interactions. Many of these parents may express a desire for the therapist to conduct counseling sessions with the child to change his or her behavior (i.e., "fix" the child). This attitude is not unexpected, because some parents have a preconceived notion about what therapy should look like (e.g., therapy sessions that merely talk about solving the problem). In this context, therapists should communicate that whereas we may not know exactly why children are noncompliant, aggressive, or defiant, the most effective way that we can change these behaviors is by altering parent–child interaction patterns at home and in other settings.

In the following sections, we provide brief descriptions of a number of highly recommended evidence-based parent training programs. These intervention programs can be characterized as *well established* or *as probably efficacious*, using the nomenclature developed by Chambless and Hollon (1998). The following discussion draws heavily from the excellent review article by Eyberg et al. (2008) published in a special issue of the *Journal of Clinical Child and Adolescent Psychology* on evidence-based psychosocial treatments for children and adolescents.

Incredible Years Parent Training

The Incredible Years Parent Training (IY-PT) was developed by Carolyn Webster-Stratton at the University of Washington and is based on years of programmatic research (Webster-Stratton & Hammond, 1997; Webster-Stratton, Reid, & Hammond, 2004). The IY-PT program is intended to reduce children's aggression and behavior problems and to increase social competence at home. The parent training program consists of a 13-session (2 hours per session) group parent training program for children ages 2–10 years who have disruptive behavior problems. In this program, parents view 250 videotape vignettes (each about 1 to 2 minutes) that demonstrate social learning and child development principles that serve as a stimulus for discussion and problem solving with the therapist and with other group members.

The IY-PT program begins with a concentration on positive parent–child interaction in which parents learn child-directed play skills, followed by a focus on effective discipline strategies such as ignoring, monitoring, commands, logical consequences, and time out. Parents are specifically instructed in how to teach problem-solving skills to their children. The IY-PT program meets established criteria for a *probably efficacious* intervention program for disruptive behavior problems.

Helping the Noncompliant Child

Helping the Noncompliant Child (HNC) is designed for children 3–8 years of age who have high rates of noncompliant behaviors (McMahon & Forehand, 2003). The program takes place in individual parent training sessions that occur weekly for 10 sessions (60–90 minutes per session). Parents are taught how to interrupt the coercive parent–child interaction cycle. The HNC approach includes use of positive feedback for appropriate child behaviors, ignoring minor negative behaviors, giving children clear directions, providing praise for appropriate behaviors, and time out for major rule violations.

The HNC program also uses modeling, coaching, role playing, and *in vivo* training in the clinic or home and the family progresses through the program as each skill is mastered. A key aspect of the program is the use of clear commands or directives for child behavior. At the heart of the HNC program is the distinction between *alpha commands* and *beta commands*. An alpha command is a clear instruction that specifies exactly what the parent wants the child to do (e.g., "Make up your bed," "Put the dishes in the sink," "Why don't you sit beside me?"). The child is given 5 seconds to comply with the command based on research that suggests most children of this age comply with these types of commands within 5 seconds. If the child does not comply within 5 seconds, he or she is given a prompt or warning that functions as a second clear instruction. If the child still does not comply, he or she is placed in time out for 3 minutes.

Beta commands are unclear directives that can take a range of forms. For example, a chain command is a combination of directives such as "Turn off the TV," "Put your plate in the sink," and "Do your homework" are best avoided—especially with very young children. In addition, vague commands that do not specify the desired behavior (e.g., "Be careful," "Act your age," "Be a good boy") should also generally be avoided. A more appropriate directive would be a question command that poses a question (e.g., "Would you like to start your homework now?"). "Let's" commands are also better in that they imply that the parent and the child will perform a task together (e.g., "Let's go clear up your room"). The HNC program meets established criteria for a *probably efficacious* treatment for disruptive behavior problems in 3- to 8-year-old children.

Multidimensional Treatment Foster Care

Multidimensional Treatment Foster Care (MTFC) is a community-based program developed as an alternative to institutional or residential-based group care placements (Chamberlain & Reid, 1998). The program is designed for youth with severe and chronic delinquent behavior problems and is often implemented with adolescent boys and girls. These youth are placed in foster homes for a period of 6 to 9 months and are provided treatment within the foster home setting. Foster parents receive a 20-hour preservice training program conducted by experienced foster parents in which they learn how to implement a daily token reinforcement system under the close supervision of an MTFC therapist. This token system consists of frequent positive reinforcement as well as clear, consistent limit setting. Foster parents award the youth points for daily expected behaviors such as getting up on time, attending school, and helping around the home. These points are exchanged for valued privileges. Minor rule violations are punished with loss of privileges (response cost) and major rule violations result in a short stay in detention. During treatment, foster parents report point levels to supervisors daily by telephone and meet weekly with supervisors for support and supervision.

Youth in the MTFC program meet weekly with individual therapists who provide support and work with them on problem-solving skills, anger management, social skills, and educational and vocational planning. They also meet once or twice a week with behavior support specialists trained in applied behavior analysis who focus on teaching and reinforcing prosocial behaviors in community settings (e.g., restaurants, sports settings). Youth also have regular appointments with consulting psychiatrists for medication management.

Concurrent with participation in this program, the child's biological parents receive intensive parent management training as well. This is designed to foster successful reintegration of the youth back into their homes and communities after treatment. The MTFC program meets established criteria for a *probably efficacious* treatment.

Multisystemic Therapy

Multisystemic therapy (MST) is an intervention for treating adolescents with serious antisocial and delinquent behavior problems that combines treatments and strategies as needed to provide an intensive family- and community-based intervention designed for individual families. These treatments include cognitive-behavioral approaches, behavior therapies, parent training, pragmatic family therapies, and pharmacological interventions that have a reasonable evidence base (Henggeler & Lee, 2003). MST takes place in natural environments (e.g., home, community, school) with a typical length of 3 to 5 months. Families are in contact with the MST therapist more than once per week either in person or by telephone and therapists are always "on call" to support families.

MST is operationalized by careful adherence to nine core principles that guide treatment planning: (1) assessing how identified problems are maintained by the family's current social environment; (2) emphasizing the positive aspects of family systems during treatment contacts; (3) focusing interventions on increasing responsible behavior and decreasing irresponsible behavior; (4) orienting interventions toward current, specific problems that can be easily tracked by family members; (5) designing interventions to target interaction sequences both within and across the systems that maintain target problems; (6) fostering developmentally appropriate competencies of youth within such systems as school, work environments, and peer groups; (7) designing daily or weekly intensive interventions that require continuing effort by the youth and family; (8) evaluating intervention plans and requiring treatment team accountability for positive outcomes; and (9) promoting generalization across time by teaching caregivers the skills to address problems across multiple contexts. The MST program meets established criteria for a *probably efficacious* treatment for severe antisocial and delinquent behaviors for adolescents.

Parent Management Training–Oregon Model

The Parent Management Training—Oregon Model (PMTO) intervention is a parent training program developed by the Oregon Social Learning Center that concentrates on teaching parents basic behavioral principles for managing and changing child behavior. It also encourages parents to monitor their child's behavior and the program assists parents in developing and implementing behavior management programs to improve targeted child problems. Therapists meet individually with parents of children between 3 and 12 years of age. Length of time in treatment varies according to the needs of the family and involves weekly treatment sessions and telephone contacts with parents.

The PMTO typically involves 10, 1-hour treatment sessions plus twice-weekly telephone contacts. The PMTO also focuses on promoting the five core principles of effective parenting that they have identified through their research: *discipline, monitoring, parent involvement, positive family management techniques,* and *crisis intervention.* In addition, the PMTO is the only parent training program to meet established criteria for a *well-established* treatment for disruptive problem behaviors (Bernal, Klinnert, & Schultz, 1980; Christensen, Johnson, Phillips, & Glasgow, 1980; Hughes & Wilson, 1988; Patterson et al., 1982).

Adjunctive Treatments for DBDs

Anger Control Training

Anger control training (ACT) is a cognitive-behavioral intervention for elementary school children with disruptive behavior problems (Lochman, Barry, & Pardini, 2002). Children meet once per week for 40–50 minutes during the school day in separate groups of about six. In these group sessions, children create specific goals and take part in exercises based on the social information processing model of anger control (Crick & Dodge, 1994; Dodge, 1986). In the group, children discuss vignettes of social encounters with peers and the social cues and possible motives of individuals in the vignettes. Children learn to use problem solving for dealing with anger-provoking social situations and they practice appropriate social responses and self-statements in response to different problem situations using behavioral rehearsal and performance feedback.

Later in treatment, children practice social situations designed to arouse their anger and the group supports their use of newly acquired anger control strategies. They also learn strategies to increase their awareness of feelings. The treatment takes place in 26–30 sessions and it meets established criteria for a *probably efficacious* treatment for anger control problems in elementary-age children.

Problem-Solving Skills Training

Problem-solving skills training (PSST) is a behavioral treatment designed for children ages 7–13 years with disruptive behavior problems (Kazdin,

2003b). Treatment consists of 25–30 sessions (40–50 minutes each) conducted individually with the child and with occasional parent contact. In the PSST program, children are taught problem-solving strategies and are encouraged to generalize these strategies to real-life problems and situations. Skills include identifying the problem, generating alternative solutions, weighing pros and cons of each solution, making a decision, and evaluating the outcome. Therapists use in-session practice, modeling, role playing, corrective feedback, and both social reinforcement and token reinforcement to gradually develop the problem-solving skills. This intervention meets established criteria for a *probably efficacious* treatment for disruptive behavior problems.

Concluding Remarks

In the past four to five decades there has been an explosion of knowledge about how to address the myriad challenges posed to parents by children who display noncompliant, explosive, disruptive, and antisocial behavior patterns. Often these behavior patterns are multiply determined and cannot be attributed to any single causal factor. However, the behavioral technology clearly exists for improving outcomes in this important socialization context. Our enduring challenge is to access and make available to parents of these children the proven strategies and techniques that will produce a meaningful difference in their lives and those of their children. It appears going forward that we know much more than we are able to implement successfully. A key purpose of this book is to try and address this gap. Additional complementary material for use by parents in the daily management of child behavior is provided in Chapter 7, which focuses on multicomponent interventions involving home and school.

Chapter Summary Points

- Children with DBDs use coercion as the key mechanism by which they control their social environment.
- Many of these children begin by exhibiting low levels of aversive behavior (e.g., noncompliance, whining) and will continue this behavior pattern into middle school, high school, and beyond.
- Some children will transform this pattern into lower-frequency but higher-intensity behaviors such as bullying, hitting, and stealing.

- Coercive behavior patterns of children with DBDs are maintained through negative reinforcement because this behavior pattern allows them to escape, avoid, delay, or reduce the demands placed on them by parents.

- Being an early starter for defiant/oppositional and antisocial behavior problems is the most important risk factor for this behavior pattern.

- Child temperamental characteristics and deficits in social-cognitive skills also contribute to the development of DBDs.

- Parent training has a distinct advantage over traditional psychotherapeutic interventions primarily because it treats the problem behavior in the naturalistic setting of the home.

- All evidence-based parent training programs consist of interventions derived from applied behavior analysis, social learning theory, and cognitive-behavioral theory.

- Although parent training is effective with most children and families, it will not be effective with about 25% of families that participate in these programs.

- Operant behavior involves the three-term contingency involving a discriminative stimulus, a behavior, and a consequence.

- Antecedents of behavior include discriminative stimuli (i.e., stimuli that signal a behavior will be reinforced), setting events (i.e., events that are temporally and physically remote from behavior but nonetheless influence its occurrence), establishing operations (i.e., any environmental event that alters the effectiveness of a reinforcer for a behavior), and prompts (i.e., events that cue the performance of certain behaviors).

- Behavior patterns can be organized into meaningful units such as a response class, which can be either a topographical response class (what the behavior looks like) or a functional response class (what functions the behaviors serve).

- Behavior patterns can also be organized into response chains whereby one behavior immediately follows another, with the first behavior functioning as a discriminative stimulus for the next behavior in the chain.

- Consequences of behavior include reinforcement (positive and negative), both of which increase behavior; punishment (positive and negative), both of which decrease behavior; and extinction, which decreases behavior.

- Schedules of reinforcement are rules that describe a contingency of reinforcement that determines the conditions by which behaviors will produce reinforcement.

- Schedules of reinforcement can be fixed or intermittent and ratio or interval-based, each producing different rates and patterns of behavior.

- Evidence-based parent training programs that meet established criteria for probably efficacious treatments include: (1) the Incredible Years Parent

Training, (2) Helping the Noncompliant Child, multidimensional treatment foster care, and multisystemic therapy.

- Only one parent training program meets established criteria for a well-established treatment for disruptive behavior problems: the Parent Management Training—Oregon Model.
- Evidence-based adjunctive treatments for disruptive behavior problems are anger control training and problem-solving skills training.

Evidence-Based
Multicomponent Interventions

This chapter focuses on multicomponent interventions for DBDs that involve intervention strategies implemented across multiple settings of home, school, and community environments. These interventions conceptualize DBDs within an ecological framework and are based on the notion that these types of behavior problems are multiply caused and maintained across a variety of social environments. Viewing behavior problems from this perspective allows for a broader conceptualization of behavioral ecologies that cause and maintain these types of behavior problems. Consistent with the views presented throughout this book, multicomponent interventions hypothesize that DBDs are initiated and maintained through social interventions of a child with his or her environment (Patterson et al., 1992). *Coercion* is the linchpin in this process whereby a child's behavior receives high rates of both positive and negative reinforcement. It occurs over a relatively long period of time and allows the child to demonstrate this coercive process with an increasingly diverse set of individuals, making this behavior pattern highly resistant to change. The earlier an intervention occurs in the development of DBDs, the less complex the reinforcement system is for these behaviors and the more likely this behavior pattern can be changed (Reid & Eddy, 2002).

Children and youth function in a context that describes the environmental factors in which the individual functions and includes interpersonal relations (e.g., peers, teachers, parents), social systems (e.g., home and school), and settings (e.g., community, neighborhood). Effective intervention must target most of these environmental contexts to lead to successful outcomes for children and youth with DBDs. In addition, a host of factors moderate the development and maintenance of these behavior problems such as socioeconomic disadvantage, high levels of stress, parental psychopathology, and marital discord. Unfortunately, we have little or no control over these moderator variables in terms of designing effective interventions.

Effective treatments for DBDs should include the family, teachers, peers, and siblings. These treatments, at a minimum, should incorporate the parent, family, and the school and may involve seeing the parents separately, meeting with the entire family, and using teachers to assess and intervene at school (Kazdin & Weisz, 2003). Contexts often change over the course of development. For example, with young children it seems logical to involve parents extensively in treatment. For school-age children, it makes sense to involve teachers quite extensively in treatments. For adolescents, it would be prudent to involve peers to some extent in treatment, given their profound influence on youths' behavior.

Rationale for Multicomponent Interventions

Operant Learning Theory

Our scientific understanding of the origins, causes, and maintenance of DBDs is most certainly incomplete. DBDs are a pressing social, educational, and mental health problem requiring multiple layers of intervention across a variety of social–ecological contexts for effective remediation of this behavior pattern. Effective remediation of DBDs requires intervention strategies drawn from several theoretical perspectives. From an operant learning perspective, current treatment of DBDs is based on the assumption that children and youth engage in this behavior pattern to the degree that it is *socially functional*. As mentioned in Chapter 1, the frequency of disruptive behavior patterns is functionally related to the extent to which it is positively and negatively reinforced in the environment. Treatment strategies based on this conceptualization entail the rearrangement of the contingencies maintaining problem behaviors and to increase the rate of reinforcement for more socially adaptive replacement behaviors (see Chapter 9).

Whereas operant learning strategies are effective in reducing disruptive behavior patterns and increasing rates of prosocial behaviors, they are not sufficient to produce lasting changes in this pattern of behavior. Principles and procedures drawn from *social learning theory* offer a more comprehensive approach to the treatment of DBDs.

Social Learning Theory

Social learning theory derives from the work of Bandura (1977, 1986) and utilizes the concept of vicarious learning and the role of cognitive mediational processes in determining which environmental events are attended to, retained, and subsequently performed when an individual is exposed to modeling stimuli. Social learning theory is based on the notion of reciprocal determinism that describes the role an individual's behavior has on changing the environment and vice versa. Social learning theory argues that vicarious learning is accounted for by four processes that occur during or shortly after observing a model of behavior: *attentional, retentional, motor reproductive,* and *motivational.*

Attentional processes deal with the individual's observation of a model's behavior and its consequences (i.e., vicarious reinforcement). If an observer does not attend to a model's behavior or attends to irrelevant aspects of a model's behavior, little learning will occur. A number of variables affect the extent to which an individual will attend to a model's behavior. One, reinforcement of a model's behavior will produce higher rates of learning (via vicarious reinforcement) than a model's behavior that is not reinforced. For example, if a model's aggressive behavior is consistently reinforced, an observer of that behavior will reproduce it. Two, characteristics of a model predict the degree to which observers learn from a model's behavior. Models that are attractive, likable, and prestigious produce more vicarious learning than less attractive, likable, and prestigious models. Three, the ability to learn from a model depends on learning experiences of an observer prior to viewing a model. For example, a child whose aggressive behavior has been reinforced on numerous occasions is more likely to imitate an aggressive model than a child with a somewhat different learning history.

After an observer has attended to a model's behavior, the observer must *retain* or *recall* key aspects of the modeled behavior. One important way that this occurs is the verbal encoding of the observed behavior. In this way, it is possible to reduce fairly complex behavior to a few words. Another important aspect of retention processes is the repeated performance of the model's behavior and/or a verbal representation of that behavior in a covert way. For example, after seeing a golf instructor demonstrate a perfect drive, an observer might covertly imitate that behavior without making any movement of the golf swing by verbally representing the modeled behavior (e.g., "Keep your left arm straight during the backswing").

Motor reproductive processes describe the physical ability to perform the modeled behavior. Some behaviors are more easily reproduced than others. For example, it is quite simple for most people to reproduce relatively simple motor acts (e.g., raising you hand or sweeping the floor with a broom). Other motor acts are quite complex and impossible for most people to reproduce (e.g., slam-dunking a basketball or turning a flip on a balance beam).

Finally, *motivational processes* are important in determining whether a modeled behavior will be imitated. An observer must expect than an imitated behavior will result in reinforcement (via vicarious reinforcement). Research has consistently shown than reinforced modeling produces greater behavior changes than nonreinforced modeling (Bandura, 1986).

Cognitive-Behavioral Theory

Interventions based on cognitive-behavioral theory are based on the premise that thoughts, emotions, and behaviors are reciprocally linked and that changing one of these will necessarily result in changes in the others. These reciprocal relationships between thoughts, emotions, and behaviors underlie all cognitive-behavioral interventions. Cognitive-behavioral interventions for child and adolescent behavior problems emphasize both the influence of external contingencies (e.g., reinforcement and punishment) as well as the individual's mediating or information processing style in resolving adjustment difficulties (Gresham & Lochman, 2009).

In cognitive-behavioral interventions, *cognitions* may be defined as sets of skills that include problem solving, coping strategies, regulation of affect, and interpersonal skills. A central assumption in all cognitive-behavioral interventions is that adaptive and maladaptive behavior from the social context in which cognitions occur. A fundamental tenet of cognitive-behavioral interventions is that one cannot successfully intervene with children and adolescents without incorporating the home and peer group at some level in the process (Lochman & Gresham, 2009).

A good example of the above principle can be found in the literature on the cognitive and attributional processes of aggressive children. Dodge and colleagues conducted seminal research on how aggressive, rejected children process social information, interpret interpersonal cues, and make decisions based on this information (see Crick & Dodge, 1994). Aggressive children frequently make errors in evaluating the motives and intent underlying social behavior directed toward them by peers and adults. They are likely to attribute hostile intentions to accidental or ambiguous behavior from others, and they respond inappropriately as a result.

Aggressive, rejected children seem to have quite abnormal standards and expectations regarding their own behavior, and these beliefs, in turn, "legitimize" much of their deviant, aversive behavior. These hostile attributional biases prevent these children from accurately decoding negative and disapproving feedback about their behavior. Smith, Lochman, and Daunic (2005) provided an in-depth analysis of cognitive behavioral interventions with problems of anger/aggression of children with DBDs.

Evidence-Based Multicomponent Interventions for DBDs

Multisystemic Therapy

MST is an intensive family- and community-based treatment for adolescent youth engaged in severe conduct problems that put them at risk for out-of-home placement and their families (Henggeler & Lee, 2003). MST has been applied to a broad range of serious clinical problems, including chronic and violent juvenile offending, adolescent sexual offenders, substance-abusing juvenile offenders, and youth in psychiatric crises (e.g., suicidal, homicidal, and psychotic). These youth create significant personal and societal costs due to the high rates of expensive out-of-home placements and consume a disproportionate share of the nation's mental health treatment resources. The long-range goals of MST are to decrease rates of antisocial behavior patterns, improve family relations and school performance, and reduce the use of expensive out-of-home placements (e.g., residential treatment and incarceration).

Theoretical Framework

MST is conceptualized from the theoretical perspective of social–ecological and family systems theories (Bronfenbrenner, 1979; Haley, 1976; Minuchen, 1974). MST sees youth as being contained within multiple interconnected systems that include the nuclear family, extended family, neighborhood, school, peer group, and community. It involves various social systems including the juvenile justice system, social services, and mental health. Effective treatment considers the risk factors occurring across these multiple systems, thereby ensuring the ecological validity of treating youth in the natural environments where skills are practiced and learned.

Conceptual Assumptions

Five conceptual assumptions are considered critical to the design and implementation of MST interventions. One, clinical problems are viewed as being *multiply determined* by the reciprocal interaction of individual, family, peer, school, and community variables. MST interventions assess and consider these potential risk factors in a comprehensive, individualized manner. Two, the *caregiver* is seen as the key to the long-term positive outcomes for youth in MST interventions. The caregiver may be a biological parent, guardian, grandparent, aunt, uncle, or sibling who has an emotional tie to the youth. The focus of treatment is the development of the caregiver's ability to parent effectively and strengthen the family's support system. Three, MST uses *empirically based treatments* that include cognitive-behavioral approaches, behavior therapies (both operant and respondent), behavioral parent training, pragmatic family therapies, and psychotropic interventions when indicated. Four, MST programs provide intensive services with the goal to *overcome barriers* to treatment access. MST therapists have a relatively low caseload to ensure quality implementation of multiple interventions and a relatively short duration of treatment (typically 3 to 5 months). Five, MST emphasizes the promotion of high levels of *treatment fidelity* to achieve desired outcomes. Treatment fidelity is ensured by a 5-day overview of the MST model, participation in weekly group supervision meetings, weekly consultation with MST consultants, and quarterly on-site consultant booster sessions.

Treatment Format

MST is delivered within the context of all-important systems in which the youth is involved, such as the peer group, school, extended family, the neighborhood, community agencies, and other agencies (e.g., social services, juvenile justice, and mental health). Early in the treatment program, specific measurable goals and functionally meaningful outcomes are decided on in collaboration with family and other stakeholders. Any person or agency with a stake in these goals is engaged by the MST therapist and caregiver with specific interventions that will lead to goal attainment.

The engagement of the family is considered essential for successful outcomes of the MST intervention. The MST treatment model uses strategies to encourage cooperative partnering, and families are treated with respect. The MST team focuses on system strengths and is responsive to families' unique needs. Barriers to successful implementation are continuously evaluated and addressed. MST is administered within a home-based model of service delivery that has been crucial to the high engagement and low dropout rates cited in recent outcome studies (see Henggeler, Pickrel, Brondino, & Crouch, 1996).

The MST intervention program addresses five major categories of interventions, including family interventions, peer interventions, school interventions, individually oriented interventions, and psychiatric interventions. As mentioned earlier, the average duration of the MST program is 3 to 5 months, and the program ends in one of two ways. First, if the goals are considered met by mutual agreement of the therapist, family, and other stakeholders the treatment is terminated. Second, if the goals are considered unmet but it is determined that the treatment has reached the point of diminishing returns, then the treatment is terminated. About two-thirds of MST cases in community settings end with successful goal attainment specified by the family and stakeholders.

Summary

MST is an effective family-based treatment for youth who present serious clinical problems including criminal behavior, violence, substance abuse, and serious emotional disturbance. The evidence base for MST is strong, with several randomized clinical trials with violent and chronic juvenile offenders showing reduction in recidivism and out-of-home placements. Research over the past 20 to 30 years across multiple disciplines has documented a variety of risk factors in the development of antisocial behavior through correlational and longitudinal research. MST interventions focus on these risk factors and have made extensive use of this evidence base. The MST model goes against much of the traditional mental health treatment model by emphasizing the importance of provider accountability for outcomes, facilitation of treatment fidelity, viewing caregivers as key players to long-term successful outcomes, and considering pragmatic commitments to overcome barriers to service access.

Anger Coping and Coping Power Programs

The Anger Coping and Coping Power programs are based on a contextual social-cognition model and are designed to prevent the development of antisocial behavior in adolescence by changing maladaptive parenting practices and children's social information processing problems associated with aggressive behavior (Lochman et al., 2002). Both programs include group sessions highlighting issues such as anger management, perspective taking, social problem solving, emotional awareness, relaxation training, social skills training, positive social and personal goals, and dealing with peer pressure. The Coping Power program adds a parent component using group sessions to deal with issues such as social reinforcement, positive attention, creation of clear home rules, behavioral expectations, monitoring procedures, use of appropriate discipline practices, family communication, positive relationships with school, and stress management. Parents are informed of the specific skills their children are working on and are encouraged to facilitate and reinforce their children for implementing these new skills at home and school.

Anger Coping Program

The Anger Coping Program (ACP) was designed to address anger arousal and social-cognitive processes associated with aggressive behavior in children. The ACP is designed for five to seven children in a group therapy format, although the sessions can be implemented on an individual basis. The program has been successfully implemented in both clinic and school settings. The program consists of 18 sessions and meets weekly for 60 to 90 minutes in a large room with a table and chairs. Poster boards and a dry-erase board are hung around the room to specify group rules, point charts for appropriate behavior, and to serve as reminders and activities in the group. The sessions for the ACP are listed below.

- Introduction and Group Rules
- Understanding and Writing Goals
- Anger Management: Puppet Self-Control Task
- Using Self-Instruction
- Perspective Taking
- Looking at Anger
- What Does Anger Feel Like?
- Choices and Consequences
- Steps for Problem Solving
- Problem Solving in Action
- Video Productions I–VIII and Review

The ACP focuses on anger arousal and social-cognitive processes and targets a number of skills that have been found to be deficient in angry and aggressive children. These skills include awareness of negative feelings, use of self-talk, distraction techniques, strategies to decrease anger arousal, perspective taking, goal setting, and social problem-solving skills. The concepts presented in Session 8 (Choices and Consequences) are seen as the most critical components of the ACP in terms of behavior change (Lochman et al., 2002). Research findings suggest that specific client characteristics are associated with greater improvement in the ACP. Aggressive children who are poor problem solvers, who have lower perceived levels of hostility, and who are more rejected by peers exhibit better treatment outcomes (Lochman et al., 2002). Also, children with a more internalized attributional style and higher levels of anxiety tend to benefit more from the ACP intervention. Approximately two-thirds of children undergoing the ACP show significant improvement, with the remaining one-third of the children requiring some type of continued involvement in treatment following the conclusion of the program.

Coping Power Program

The Coping Power Program (CPP) extends the ACP by including 33 child sessions and 16 parent sessions delivered over a 15-month period. The additional 15 child sessions allow for coverage of other problem areas associated with aggressive behavior in children, such as relaxation training, advanced emotional awareness skills, and setting positive social and personal goals (see Lochman & Wells, 1996). The additional child sessions also focus on improving social skills, entering positive peer networks, and working on negotiating and cooperative skills in the peer group.

The parent group sessions focus on social learning techniques such as identifying prosocial and disruptive behavioral targets in specific operational terms, rewarding and attending to appropriate child behaviors, issuing effective instructions or directives, establishing age-appropriate rules and expectations in the home, and applying effective consequences for negative child behaviors (Lochman & Wells, 1996). Parents learn strategies for managing child behavior outside the home and ways of establishing ongoing family communication structures via weekly family meetings. Parents also learn techniques that support social-cognitive and problem-solving skills that their children are learning in the group sessions. Parents also learn stress management skills to cope with problems in dealing with stressful disciplinary interactions with their children.

An enhanced version of the CPP includes a third teacher component that involves five 2-hour teacher inservice meetings and ongoing teacher consultation. Teachers learn about the CPP and how they can prompt and reinforce the skills being taught in the group sessions. Each teacher meeting includes a combination of didactic presentation of information on the topic of the day and problem solving around that topic.

Outcome analyses of the CPP indicate that the program produced lower rates of delinquent behavior and of parent-rated substance abuse at 1-year follow-up than did the control group. Children also displayed teacher-rated behavioral improvements in school. The CPP moved at-risk children into normative ranges for substance use, delinquency, and school behavior compared to controls. Mediator analyses showed that the intervention effects were mediated by changes in social-cognitive processes, schemas, and parenting processes (Lochman & Wells, 1996).

Summary

Controlled research using the ACP and CPP indicates that these cognitive-behavioral interventions have immediate effects at postintervention on children's aggressive behavior at home and school using independent parent and teacher ratings of behavior. Effect sizes are typically in the moderate range, and these programs can have lasting preventive effects on children's later substance use up to 3 years after treatment. It appears necessary to include the parent component (CPP) to have longer-term effects on children's delinquent behavior. The addition of the teacher component appears to produce the most robust effects on children's aggressive behavior.

Fast Track

The Fast Track program is a comprehensive prevention and remediation strategy designed for children and youth having severe and chronic conduct problems and was developed by the Conduct Problems Prevention Group (CPPG, 1992) for at-risk children identified in kindergarten and extending up to 10th grade. The Fast Track program was based on longitudinal research on the development and maintenance of serious adolescent conduct problems that suggested these problems develop from a combination of child, family, and community risk factors that interact from childhood through adolescence. The CPPG indicated that interventions should take time and must develop social and self-regulation skills. These interventions focus on building behavioral and cognitive skills in school and family environments by changing the patterns of interaction among members of the child's social ecology. Fast Track also provides a program of universal prevention education based on the Promoting Alternative Thinking Strategies (PATHS) curriculum (Kusche & Greenberg, 1994).

Fast Track consists of five integrated component activities for at-risk children. The first component is parent training that utilizes a social learning approach to teach effective parenting skills. Parents of first-grade children meet for 22 sessions to address the development of a more positive relationship between the school and the family and to learn specific skills to decrease coercive interactions and to facilitate more positive parent–child relationships. Sessions early in the year concentrate on helping children succeed in school by creating organized learning times at home and helping parents become more involved in the educational process. Parents are introduced to the PATHS curriculum in which they are taught ways to coach their children in anger control and problem-solving strategies. The remaining sessions focus on developing positive parent–child interactions and decreasing noncompliance and aggression.

The second component of the Fast Track program is home visiting. Home visits and phone calls are used twice weekly to practice skills taught in the parenting groups, to apply concepts to the actual family environment, and to respond to difficulties parents have in implementing skills. The home visits are designed to teach parents problem-solving skills, to promote feelings of efficacy, and to enhance family organization to create a safe and supportive environment. During the home visits, parents are asked a series of questions and to work collaboratively to solve problems in their current lives. Home visits continue during the summer after the first grade.

The third component is social skills training for the child to improve peer relations, including reducing aggressive interactions with peers, parents, and teachers. Self-control skills and anger management as well as interpersonal social problem-solving skills are taught in the group. Social skills strategies include modeling, coaching, performance feedback, and role playing.

The fourth component of Fast Track is academic tutoring related primarily to reading. Fast Track uses phonics and phonemic awareness training implemented by paraprofessionals who meet twice a week and once on Saturday with parents present to demonstrate the child-paced aspects of the program and to help parents see their child's progress.

The fifth component is classroom intervention to increase reinforcement for positive behaviors and to improve classroom behavior management practices. Teachers are also trained in the PATHS curriculum. Teachers present the PATHS material to all students in their classrooms three times per week using didactic instruction, modeling, and role playing.

Outcome Research

A multisite evaluation involved schools in four areas of the country that were selected as high risk based on local neighborhood crime and poverty statistics (CPPG, 1999, 2002). Fifty-four elementary schools were randomly assigned to intervention or control conditions with 445 children in the intervention condition and 446 in the control condition. At the end of first grade, behavioral observations indicated lower rates of problem behavior among target children in the intervention schools. Fewer intervention-group children spent time in special education and peer relations improved. Results at the end of 3 years indicated that more intervention-group children were rated as free of conduct problems than children in the control group. Parent ratings provided additional support for these findings and extended the behavioral improvements to the home. Effect sizes were moderate but consistent across measures for the intervention group.

Problem-Solving Skills Training

This treatment program was developed at the Yale Child Conduct Clinic as an outpatient service for children and families (Kazdin, 2003b). This clinic, affiliated with the Yale Child Study Center, addresses multiple clinical issues including inpatient and outpatient services, psychiatric evaluation, and medication evaluation. Children between the ages of 2 to 13 years are referred to this clinic for aggressive and antisocial behavior. Most of these children meet the criteria for a primary diagnosis of conduct disorder or oppositional defiant disorder using the DSM-5 (American Psychiatric Association, 2013).

The treatments provided at the clinic consist of cognitive problem-solving skills training (PSST) and parent management training (PMT). Both of these treatments are provided individually to children and families rather than in a group format. The group format was abandoned by the clinic due to several logistical problems such as missed appointments, coming to treatment on incorrect days, and varied pace in learning and using the treatment material. The two treatments were differentiated based on several considerations. Many times parents are not available because they either will not or cannot participate in treatment. Reasons for this lack of participation range from parental mental illness, engagement in prostitution, incarceration, mental retardation, or unwillingness to participate in the treatment program. Children's parents who fall into this category are given the PSST as a standalone treatment for conduct problems. Parents who can and do participate in treatment are given the PMT program and the children also receive the PSST treatment program.

Cognitive Problem-Solving Skills Training

The PSST program is predicated on the notion that cognitive processes underlie how an individual perceives, codes, and experiences the world. Children with DBDs, particularly aggressive behavior, exhibit distortions and deficiencies in a number of these cognitive processes. Some examples include generating alternative solutions of interpersonal conflict, identifying ways to obtain social goals (e.g., entering a peer group or making a friend), consequences of one's behaviors, making attributions of others' motivations, perceiving how others feel, and expectations of the effects of one's own behavior (Lochman, Whidby, & FitzGerald, 2000; Shure, 1997).

A salient example of the distorted cognitive processes in DBDs is evidenced in the work on attributional style and aggressive behavior. In this view, aggressive behavior is not triggered by environmental events, but through how these environmental events are perceived and processed by the individual. Attribution of the intent of others in a social interaction is an important cognitive disposition that helps us understand aggressive behavior. Aggressive children tend to attribute *hostile intent* to others in social situations wher the cues of actual intent are ambiguous (see Crick & Dodge, 1994). When situations are misperceived as hostile, children are more likely to engage in aggressive behavior. Research on these cognitive processes with aggressive children has served as a key basis for conceptualizing treatment and developing specific treatment strategies (Dodge, Dishion, & Lansford, 2006).

The PSST consists of weekly therapy sessions with the child, with each session lasting 30–50 minutes. The basic treatment program involves 12–20 sessions that may be supplemented with optional sessions depending on the child's needs in mastering the content. The basic treatment tenet is the use of *problem-solving steps* to dissect interpersonal situations into units that allow identification and use of prosocial behaviors. These problem-solving steps are listed below.

- "What am I supposed to do?" (Identify and define the problem.)
- "I have to look at all my possibilities." (Delineate or specify alternative solutions to the problem.)
- "I'd better concentrate and focus in." (Concentrate and evaluate solutions he or she has generated.)
- "I need to make a choice." (Choose the answer he or she thinks is correct.)
- "I did a good job or I made a mistake." (Verify whether the solution was best among alternatives, whether problem solving was correctly followed, or whether a mistake or less desirable solution was selected.)

These steps are taught via modeling, with the therapist and the child taking turns using and applying the steps. The therapist uses prompting, shaping, performance feedback, and specific praise the child's mastery of these skills. The problems and solutions are practiced in each session via role playing and behavioral rehearsal. The treatment focuses of the child's use of the problem-solving steps to generate and enact prosocial solutions to interpersonal problems in a range of social situations. Role playing is used extensively throughout the program to provide opportunities to enact prosocial solutions to potential interpersonal conflict situations.

A crucial aspect of the treatment program is the use of the problem-solving steps outside treatment (i.e., generalization across settings). The program makes use of *in vivo* practice in which assignments are designed to extend the child's use of the problem-solving skills to everyday situations. When possible, parents are included in some of the treatment sessions to learn the problem-solving steps and practice their implementation in real-life situations.

Parent Management Training

PMT consists of a set of procedures in which parents are trained to change their child's behavior at home. Parents meet with a therapist or trainer who teaches them to use procedures to alter their interactions with their child, to promote prosocial behavior, and to decrease deviant behavior. Much of the PMT program is based on the conceptualization of antisocial behavior developed by the OSLC group (Patterson et al., 1992). You will recall from Chapter 1 that much of antisocial behavior is developed via parent–child interactions in the home through a *coercive family process*. Coercion refers to deviant behavior on the part of the child that is reinforced by the parent. These coercive behavioral interchanges between a parent and child operate in such a way as to reinforce aggressive child behavior. Parent–child interaction sequences are crucial in understanding how and why aggressive behavior occurs and serve as the basis for all evidence-based parent training programs (Reid et al., 2002).

The PMT program draws heavily from the applied behavior analysis literature that is based on operant learning theory. Recall from Chapter 6 the extensive discussion of *contingencies of reinforcement* that refer to the relationship between behaviors and environmental events that influence these behaviors. The three-term contingency consists of antecedents (discriminative stimuli, setting events, or motivation operations), behaviors (focus of change), and consequences (reinforcement and punishment). The three-term contingency model underlies the majority of what is taught in the PMT program to change deviant child behavior.

The PMT consists of 12–16 weekly sessions, with each session lasting 45–60 minutes. The program starts with relatively simple tasks for the parent and increases in complexity over the course of treatment. Individual sessions are designed to teach content and skills in behavior management strategies. A typical session would begin with teaching a basic concept such as positive reinforcement and how it might be implemented in the home to facilitate appropriate behavior. Therapists model, role-play, and rehearse specific behavior management strategies, alternating roles of the parent and the child. A token reinforcement system is used in the home to provide parents with a structured way of implementing reinforcement contingencies.

The PMT program also includes attention to the child's performance in school. The therapist contacts the child's teacher to discuss individual problem areas, including conduct problems, grades, and homework completion. A home-based reinforcement system is created in which child performance at school is monitored and contingencies are provided at home by parents. Teachers also implement specific interventions in their classrooms.

Studies have shown that significant improvements are made with both the PSST and PMT programs as indexed by rather large effect sizes (>1.2) (see Kazdin & Wassell, 2000). An effect size of 1.2 indicates that approximately 76% of children in the treatment group improve compared to only 24% of children in the control group using the binomial effect size display or BESD. Also, follow-up assessments of both programs have shown that therapeutic changes at both home and school are maintained over 1 year.

Chapter Summary Points

- Effective interventions should target most of the environmental contexts in which children and youth with DBDs function (home, school, community, peer group).

- Multicomponent interventions for DBDs are based on a combination of operant learning theory, social learning theory, and cognitive-behavioral theory.

- Interventions based on operant learning theory are based on the assumption that children and youth engage in disruptive behavior patterns to the extent to which these behaviors are socially functional (i.e., these behaviors are positively and/or negatively reinforced).

- Interventions based on social learning theory are based on the notion of reciprocal determinism that describes the role an individual's behavior has on the environment and the role that the environment has on the individual's behavior.

- Interventions based on cognitive-behavioral theory are based on the premise that thoughts, emotions, and behaviors are reciprocally linked and that changing one of these will result in changes in the others.

- MST is an intensive family- and community-based treatment for adolescent youth engaged in severe conduct problems that put them at risk for out-of-home placement.

- MST has been successfully used in treating a broad range of serious clinical problems, including chronic and violent juvenile offending, adolescent sexual offenders, substance-abusing juvenile offenders, and youth in psychiatric crises (suicide, homicide, psychoses).

- MST is based on the theoretical perspective of ecological and family systems theories that sees youth as being embedded within multiple, interconnected systems that include the nuclear family, neighborhood, school, peer group, and community.

- MST is based on five conceptual assumptions: (1) multiply determined problem behaviors, (2) the caregiver as the pivotal player in successful long-term successful outcomes, (3) use of empirically based treatments, (4) overcoming barriers to treatment access, and (5) promotion of high levels of treatment fidelity.

- The evidence base for MST is strong, with several randomized clinical trials with violent and chronic juvenile offenders showing reductions in recidivism and out-of-home placements.

- The Anger Coping Program is designed to address anger arousal and social-cognitive processes with aggressive behavior in children.

- Research findings suggest that aggressive children who are poor problem solvers and who have lower levels of hostility exhibit better treatment outcomes than children with higher levels of hostility.

- Children with a more internalized attributional style and higher levels of anxiety also respond better to the Anger Coping Program.
- The Coping Power Program extends the Anger Coping Program by including 33 child sessions and 16 parent sessions delivered over a 15-month period.
- Outcome analyses of the Coping Power Program show that the program lowers rates of delinquent behavior and parent-rated substance abuse at 1-year follow-up.
- The Fast Track program is a comprehensive prevention and remediation strategy for children and youth exhibiting severe and chronic conduct problems.
- Fast Track consists of five integrated component activities: (1) parent training, (2) home visiting, (3) social skills training, (4) academic tutoring in reading, and (5) classroom intervention.
- Multisite evaluation of the Fast Track program showed it produces lower rates of observed problem behavior, fewer special education placements, and improved peer relations.
- Problem-solving skills training is based on the notion that cognitive processes underlie how an individual perceives, codes, and experiences the world.
- Children with aggressive behavior patterns often attribute hostile intent to others in social situations in which the cues of actual intent are ambiguous and, in turn, they behave aggressively.
- Problem-solving skills training uses problem-solving steps to dissect interpersonal situations into units that allow for the identification and use of prosocial behaviors.
- Parent management training consists of a set of procedures in which parents are trained to change their child's behavior at home using principles based on operant learning theory.
- Outcome studies have shown that the parent management training program and the problem-solving skills training program leads to improvement of 76% of children in the treatment group and only 24% of children in the control group.

Primary Prevention Strategies

This chapter focuses on best practices in the primary prevention of DBDs by identifying and modifying risk factors known to lead at-risk children down a destructive path of poor social, emotional, mental health, and educational outcomes. Prevention science tells us that these risk factors operate within and across different environmental contexts such as school, home, and community to produce these negative outcomes. Recall from Chapter 4, the goal of primary prevention efforts is to *prevent harm* and rather than to reverse (secondary prevention) or reduce harm (tertiary prevention). Primary prevention efforts are common in medicine. Procedures such as taking a low-dose aspirin daily, maintaining a healthy weight, and abstinence from smoking are all primary prevention strategies aimed at preventing cardiovascular disease. Primary prevention efforts for DBDs necessarily should involve parents, teachers, and peers in coordinated intervention efforts that target the child's behavior and addresses the risk factors surrounding this behavior pattern.

Kellam (2002) made the following observations about prevention science:

- Effective prevention interventions are often based in schools, and many of these programs involve family members as part of the intervention team.
- Prevention is based on knowledge of risk factors and directing interventions at these specific risk factors to produce positive outcomes and prevent negative outcomes.

- Prevention efforts are best viewed from a public health perspective to (1) promote social adaptation and psychological well-being and (2) reduce maladaptive behaviors over the life span.
- Effective primary prevention requires that we address those specific features of social contexts that either help (protective factors) or hinder (risk factors) the development of individuals and their abilities to meet the demands of social adaptation.
- Risk factors reside in the physical environment and within the individual and are manifested when individuals respond to the environmental demands.

Kellam's observations have substantial value in guiding the achievement of prevention outcomes for students with DBDs, particularly within the context of schooling. The most informative way for conceptualizing primary prevention outcomes is from a social-ecological approach perspective. A key feature of social ecology is the notion of person–environment fit (P-E fit). A P-E fit or match occurs when the demands of the environment are consistent with the abilities, skills, resources, and motivations of the individual. If an individual is able and willing to respond appropriately to task demands of the environment and if the environmental demands are appropriate, a P-E fit is highly likely and should produce positive outcomes. A cardinal feature of children and youth with DBDs is that they consistently either do not respond to these demands at all or respond to them inappropriately. Numerous studies conducted in school settings have shown that students with DBDs are more likely to (1) behave inappropriately to escape from teacher-imposed task demands and/or (2) engage in maladaptive behavior in order to seek attention (see Gresham, Watson, et al., 2001).

Walker and Severson (2002) have identified the following characteristics of effective primary prevention programs:

- These efforts must address known risk factors and the precursors to destructive outcomes.
- These efforts must be applied as early as possible in a child's life and school career.
- These efforts must be carefully coordinated and delivered with integrity.
- These efforts must be adequately funded.
- These efforts must establish benchmarks and outcomes to gauge progress.

The Importance of Identifying Risk Factors

Children and youth with DBDs are at risk for a number of short-term and long-term negative outcomes, including, but are not limited to, poor academic achievement, school dropout, retention in grade, referral to mental health agencies, contact with the juvenile justice system, substance abuse, and suspension or expulsion from school (Hinshaw, 1992; Loeber & Farrington, 1998; Parker & Asher, 1987). A number of risk and protective factors operating within the family, school, and community have been associated with severe DBDs. However, the extent to which these risk and protective factors within these interlocking systems moderate or mediate the development of DBDs is unclear.

Understanding risk and protective factors in the development of DBDs is important for at least three reasons. First, significant numbers of these students experience short-term and long-term negative outcomes and/or fail to achieve positive outcomes (Walker et al., 2004). Second, current policy imperatives dictate a consideration of risk and protective factors as primary prevention strategies (Kellam, 2002). Three, a consideration of risk and protective factors may moderate children's response to intervention (Sugai & Horner, 1997; Walker et al., 1997).

Much of the prior meta-analytic risk/protection research has focused on single outcomes or single risk/protective factors; thus the interrelationships that do exist between the entire range of outcomes and contributing factors are not apparent. Research prompted by risk and protection theory suggest that risk and protective factors can be distinguished and quantified and that risk and protective factors that affect multiple outcomes may exist. The identification of risk and protective factors has three implications. One, if risk and protective factors can be distinguished and quantified, the effects of primary prevention efforts may be maximized. Two, if risk and protective factors that affect multiple outcomes can be identified, then primary prevention interventions might address these factors for maximum effectiveness. Three, if the risk and protective factors arise in multiple contexts, then multisystem primary prevention interventions should constitute the best intervention practices.

Mechanisms of Action in Risk and Protective Factors

The etiology of specific behavior patterns for individuals with DBDs is complex. A single risk factor is not likely to be responsible for any given behavior pattern, nor is any single protective factor likely to be sufficient to prevent the development of problematic behavior patterns (Greenberg et al., 2001). No single factor, whether considered risk or protective, can account for children's DBDs. Moreover, not all children experiencing the same risk factors develop DBDs. The presence of a single behavioral marker may be important in the school context, depending on frequency or intensity of the behavior pattern in question. Researchers typically find a nonlinear relationship between risk factors and outcomes, suggesting that a single risk factor may have a small effect, but find that rates of behavior problems increase rapidly with the accumulation of additional risk factors (Rutter, 1979; Sameroff et al., 1987). In addition, risk and protective factors are not equal in importance; therefore, a primary challenge is to identify and target those risk and protective factors that have the greatest influence in promoting positive outcomes and preventing negative ones (Nash & Bowen, 2002).

Coie et al. (1993) suggested that protective factors may work in one or more of the following four ways: (1) they directly decrease dysfunction, (2) they interact with risk factors to buffer their effects, (3) they disrupt the mediational chain by which risk factors lead to disorder, and (4) they prevent the initial occurrence of risk factors. In the same way reinforcers and punishers are distinguished on the basis of their effects on the probability of future behavior, risk and protective factors can be distinguished only by the effect exerted on the probability of future positive and negative outcomes. A priori assumptions regarding the effects of risk and protective factors often can be erroneous or misleading (Nash & Bowen, 2002).

Risk Factors

A central idea of risk factor theory is that many individual and contextual risk factors are associated with poor developmental outcomes or with the failure to achieve positive outcomes. Many developmental risk factors are not disorder specific, but rather may be related to multiple maladaptive outcomes. Given that single risk factors may predict multiple outcomes and that a great deal of overlap occurs between behavioral markers, interventions focusing on risk reduction of interacting risk factors may have direct effects on multiple outcomes (Coie et al., 1993). Because risk factors arise in diverse contexts within an ecological model, interventions addressing risks in a single context are unlikely to be sufficient to eliminate or significantly ameliorate problem behaviors (Rutter, 1982).

Protective Factors

Protective factors are variables that reduce the likelihood of maladaptive outcomes, given conditions of risk. Positive developmental outcomes are more likely when protective factors are present at multiple system levels (Nash & Bowen, 2002). Three contexts in which protective factors arise have been identified: (1) within child, (2) family, and (3) community (Kazdin, 1991; Rutter, 1985). The within-child context includes characteristics of the individual such as social-cognitive skills, temperamental characteristics, and social skills. The family context includes the child's interactions with the environment such as secure attachment and positive parent–child relationships. The community context includes attachment to prosocial peers and other adults.

Previous Research on Risk and Protective Factors

The term *risk factor* was first used by Stamler in 1958 and was initially applied to cardiovascular disease prevention (Stamler, 1978). Given its origins in the medical literature, specifically in the discipline of epidemiology, analyses revolved around odds-risk or relative-risk ratio predictors of dichotomous variables (e.g., sick or not sick) (Hennekens & Buring, 1987). The risk-factor model was originally directed at identifying psychological, social, and biological factors related to the emergence of a health problem (Arnold, Kuller, & Greenlick, 1981). Risk factors have been used extensively to depict increased risk for drug abuse using correlational research (Bukowski, 1991). Risk factors and protective factors are increasingly linked with notions of resilience in theoretical and practice literature in the field of psychology, social work, education, and public health. Risk and protection theory has emerged as the dominant theoretical framework in the field of prevention research

At least four divergent approaches to understanding risk and protective factors have been suggested in the literature (Stouthamer-Loeber et al., 1993). First, some researchers suggest that variables are uniquely risk or protective related. A single variable is thus best considered as contributing to an increased risk or an increase in protection from the development of problematic outcomes (Rae-Grant, Thomas, Offord, & Boyle, 1989). Second, other researchers treat protective and risk factors as opposite extremes of the same single variable (Kandel et al., 1988; White, Moffit, & Silva, 1989). Most researchers have favored dichotomization on the risk side of variables; therefore, the distribution extant knowledge base is tilted toward knowledge about risks rather than protective factors. Third, the protective and risk tails of the variable distribution are not necessarily mirror images of each other, but may differ in magnitude of relationship to outcomes. The relationship is therefore best described as nonlinear. Fourth, protective factors are processes that interact with risk factors in reducing the probability of reducing negative outcomes (Rutter, 1985).

Risk and protective factors have also been discussed in relation to resilience research (Stouthamer-Loeber et al., 1993). Risk and protective factors can be statistically evaluated using bivariate correlations between a variable and an outcome, whether that outcome is measured dichotomously (risk or not at risk) or on a continuous scale of measurement. Resilience must be statistically evaluated using a multivariate approach.

Implications of Identifying Risk and Protective Factors

If risk and protective factors can be distinguished and quantified, the effects of intervention, theoretically, can be maximized. The risk and protective factors can be used to identify individuals considered to be at risk for problem behaviors in order to initiate preventive interventions. Risk and protective factors can also be targets of intervention. Interventions are likely to be more effective if risk and protective factors can be identified and successfully used to influence variables that are strongly related to targeted outcomes (Fraser & Galinsky, 1997). Although research indicates that sociological factors (e.g., low socioeconomic status) are powerful predictors of developmental outcomes, many of these variables are not amenable to change by cognitive or behavioral interventions. It is true, however, that behavioral difficulties arise within the ecological context of low socioeconomic status that may moderate or mediate the effects of interventions (Reid, 1993).

Bukowski (1991) suggested that the onset of maladaptive behavior is determined by the interaction between risk factors that predispose an individual to the development of DBDs and protective factors that predispose an individual to the development of positive outcomes, thereby buffering individuals against the development of severe DBDs. Protective factors exert both a direct positive influence on behavior and a moderating influence on the relation between risk factors and behavior (Jessor, Van Den Bos, Vanderryn, Costa, & Turbin, 1995). Risk and protection theory argues that risk and protective factors arise in multiple contexts and that complex behavioral problems do not stem from a single causal variable or a fixed set of specific precursors (Reid, 1993).

Multiple pathways can be taken to the development of DBDs and various risk and protective influences can be identified.

"Mega-Analysis" of Risk and Protective Factors

Crews et al. (2007) conducted a "mega" analysis of 18 meta-analyses of risk and protective factors related to the development of externalizing behavior disorders (conduct disorder, oppositional defiant disorder, ADHD) for children and adolescents 0 to 18 years of age. More than 500 primary studies were analyzed, involving over 30,000 subjects.

All effect sizes were reported in terms of Pearson r so as to have a standard unit of effect size. Meta-analyses reported in terms of Cohen's d were transformed into Pearson r using the formula reported by Rosenthal, Rosnow, and Rubin (2000). The desirable or problematic nature of an outcome and the direction of the relationship between and a factor of interest distinguished risk from protection. *Protection* implies either a positive relationship with a desired outcome or a negative relationship with a problematic outcome. *Risk* implies a positive relationship with a negative outcome or a negative relationship with a desirable outcome. The magnitude of the relationship is an indicator of the relative importance of a particular risk or protective factor.

Table 8.1 shows that the risk factors most highly correlated with externalizing behavior problems are lack of bonding to school ($r = .86$), having delinquent peers ($r = .49$), and having an internalizing comorbid disorder ($r = .47$). Five risk factors showed identical correlations with externalizing behavior problems ($r = .41$) and included prior history of antisocial behavior, low academic achievement, nonsupportive home environments, corporal punishment by parents, and controversial sociometric status. Interestingly, several risk factors showed virtually no association with externalizing behavior problems such as low socioeconomic status, substance abuse, poor social skills, racial minority status, and being male (median $r = .06$).

Table 8.2 depicts the protective factors associated with externalizing behavior problems. Age at first juvenile justice commitment ($r = .34$), adequate academic performance ($r = .33$), and positive play activities with peers ($r = .26$) were the three highest protective factors for externalizing behavioral difficulties. Being popular with peers, having a high IQ, and having high socioeconomic status did not operate as substantial protective factors for externalizing behavior problems (median $r = .14$).

The breadth of contexts in which risk and protective factors arise

TABLE 8.1. Risk Factors Correlated with Externalizing Disorders

Risk factor	Median Z^r	Median r
Lack of bonding to school	1.29	.86
Delinquent peers	0.53	.49
Internalizing comorbidity	0.50	.47
Prior antisocial behavior	0.44	.41
Low academic achievement/IQ	0.44	.41
Nonsupportive home environment	0.44	.41
Corporal punishment by parents	0.44	.41
Controversial sociometric status	0.44	.41
Violent video games/media violence	0.30	.29
Rejected sociometric status	0.25	.25
Victim of abuse	0.14	.14
Substance abuse	0.14	.14
Poor social skills	0.14	.14
Low socioeconomic status	0.12	.12
Criminal commitment	0.12	.12
Nonsevere psychopathology	0.12	.12
Neglected sociometric status	0.10	.10
Male	0.10	.10
Racial minority	0.03	.03

suggests that interventions targeting factors beyond the individual student may be more effective than focusing solely on building students' strengths or remediating areas of risk. This "mega" analysis focused on problematic outcomes; it defined risk factors as exhibiting a negative relationship with problematic outcomes. An important consideration was to extend the overall scope of research to include risk factors defined as exhibiting a negative relationship with desirable outcomes and protective factors that exhibit a positive relationship with desirable outcomes.

Simply examining the number of effect sizes having positive correlation with problematic outcomes leads to the conclusion that dealing with risk factors should dominate the field of intervention, but that conclusion may be unwarranted. Many, if not most, behavior support plans begin with problem behaviors and then proceed to specify and address risk factor antecedents of those problem behaviors (Sugai & Horner, 1999). Protective factors are frequently ignored in behavior support

TABLE 8.2. Protective Factors with Externalizing Disorders

Protective factor	Median Z^r	Median r
Age at first commitment	0.23	.34
Adequate academic performance	0.35	.33
Play activities	0.34	.26
Corporal punishment	0.27	.24
Intact family structure	0.24	.24
Popular sociometric status	0.18	.18
High IQ	0.14	.14
Neglected sociometric status	0.10	.10
High socioeconomic status	0.10	.10

planning. The failure to utilize these preexisting protective factors may be one factor that unnecessarily complicates the planning process for behavior support.

Addressing these protective factors may substantially and positively affect future behavior. For example, positive play activities with peers and academic achievement were significantly correlated with positive outcomes for externalizing behavior problems. These protective factors appear to be natural targets of focus in school settings to moderate the effects of externalizing behavior problems.

Evidence-Based Primary Prevention Interventions

Positive Behavioral Interventions and Supports

Positive behavioral interventions and supports (PBIS) refers to the systematic application of effective instructional and behavioral supports designed to attain desirable social and learning outcomes by *preventing* problem behaviors (Sugai & Horner, 2008). PBIS is based on three fundamental principles that facilitate student success: (1) promoting evidence-based practices, (2) supporting change in discipline practices, and (3) building local capacity to sustain effective practices over time. When PBIS is embraced and used across the entire school, it is referred to as schoolwide positive behavioral interventions and supports (SWPBIS). SWPBIS is a systems approach to creating the social culture and behavioral supports required for all children in a school to attain both social and academic success that can be achieved through a variety of strategies (Horner et al., 2009).

SWPBIS is currently being implemented in more than 9,000 schools within the United States and demonstrates positive effects on student behavior and the school climate (Horner et al., 2009; Sugai & Horner, 2008). SWPBIS involves four central elements: (1) focus on student outcomes relative to desired changes in student academic and social behavior, (2) use of research-validated practices to support student behavior, (3) using a systems approach to support staff behavior, and (4) use of data-based decision making to evaluate the effects of the SWPBIS program. Several features that distinguish SWPBIS from traditional approaches to student discipline in schools include:

- Emphasis on *preventing* problem behaviors.
- Active instruction of behavioral skills.
- Specifying a continuum of consequences for problem behaviors.
- Using a systematic approach to supporting effective behavioral interventions in the school.
- Using data to guide decisions regarding the integrity and effectiveness of interventions being implemented.

SWPBIS and the RTI approach are both based on a multi-tiered model of prevention and intervention. My focus in this chapter is on Tier 1, or primary prevention, strategies for DBDs using the SWPBIS model. Tier 1 practices concentrate on supporting academic success and desirable behavior and in preventing initial occurrence of academic failure and problem behavior. These interventions apply to *all students* and are used by all staff in the school setting. Some examples of Tier 1 interventions include the use of effective, evidence-based instructional practices, establishing and teaching behavioral expectations to all students, modifying environmental arrangements by altering the physical or interactional features of locations where problem behavior is most likely to occur, and by applying positive consequences to increase desired behavior and negative consequences to decrease undesirable behavior. Tier 1 practices also develop linkages between the school and community and the students' homes.

Implementation of SWPBIS

Concerns regarding school safety with regard to student behavior set the occasion for researchers and practitioners to address these behaviors in terms of preventive practices. In the SWPBIS approach, schools are considered to be the host environment that adopts and utilizes effective, evidence-based practices. Outcomes of these practices are measured by analyzing data such as office discipline referral (ODR) rates, suspensions and expulsions, behavior rating scales or checklists, and the use of state-and/or districtwide high-stakes test scores.

An extremely important aspect of SWPBIS implementation is the formation of a leadership team whose purpose is to guide and oversee implementation efforts in the school. This team functions as the representative of various stakeholders within the school and community. Principals are seen as essential team members because of their authority in decision making, and parents are also viewed as essential team members. It is recommended that the team meet at least monthly and use a problem-solving approach in dealing with behavioral issues in the school.

Tier 1 Primary Prevention

The goal of Tier 1 primary prevention interventions is to support appropriate behaviors of all students by designing safe and supportive school environments and to prevent the onset of academic and social failure among all students. The fundamental criteria for Tier 1 interventions are that they are evidence based, possess high quality, and can be applied to all students, by all school personnel, using available school resources. Associated outcomes of this goal are higher academic achievement for all students and fewer students needing support at the Tier 2 (secondary prevention) and Tier 3 (tertiary prevention) levels.

Tier 1 interventions are applied throughout the entire school in both classroom and nonclassroom settings (e.g., hallways, cafeteria, and common areas of the school). Some helpful Tier 1 strategies can be summarized as follows:

- Establishing and teaching behavioral expectations to all students.
- Making environment arrangements and providing active supervision.
- Applying consequences to encourage desirable behavior and to decrease undesirable behavior.
- Developing school and community linkages.
- Developing school and home linkages.

There is a plethora of evidence for many of the Tier 1 intervention strategies discussed in this chapter. Research supports the use of instructional practices that increase academic engaged time, produce high rates of correct academic responding, and increase the academic content covered (Darch & Kame'enui, 2004; Landrum, Tankersley, & Kauffman, 2003; Rosenshine, 2008; Yell, 2009). In terms of behavior, several strategies for increasing desirable behavior and preventing or reducing undesirable behavior have received empirical support. These strategies include structuring the environment, clarifying behavioral expectations, providing active supervision, using contingent praise, giving precision requests, and using group-oriented contingencies (to be discussed later in this chapter) (Alberto & Troutman, 2009; Kerr & Nelson, 2010; Yell, Meadows, Drasgow, & Shriner, 2009).

While this evidence base is encouraging, the integrity and effectiveness of SWPBIS when implemented in settings without external consultants and funding is uncertain. It appears that the core features of SWPBIS must include obtaining administrative and district support, systematically rewarding students and staff, securing staff buy-in prior to implementation, using data-based decision making, encouraging cooperative teamwork, and including families and the community in implementation efforts (Johns, Patrick, & Rutherford, 2008; McKevitt & Braaksma, 2008).

The Good Behavior Game: A Universal Behavioral Vaccine

A vaccine is a simple, scientifically proven practice that is widely used to reduce morbidity and mortality (Embry, 2002). Prior to 1955, polio was a highly feared crippling disease that affected both children and adults. In 1949, close to 40,000 cases of polio were reported in the United States, one for every 3,775 people (Oshinsky, 2005). Victims of polio ranged from unknown children to the President of the United States (Franklin D. Roosevelt). Jonas Salk headed the Salk Vaccine Trials of 1954, in which 221,998 individuals were vaccinated with the Salk vaccine and compared to 200,725 individuals who received a placebo vaccination. The results were staggering. Of the 221,998 individuals who were vaccinated, only 38 developed polio (0.01%) compared to 115 cases in the placebo condition (0.05%). Today, polio vaccinations have virtually eliminated the prevalence of polio worldwide.

In terms of behavior problems, substance abuse, ADHD, oppositional defiant disorder, antisocial behavior, depression, and teen suicide have adversely affected the lives our children and youth. Could we develop a *behavioral vaccine* similar to the Salk vaccine to reduce the prevalence of these myriad behavior problems? Embry (2002) defined a behavioral vaccine as a simple procedure that can dramatically reduce or eliminate adverse outcomes. Unlike many primary prevention programs that are implemented over a period of time, a behavioral vaccine is used routinely in daily life. Behavioral vaccines are simple actions that produce large results, are inexpensive, and do not require a high level of expertise.

Behavioral vaccines share many common elements found in the risk and protective factors literature (see Crews et al., 2007). Behavioral vaccines and the risk/protection literature are based on empirical data. Behavioral vaccines can produce substantial benefits for individuals, classrooms, schools, families, and communities. Are there behavioral vaccines that could be used to address multiproblem behavior?

The Good Behavior Game (GBG) is based on the use of group-oriented contingencies that consist of delivering a reinforcer contingent on the behavior of a group (Cooper et al., 2007; Litow & Pumroy, 1975). Target behaviors, reinforcers, and criteria for reinforcement are common across the group. Group contingencies are more efficient and simpler to implement than individual contingencies and have been shown to be equally effective (Gresham & Gresham, 1982; Stage & Quiroz, 1997; Tingstrom, Sterling-Turner, & Wilczynski, 2006).

The GBG is one of the most well-known and empirically supported interventions using group contingencies to reduce disruptive behavior. The first published study using the GBG was conducted by Barrish, Saunders, and Wolf (1969), using a multiple baseline design in a fourth-grade classroom that had high rates of disruptive behavior. The GBG was played every day during the math instructional period with the class divided into two teams. One or both teams could earn privileges (e.g., free time, victory tags, being first in the lunch line) by having the lowest number of marks for disruptive behavior. Teams with fewer than 20 marks for the week could earn additional special privileges at the end of the week. The rate of disruptive behavior decreased from 90% of the intervals observed to about 10% of the intervals during math.

The effects of the GBG on disruptive behavior have been replicated and the components of the intervention have been analyzed (see meta-analysis by Tingstrom et al., 2006). A randomized controlled trial of the GBG was conducted in the Baltimore Prevention Project using 864 first-grade children in 19 public schools (Kellam, Mayer, Rebok, & Hawkins, 1998). Results indicated that the GBG reduced the aggressive behavior in students who began the year with high aggressive ratings, suggesting that it is a viable behavioral vaccine. The GBG also reduced peer ratings of aggressive behavior and increased students' on-task behavior in the classroom.

Six years later, Kellam et al. (1998) found that the effects of the GBG continued into the sixth grade, with aggressive behavior decreasing over 30% then. Boys were less likely to initiate smoking (a 50% reduction) in the early teens, and teacher ratings showed that boys were better behaved than controls. Overall, it appears that the GBG functions as a powerful long-term behavioral vaccine for aggressive and disruptive behavior.

Embry (2002) reviewed the literature on the GBG and found the following:

- The GBG showed a 5% reduction in special education placement, resulting in a cost savings of $2–4 million per year.
- The GBG reduced involvement with corrections by 2%, resulting in a savings of $3–10 million per year by reducing juvenile arrests for serious drug offenses.
- The GBG created a 4% reduction in lifetime prevalence of tobacco use that could save millions of dollars in medical costs associated with tobacco-related diseases.

These savings sum to approximately $15–20 million per year over time. The cost of implementing the GBG is estimated to be about $200 per child. If the GBG was implemented with 5,000 children, then the cost–benefit ratio would be about $15–20 million to $1 million.

The notion of behavioral vaccines that are defined as simple actions that can be repeated on a daily basis with positive behavioral benefits is entirely possible. A behavioral vaccine for DBDs should have a strong history of efficacy and effectiveness, be adaptable to different situations and circumstances, and be relatively inexpensive. The GBG is a powerful candidate for a behavioral vaccine based on its simplicity and multiple replications of positive outcomes in short- and long-term effectiveness studies.

Concluding Remarks

The developmental trajectory and prognosis of children having DBDs early in life is bleak. Longitudinal studies have shown that these behavior problems that are evident in the preschool years have considerable stability over time and continue to be problematic through the elementary school years and adolescence (Dunlap & Fox, 2014). In addition, other longitudinal studies have shown that early aggression has a predictive relationship to low academic achievement (see Hinshaw, 1992), with many of these children being placed into special education. Studies have also shown that aggressive and oppositional behavior patterns in preschool are among the best predictors of juvenile delinquency, gang membership, and criminal activity in adulthood (Dishion & Stormshak, 2007; Reid, 1993).

Universal or primary prevention practices are essential in addressing these social behavioral challenges early in life. Universal interventions can be delivered broadly by multiple programs, treatment agents, and within multiple settings. The overwhelming majority of children (>80%) will respond adequately to Tier 1 strategies. Intervention programs that help parents learn parenting skills, approaches to control disruptive behavior in schools, and community-based programs all can be effective universal intervention strategies.

This chapter focused on various risk and protective factors that influence the development of DBDs. By targeting these risk and protective factors, more effective interventions can be developed and implemented. This chapter highlighted two well-established, cost-effective, and evidence-based school interventions: SWPBIS and the Good Behavior Game. SWPBIS reduces ODRs, decreases referrals to special education, and dramatically reduces school suspensions and expulsions. It also creates an increased positive bonding to school that is the overall best predictor of an externalizing behavior pattern (see Crews et al., 2007). The Good Behavior Game, on the other hand, functions as a *behavioral vaccine* inoculating children from the long-term negative effects of aggressive and oppositional behaviors. Well-established, empirically based primary prevention strategies are an essential practice in the prevention or moderation of DBDs.

Chapter Summary Points

- The goal of primary prevention efforts is to *prevent harm* rather than to reverse or reduce harm.

- Effective primary prevention efforts often are based in schools and many of these efforts involve parents as part of the intervention team.

- Prevention is based on knowledge or risk and protective factors that are used to prevent negative outcomes and to promote positive outcomes.

- Risk factors reside in the physical environment and within the individual and are manifested when individuals respond to the demands of the environment.

- The most informative way of conceptualizing primary prevention outcomes is from a social-ecological perspective that is based on the notion of person–environment fit (P-E fit).

- A P-E fit or match occurs when the demands of the environment are consistent with the abilities, skills, resources, and motivations of the individual.

- A single risk factor is not likely to be responsible for any given behavior pattern, nor is any single protective factor likely to prevent the development of problematic behavior.

- Typically, there is a nonlinear relationship between risk factors and outcomes that become more predictive as risk factors accumulate over time.

- A central idea of risk factor theory is that a range of individual and contextual risk factors are associated with poor developmental outcomes or with the failure to achieve positive outcomes.

- Protective factors are variables that reduce the likelihood of maladaptive outcomes, given conditions of risk.

- Research suggests that many sociological factors (e.g., low socioeconomic status) are associated with poor developmental outcomes, but many of these variables are not amenable to change by cognitive or behavioral interventions.

- Risk and protection theory suggests that risk and protective factors arise in multiple contexts and that complex behavior problems do not stem from a single causal or fixed set of specific precursors.

- The three risk factors showing the highest correlations with an externalizing behavior pattern are lack of bonding to school, having delinquent peers, and having a comorbid internalizing disorder.

- Five risk factors showed identical moderate correlations with externalizing behavior pattern (prior history of antisocial behavior, low academic achievement/IQ, nonsupportive home environment, corporal punishment by parents, and controversial sociometric status).

- Several risk factors show virtually no relationship to externalizing behavior (low socioeconomic status, substance abuse, poor social skills, racial minority status, and being male).

- Protective factors show lower correlations with outcomes than risk factors with age at first juvenile commitment, adequate academic performance, and positive play activities with peers showing the highest correlations.

- Positive behavioral interventions and supports (PBIS) refers to the systematic application of effective instructional and behavioral supports designed to attain desirable social and learning outcomes by preventing problem behaviors.

- When PBIS is embraced and used across an entire school, it is known as schoolwide positive behavioral interventions and supports or SWPBIS.

- SWPBIS an be characterized by: (1) an emphasis on prevention of problem behaviors, (2) active instruction of behavioral skills, (3) specification of a continuum of consequences for problem behaviors, (4) use of a systematic approach to supporting effective behavioral interventions, and (5) use of data to guide decisions regarding the integrity and effectiveness of interventions.

- There is a plethora of empirical research to support the use of interventions developed within the context of SWPBIS to increase academic engaged time, improve academic performance, decrease problem behaviors, and reduce school suspensions and expulsions.

- The Good Behavior Game is based on the use of an interdependent group contingency that consists of delivering a reinforcer contingent on the behavior of a group.

- The Good Behavior Game has a plethora of research supporting its use in elementary, middle school, and high school settings and functions as a *behavioral vaccine* inoculating students from the long-term negative effects of aggressive and oppositional behaviors.

Replacement Behavior Training Strategies

An important consideration in the conceptualization of interventions for DBDs is the contribution of *competing problem behaviors* prevent these individuals from acquiring and performing prosocial behaviors. Children and youth with conduct problems and oppositional defiant problems display high rates of competing problem behaviors such as aggression, noncompliance, defiance, and impulsivity that effectively compete with the development of prosocial behavior patterns. For example, a child with a history of noncompliance, coercive interactions, and impulsivity may *never* learn prosocial behavior alternatives such as sharing, cooperation, and self-control because of the absence of opportunities to learn these behaviors (Eddy, Reid, & Curry, 2002).

As children make the transition from the home to day care, preschool, and school environments, they are systematically exposed to many peers. Peer relationships are important to the young child, and these relationships assume increasing importance as they grow older. This transition provides children's first peer culture, and those who fail to acquire social skills and a rule-following pattern at home are likely to exhibit deficits in their social competence and display aggressiveness toward peers (Snyder, 2002). This often results in these children being disliked and socially rejected by peers, which is established as early as the preschool years and continues throughout their school careers (Dishion, 1990). Due to their noncompliance, lack of social skills, poor academic performance, and aggressiveness, teachers and other nonfamilial adults also tend to view these children in a negative light.

Peer dislike, rejection, academic deficits, and rejection by teachers are early social failures that increase children's risk for a number of concurrent and later forms of social and personal maladjustment such as antisocial behavior, early drug use, and depression (Dishion, 1990; Kupersmidt & Patterson, 1991). Rejection by normative peers often leads to association with deviant peers, which, in turn, governs the metastasizing of peer rejection into multiple forms of later maladjustment (Dishion, Patterson, Stoolmiller, & Skinner, 1991).

The number of children found to have serious peer relationship problems can vary depending on the type of assessment procedures used. When elementary school students are asked to nominate their three best friends in their class, about 10% of class members are not named by anyone (Hymel & Asher, 1977). When using reciprocal peer nominations, this percentage is even higher, suggesting that these children have no friends at all among their classmates. The number of children having few or no friends in school is even higher in samples of those having conduct problems and oppositional defiant problems.

As I have discussed earlier, *coercion* and *negative reinforcement* are key processes by which peer dislike and rejection increase risk for the development of antisocial and oppositional defiant behavior patterns. The peer environment and the school classroom present a large number of aversive social events. A key developmental task children must accomplish in making the transition to school requires learning how to deal with disagreement, conflict, and competition in a way that promotes positive peer relationships and friendships.

Snyder (2002) presents data showing that antisocial children have great difficulty in accomplishing the above tasks. Comparisons of aggressive and nonaggressive children's observed social interactions with peers and teachers show that aggressive children are much more likely to initiate unprovoked verbal and physical aggression toward peers and to continue in aggression once they have initiated it. This behavior pattern conflicts with the establishment of constructive, cooperative peer relationships and results in peer dislike and rejection. In addition, aggressive children are much more likely to be *recipients* of peer-initiated verbal and physical aggression. Over time, aggressive children acquire a negative reputation among peers (i.e., reputational bias), and peer interactions between aggressive and nonaggressive children become organized around mutually contributed aversive behavior exchanges (Snyder, 2002).

Peer Rejection and Maladjustment

Much of the research that points to a predictive connection between peer rejection and psychosocial maladjustment outcomes has been based on archival data that were not originally designed to explore moderators or mediators of this relationship (Kupersmidt, Coie, & Dodge, 1990). We have few empirical data to establish whether being rejected by one's peers causes or mediates the development of DBDs. Several plausible hypotheses can be stated regarding the role of peer rejection in the development of DBDs. One hypothesis is that peer rejection is a marker or predictor variable indicating that risk has resulted from a more fundamental or basic factor. An example of this might be that social skills deficits (e.g., lack of cooperative behavior, lack of self-control, and poor social problem solving) lead to peer rejection, and these same deficits account for the development of DBDs later in a child's life. This suggests that peer rejection moderates (correlates) with the development of DBDs, but does not mediate (cause) onset.

A second hypothesis suggests that the experience of being accepted by peers may play a moderating role in the development of DBDs. As such, social support from peers might operate as a protective factor that buffers a child from the development of DBDs by enhancing self-efficacy and providing opportunities for the acquisition of prosocial behaviors from the peer group. In contrast, a vulnerable child might experience the additional stress of social isolation (Kupersmidt et al., 1990). A third hypothesis might be that the experience of peer rejection is causally related to the development of DBDs. This suggests two developmental trajectories that may add clarity to this hypothesis.

One possibility is that peer acceptance exposes the child to opportunities for prosocial interaction in the peer group, thereby providing the child with peers who promote social skills development. Children who are rejected by peers would be deprived of these beneficial experiences and would fail to develop appropriate social skills, leading to the development of DBDs. A second developmental trajectory suggests that being rejected by peers leads to internal reactions in the child that are associated with antisocial and oppositional/defiant outcomes. The child comes to feel personally inadequate, lonely, and shows anger/resentment that can lead to maladaptive outcomes (Coie, Dodge, & Coppotelli, 1982). Those children who turn against the peer group and who show anger and resentment toward its members are at heightened risk for developing DBDs.

The Role of Competing Problem Behaviors

As discussed in Chapter 1, a conceptually powerful learning principle, the matching law, states that the relative rates of any behavior will match the relative rate of reinforcement for that behavior (Herrnstein, 1961). Matching is studied experimentally in what are known as concurrent schedules of reinforcement, which are experimental arrangements involving two or more behaviors being reinforced according to two or more schedules of reinforcement that are available concurrently. In other words, the individual has the "choice" of which schedule of reinforcement he or she will respond to more frequently. The concept of matching predicts that the behavior, which is reinforced more frequently, will be performed at a higher rate. For example, if arguing with teachers or parents is reinforced every five times it occurs and staying calm when disagreeing with teachers or parents is reinforced every 20 times it occurs, then arguing will be performed *four times* more frequently than staying calm in disagreements.

Children and youth with DBDs have a choice between engaging in behaviors that coerce or harm others and engaging in prosocial forms of behavior. This "choice" depends directly on the relative rate of reinforcement that is concurrently available for each behavior. Based on the learning histories of children with DBDs, coercive, defiant behaviors typically receive reinforcement more frequently than prosocial behaviors, and therefore these behaviors will occur more frequently. In short, coercive and defiant behaviors have greater *utility* in generating reinforcement to an individual than prosocial behaviors (Snyder & Stoolmiller, 2002).

Maag (2005) has suggested that a potentially effective way of decreasing competing problem behaviors is to teach *positive replacement behaviors*, or what has been called replacement behavior training (RBT). RBT is based on the matching law described above. The goal of RBT is to identify a prosocial behavior that will result in more frequent reinforcement relative to a competing problem behavior. Table 9.1 shows potential replacement behaviors for competing problem behaviors. Conceptually, RBT depends on identifying *functionally equivalent behaviors*. Behaviors are considered to be functionally equivalent if they produce similar or greater amounts of reinforcement from the environment (Horner & Billingsley, 1988). Also, functional equivalence of behavior is based on the notion of *differential reinforcement of incompatible behaviors* (DRI), a procedure in which a behavior that is incompatible with the problem behavior is reinforced. Behaviors are considered incompatible if they *cannot* occur simultaneously. For example, arguing and calmly resolving conflicts cannot occur at the same time. A practitioner using DRI would increase the rate of reinforcement for a prosocial, incompatible behavior and decrease the rate

TABLE 9.1. Evidence-Based Social Skills Intervention Strategies

Promoting skill acquisition

1. Modeling
2. Coaching
3. Behavioral rehearsal
4. Social problem solving

Enhancing skill performance

1. Manipulation of antecedents
   a. Peer-mediated interventions
   b. Cuing or prompting
   c. Precorrection
   d. Choice
2. Manipulation of consequences
   a. Social praise
   b. Error correction
   c. Performance feedback
   d. Behavioral contracts
   e. Token/point systems
3. Removal of competing problem behaviors
   a. Differential reinforcement of incompatible behavior (DRI)
   b. Differential reinforcement of alternative behavior (DRA)
   c. Differential reinforcement of other behavior (DRO)
   d. Anger control training
   e. Self-instruction training
   f. Social problem solving

of reinforcement (i.e., adult negative attention) for the disruptive behavior alternative (Cooper et al., 2007).

Conceptualization of Positive Replacement Behaviors

Positive replacement behaviors can be conceptualized as socially skilled behaviors that compete with and replace disruptive behavior patterns based on the principle of matching. An important issue in the theoretical conceptualization of positive replacement behaviors is the distinction among the concepts of *social skills, social tasks,* and *social competence.* Social skills can be conceptualized as a specific class of behaviors that an individual displays in order to successfully complete a social task. Social tasks might include such things as peer group entry, having a conversation, making friends, or playing a game with peers. Social competence, in contrast, is an evaluative term based on the *judgments* of others (given certain criteria) that an individual has successfully performed a social task. Key social agents (e.g., peers, teachers, parents) make these judg-ments based on numerous social interactions with individuals occurring within natural environments (e.g., school, home, community). Given this conceptualization, social skills are specific behaviors exhibited in specific situations that lead to judgments by others that these behaviors are competent or incompetent in accomplishing social tasks (Gresham & Elliott, 2014).

Competence does not necessarily imply *exceptional* performance; it only indicates that a social performance was adequate (McFall, 1982). Gresham (1986) suggested that evaluations of competence should be based on three criteria: (1) relevant judgments about an individual's social behavior (e.g., peers, teachers, parents); (2) evaluations of social competence relative to explicit established criteria (e.g., number of steps successfully performed in the completion of a social task); and (3) social behavioral performances relative to a normative standard (e.g., scores on norm-referenced social skills rating scales). It is important to note that social behaviors cannot be considered "socially skilled" apart from their impact on judgments of social agents in a social environment or context.

Social Skills as Academic Enablers

Researchers have documented meaningful and predictive relation-ships between children's social behaviors and their long-term academic achievement (DiPerma & Elliott, 2002; Malecki & Elliott, 2002; Wen-tzel, 2009). It has been documented that children who have positive social interactions and relationships with their peers are more academi-cally engaged and have higher levels of academic achievement (Went-zel, 2009). The notion of *academic enablers* evolved from the work of researchers who explored the relationship between students' nonaca-demic behaviors (e.g., social skills and motivation) and their academic achievement (Gresham & Elliott, 2008; Wentzel, 2005, 2009; Wentzel & Watkins, 2002).

Researchers often make a distinction between academic skills and academic enablers. Academic skills are viewed as the basic and complex skills that are the primary focus of academic instruction. In contrast, academic enablers are the attitudes and behaviors that allow students to participate in and ultimately benefit from academic instruction in the classroom. Research using the Academic Competence Evaluation Scales (ACES; DiPerma & Elliott, 2000) showed that academic enablers were moderately related to students' academic achievement as measured by standardized achievement tests (*median r* = .50). In a major longitudinal study, Capara and colleagues found that teacher ratings of prosocial behavior in third grade were *better* predictors of eighth-grade academic achievement than academic achievement in third grade (Caprara, Barbarnelli, Pastorelli, Bandura, & Zimbardo, 2000).

Most researchers have concluded that positive peer interactions promote displays of competent forms of social behavior that, in turn, prompt successful academic performance. Behaviors such as cooperation, following rules, and getting along with others are related to efficient classrooms and allow students to benefit from academic instruction (Gresham & Elliott, 2008; Walker, Irvin, Noell, & Singer, 1992). Displays of prosocial behavior patterns and restraints from disruptive and antisocial forms of behavior have been consistently and positively related to peer acceptance, achievement motivation, and academic success (Wentzel, 2009). Socially competent behavior provides the essential basis for learning that allows students to benefit from classroom instruction (DiPerma & Elliott, 2002; Elliott & Gresham, 2007; Wentzel & Looney, 2007).

Disruptive Behaviors as Academic Disablers

Whereas social skills function as academic enablers, it has been documented that disruptive problem behaviors interfere or compete with acquiring and performing both social and academic skills (Gresham & Elliott, 2008; Walker et al., 1992). In other words, these competing problem behaviors function as *academic disablers* in that they are associated with decreases in academic performance. Children with disruptive behavior patterns such as defiance, noncompliance, and aggression often have moderate to severe academic skill deficits that are reflected in below-average academic achievement (Coie & Jacobs, 1993; Hinshaw, 1992; Offord, Boyle, & Racine, 1989; Reid, 1993). It is unclear whether these academic disablers are primarily the correlates (moderators), causes (mediators), or consequences of academic underachievement, but there is little doubt that these behaviors contribute substantially to academic performance difficulties. As these children progress through their school careers, their academic deficits and achievement problems become even more severely affected (Walker et al., 2004).

Types of Social Skills Deficits

An important conceptual consideration in designing and delivering social skills interventions is distinguishing between different types of social skills deficits. Gresham (1981a) first distinguished between social skill *acquisition deficits* and *performance deficits*. Since that time, other researchers have supported this distinction (Elliott & Gresham, 2008; Gumpel, 2007; Maag, 2005; Walker et al., 2004). This distinction is important because different intervention approaches are called for in remediating these differing social skills deficits. They also dictate differing instructional contexts (e.g., general education classrooms vs. pullout groups).

Acquisition deficits, for example, result from a lack of knowledge about how to perform a social skill, an inability to fluently enact a sequence of social behaviors, or difficulty in knowing which social skills are appropriate in specific situations (Gresham & Elliott, 2014). Based on this conceptualization, acquisition deficits can result from deficits in social-cognitive abilities, difficulties in integrating fluent behavior patterns, and/or deficits in appropriate discrimination of social situations. Acquisition deficits can be characterized as "can't-do" problems because the child cannot perform the social skill under the most optimal conditions of motivation. Remediation of these types of deficits requires direct instruction of social skills in protected settings that will promote the acquisition of socially skilled behaviors.

Performance deficits can be conceptualized as the failure to perform a social skill at an acceptable level even though the child knows how to perform it. These types of social skills deficits can be thought of as "won't-do" problems because the child knows what to do, but chooses not to perform a particular social skill in given situations. These types of social skills deficits can best be thought of as *motivational* or performance problems rather than learning or acquisition problems. As such, remediation of these types of deficits requires the manipulating antecedents and consequences in naturalistic settings to increase the frequency of these behaviors.

Gresham and Elliott (1990) provided the first empirical attempt to quantify this distinction using the Social Skills Rating System (SSRS). Each SSRS item is rated on a 3-point frequency dimension (0—Never, 1—Sometimes, 2—Very Often) and a 3-point importance dimension (0—Not important, 1—Important, 2—Critical). Social skills considered acquisition deficits received a frequency rating of 0 (Never) and an importance rating of 1 (Important) or 2 (Critical), whereas performance deficits received a frequency rating of 1 (Sometimes) and an importance rating of 2 (Critical). This approach enjoyed widespread acceptance and use over the next 18 years until the revision of the SSRS to the Social Skills Improvement System Rating Scales (SSIS-RS) was published (Gresham & Elliott, 2008). Social skills on the SSIS-RS are rated on a

4-point frequency dimension (0—Never, 1—Rarely, 2—Sometimes, 3—Very Often) and a 3-point importance dimension (0—Not important, 1—Important, 2—Critical). Using this method, social skills acquisition deficits receive a frequency rating of 0 (Never) and an importance rating of 2 (Critical), whereas performance deficits receive a frequency rating of 1 (Rarely) and an importance rating of 2 (Critical).

More recently, Gresham and colleagues investigated the base rates of social skills acquisition and performance deficits using the national standardization data of the SSIS-RS (Gresham, Elliott, & Kettler, 2010). Participants were 4,550 children and adolescents ages 3–18 with equal numbers of males and females and matched to the U.S. population with regard to race/ethnicity, socioeconomic status, and geographic region. Using the SSIS-RS methodology for identifying social skills acquisition and performance deficits, the base rates for acquisition deficits across teacher, parent, and student raters was extremely low, with less than 1% of the standardization sample showing these types of deficits. In short, social skills acquisition deficits appear to be a rare phenomenon in a representative normative sample of children and adolescents.

Based on the results of the Gresham et al. (2010) study, an alternative method of operationalizing social skills acquisition deficits was developed by Gresham and Noell (1993). In this method, using only the SSIS-RS frequency ratings identifies social skills acquisition deficits. Individuals are identified as having social skills acquisition deficits if they receive a Total Social Skills standard score of 80 or lower (10th percentile or lower). The SSIS-RS contains 46 social skills items, and a standard score of 80 corresponds to a raw score of 59 indicating that overall, the child *rarely* exhibits most of the 46 rated social skills.

Based on the finding of extremely low base rates for social skills acquisition deficits in the general population, we concluded that the majority of children and youth with DBDs will have primarily social skills *performance deficits*. The few who have primarily social skills acquisition deficits will require social skills interventions using direct instruction techniques in small-group settings. The vast majority of children will benefit from RBT strategies based on the principle of differential reinforcement described earlier in this chapter.

Efficacy of Social Skills Interventions

The importance of social competence for children with or at risk for DBDs has been translated into various service delivery and instructional approaches to remediate deficits in social skills functioning. Social skills interventions (SSIs) are designed to remediate children's acquisition and performance deficits and to reduce or eliminate competing problem behaviors (Elliott & Gresham, 2008; Gresham, Sugai, & Horner, 2001). Between the late 1970s to early 1980s, SSIs targeted poorly accepted or rejected children and linked these interventions to the developmental literature, research on interpersonal dynamics, and the longitudinal course of poor peer relations (Bierman & Powers, 2009; Parker & Asher, 1987). By the early 1990s, SSIs were incorporated into epidemiologically based, long-term, multicomponent interventions targeting children with significant behavior problems such as conduct disorders and ADHD (Conduct Problems Prevention Group, 1992; MTA Cooperative Group, 1999). From 2000 to the present, SSI research has focused primarily on promoting behavior change in special needs populations and has often been embedded in disorder-specific, multicomponent intervention models. Despite these advances, a comprehensive framework that facilitates the identification of theoretical and methodological common ground across SSI studies is currently lacking, thereby creating a disparate empirical literature on social skills interventions (Bierman & Powers, 2009).

Literature Reviews of SSIs

There have been at least 12 SSI narrative literature reviews using both group and single-case experimental designs over the past 30 years (Ager & Cole, 1991; Coleman, Wheeler, & Webber, 1993; Gresham, 1981b, 1985; Hollinger, 1987; Landrum & Lloyd, 1992; Mathur & Rutherford, 1991; McIntosh, Vaughn, & Zaragoza, 1991; Olmeda & Kauffman, 2003; Schloss, Schloss, Wood, & Kiehl, 1986; Templeton, 1990; Zaragoza, Vaughn, & McIntosh, 1991). These narrative reviews reached the following conclusions:

- The most effective SSI strategies appear to be a combination of modeling, coaching, behavioral rehearsal, and procedures derived from applied behavior analysis.
- Evidence for cognitive-behavioral approaches (e.g., social problem solving and self-instruction) appear to produce weaker effects.
- The greatest weakness in the SSI literature was the absence of consistent and durable gains in prosocial behavior across situations, settings, and over time.

Nine meta-analyses of the SSI literature have been conducted since 1985 (Ang & Hughes, 2001; Beelman, Pfingsten, & Losel, 1994;

Chenier et al., 2011; Cook et al., 2008; Schneider, 1992; Schneider & Byrne, 1985). These meta-analyses focused on children and youth with behavioral difficulties and involved 464 studies and included over 28,000 children and youth 3 to 18 years of age. Based on these meta-analyses, there appears to be consistency in how the construct of social skills has been defined for research purposes. These meta-analyses suggest that the construct of social skills can be divided into three major categories: *social interaction, prosocial behavior,* and *social-cognitive skills.* Correlates of social skills fall into two major categories: problem behaviors (externalizing and internalizing) and academic achievement/ performance. These social skill categories and behavioral correlates are consistent with other work in the area of social skills conducted by other researchers (Caldarella & Merrell, 1997; Coie et al., 1982; Dodge, 1986; Gresham, 2010; Gresham & Elliott, 2008; Walker & McConnell, 1995; Walker et al., 1992).

Eight of the nine meta-analyses used group experimental designs that showed a grand mean effect size of $r = .29$ ($g = 0.60$), suggesting that about 65% of the participants in the SSI groups improved compared to only 35% of those individuals in control groups based on the binomial effect size display (BESD; Rosenthal & Rosnow, 1991). A recent meta-analysis by Godbold et al. (2010) of 34 studies published between 2000 and 2008 found that studies using random assignment to groups produced the largest effect size ($g = 0.67$) compared to studies not using random assignment (quasi-experimental designs) ($g = 0.16$). In short, better-controlled studies with high internal validity appear to produce the largest effect sizes, with the randomized studies showing that 82% of children receiving SSI improve compared to only 58% of children in the nonrandomized studies using the BESD.

The single-case design meta-analysis by Chenier et al. (2011) of 40 studies showed a large overall effect size ($g = 3.06$), with effect sizes varying by type of social skills intervention procedures. Specific SSI procedures ranged from 2.17 (reinforcement-based procedures) to 3.94 (social stories). The largest effect sizes were observed for children with autism spectrum disorders ($g = 4.04$) and the smallest effect sizes for children with disruptive behavior disorders ($g = 2.31$).

Summary

Both narrative and meta-analytic reviews of the SSI literature over the past 30 years suggest that it is an efficacious intervention for children and youth with social-behavioral difficulties. Quantitative reviews of this literature suggests that approximately two-thirds of children and youth receiving SSI improved compared to only one-third of individuals in control groups. This estimate is substantially higher in randomized SSIs than in nonrandomized, quasi-experimental deign studies. Depending on the degree of internal validity, SSI studies produce medium to large effect size estimates using conventional standards for interpreting effect sizes (Cohen, 1988).

It should be noted that all of the above studies in these meta-analyses should be considered Tier 2, or selected intervention, studies. No studies in the above syntheses could be considered Tier 1, or universal interventions, and none of the studies could be considered Tier 3, or intensive interventions.

As noted earlier, SSIs produce moderate to large effect sizes depending on the degree of internal validity in the experimental design using conventional standards for effect sizes. The nine meta-analyses indicate that about two-thirds of children receiving SSIs will improve. As mentioned earlier, most of the studies in these meta-analyses should be considered Tier 2 or selected interventions because they are typically delivered to at-risk samples on an individual or small-group basis. However, we think this is a limitation in the SSI literature, as universal intervention approaches (1) can have a positive impact on classroom ecology and (2) provide an important foundation for implementing Tier 2 interventions. The following section reviews three Tier 1 SSI intervention programs that have varying levels of empirical support.

Tier 1 (Universal) Interventions

Over the past decade, a number of Tier 1 social skills programs have begun to emerge, with the primary goal of promoting positive social behavior in school settings. Most of these programs have a strong theoretical evidence base and include intervention strategies and tactics based on empirical evidence. A smaller number of these Tier 1 intervention programs have yet to be empirically tested using strong experimental designs. These universal intervention programs include (1) Promoting Alternative Thinking Strategies (PATHS; Kusche & Greenberg, 1994), (2) the Incredible Years (Webster-Stratton & Hancock, 1998), and (3) the Social Skills Improvement System Classwide Intervention Program (SSIS-CIP; Elliott & Gresham, 2007). In this chapter, I will restrict discussion to the two school-based universal intervention programs: PATHS and SSIS-CIP.

Promoting Alternative Thinking Strategies

The PATHS curriculum (Kusche & Greenberg, 1994) is designed for children in grades 3–12 and promotes emotional/social competency and reduces aggressive and other behavior problems. PATHS is based on an ABCD model (affective, behavior, cognitive, and dynamic). The curriculum is delivered in 36 to 52 lessons over about 22 weeks, depending on the grade level. It covers three major conceptual domains: *self-control, feelings and relationships,* and *social problem solving.*

PATHS has been evaluated in three randomized controlled trials across grades 1–6. Achieved outcomes were improved understanding of social problems, generating alternative solutions to social problems, and violence reduction. The average effect size across these three studies was $d = 0.40$. This effect size indicates that about 60% children receiving the curriculum will improve and 40% will not improve using the binomial effect size display (BESD).

Social Skills Improvement System Classwide Intervention Program

The SSIS-CP (Elliott & Gresham, 2007) is designed to teach the following 10 social skills:

1. Listening to others
2. Following directions
3. Following classroom rules
4. Ignoring peer distractions
5. Asking for help
6. Taking turns in conversations
7. Cooperating with others
8. Controlling temper in conflict situations
9. Acting responsibly with others
10. Showing kindness to others

These skills were chosen on the basis of research conducted with teachers who rated them as the most critical to classroom success from preschool to early adolescence (Gresham & Elliott, 2008). The general education teacher teaches the SSIS-CIP skills with support provided by a behavioral coach who helps with program implementation and trouble-shooting. Appendix 9.1 contains scripted lessons for one of the skills (staying calm with others) to illustrate the instructional process. Similar scripts are provided in the SSIS-CIP program for the other nine skills.

Three versions of the SSIS-CIP accommodate different developmental levels—preschool (ages 3–5), early elementary (grades 1–3), and upper elementary (grades 4–5)—in teaching these critical skills. The content of the SSIS-CIP units at each of these developmental levels focuses on helping students acquire and apply the same 10 social skills. However, the program content at each level was customized to accommodate (1) developmental differences in the amount of required reading, (2) the ages of the social models used in the video vignettes, and (3) the nature of interactions students are expected to engage in when applying the social skills.

The SSIS-CIP skill units are supported with student booklets, video vignettes, and several other resources to promote student and parent involvement. Each of the units is taught across three 20- to 25-minute lessons per week for about 10 weeks, for a total of 30 lessons. Each lesson follows a six-phase instructional model: *tell* (coaching), *show* (modeling), *do* (role playing), *practice* (behavioral rehearsal), *monitor progress* (feedback), and *generalize* (application in multiple settings). An additional 2 weeks are built into the SSIS-CIP program in order to ensure that all skills are mastered to the maximum extent possible. The teacher's program guide instructs teachers in how to review their classwide progress monitoring data and to identify priority skills that need reteaching. The entire SSIS-CIP program takes about 12 weeks to complete. The teacher's guide provides detailed plans for each lesson, including instructional objectives, suggested instructional scripts (detailed use of video vignettes and integration of student activity booklets), and take-home activities for students.

The SSIS-CIP was evaluated via an Institute of Educational Sciences research grant directed by Gresham (2008–2011). In the first year of the program, 450 students in 22 classrooms were exposed to the SSIS-CIP. At the conclusion of the program, classroom teachers rated students in their classrooms on the Performance Screening Guide (PSG), a criterion-referenced measure on which students' prosocial behavior is rated on a 5-point Likert scale (1=Very limited to 5=Excellent). After receiving the SSIS-CIP, approximately 87% of students responded adequately to the program as measured by the PSG. The 13% of students who did not respond adequately to the program were given a more intense, Tier 2 (selected) intervention program (to be described later).

In summary, both the PATHS and the SSIS-CIP show promise for improving students' prosocial behaviors as evidenced by observed changes in social skills and reductions in problem behaviors. The PATHS and SSIS-CIP are based on effective intervention components identified in the empirical literature and represent the next generation of widely used and commercially available social skills intervention programs with a strong theoretical and empirical evidence base.

Tier 2 (Selected) Interventions

Several randomized controlled trials (RCTs) have demonstrated the efficacy of selected Tier 2 social skills interventions in changing peer relations and social competence. One of the first of these studies to use a randomized controlled group comparison approach to evaluate the impact of a *coaching intervention* on sociometric status was conducted by Oden and Asher (1977). Relative to a peer play condition and a no-treatment control condition, unaccepted third- and fourth-grade children who received five coaching sessions showed significant gains in "play with" sociometric ratings at posttreatment. Following this initial study, several other RCT studies used social skills training to enhance the prosocial behavior and peer acceptance of children selected on the basis of low peer acceptance scores. Gresham and Nagle (1980) used an RCT in which they compared the impact of social skills training components (e.g., coaching only, modeling only, and coaching + modeling). LaGreca and Santogrossi (1980) conducted an RCT in which they varied the timing of coaching sessions using longer sessions after school.

Generally speaking, the results of these studies were promising but the results were mixed. Some studies produced significant improvements in peer ratings (Gresham & Nagle, 1980; Oden & Asher, 1977), but some did not (LaGreca & Santogrossi, 1980). Most demonstrated some behavior changes (Gresham & Nagle, 1980; LaGreca & Santogrossi, 1980), but some did not (Oden & Asher, 1977). Overall, these studies demonstrated the efficacy of social skills training for improving peer relations, but their results suggested further refinements were needed to strengthen the consistency and size of effect, as well as to promote generalization and maintenance of behavioral and sociometric gains.

A meta-analysis by Chenier et al. (2011) of 40 studies using single-case experimental designs showed a large overall effect ($g = 3.06$), with effect sizes varying by type of social skills intervention procedures. Effect size estimates for SSI for children with *disruptive behavior problems g = 2.31*. Effect sizes varied by type of intervention procedure and ranged from 2.17 (reinforcement-based procedures) to 3.94 (social stories). Effect sizes also varied by type of outcome measure with academic engaged time showing the smallest effect ($g = 1.57$) and cooperative play showing the largest effect size ($g = 5.54$).

Table 9.1 shows various evidence-based social skills intervention strategies based on both narrative and meta-analytic reviews of the literature. As can be seen in Table 9.1, some social skills intervention strategies are more effective in remediating social skills acquisition deficits (e.g., modeling, coaching, behavioral rehearsal), whereas other strategies are more effective in remediating social skills performance deficit (e.g., reinforcement, behavioral contract, differential reinforcement). In the following section, I describe a commercially available Tier 2 social skills intervention program designed to remediate social skills acquisition deficits.

Social Skills Improvement System Intervention Guide

The Social Skills Improvement System Intervention Guide (SSIS-IG; Elliott & Gresham, 2008) is a manualized, commercially available Tier 2 selected intervention program conceptualized as teaching social skills across the following domains: communication, cooperation, assertion, responsibility, empathy, and self-control. These six domains were derived, in part, from research using the SSIS-RS (Gresham & Elliott, 2008).

Instructional strategies in the SSIS-IG are based on principles derived from social learning theory and cognitive behavior therapy. Specifically, instructional strategies rely on modeling, coaching, behavioral rehearsal, performance feedback, and social problem solving. The theory of change for these intervention procedures and how they affect intervention outcomes is presented in Figure 9.1.

The theory of change model derives, in part, from social learning theory (Bandura, 1977, 1986) that utilizes the concept of vicarious learning and the role of cognitive-mediational processes in determining which environmental events are attended to, retained, and subsequently performed. Social learning theory is based on the idea of reciprocal determinism, which describes the role an individual's behavior has on changing the environment and vice versa. The above model utilizes strategies from social learning theory, including modeling (vicarious learning), coaching (verbal instruction), behavioral rehearsal (practice) to enhance fluency of instructed social skills, and feedback/generalization programming strategies to facilitate transfer of social skills to naturalistic environments and situations outside the group instructional setting.

Social skills are taught in this theory of change model using a six-step instructional sequence: Tell (coaching), Show (modeling), Do (role playing), Practice (behavioral rehearsal), Monitoring Progress

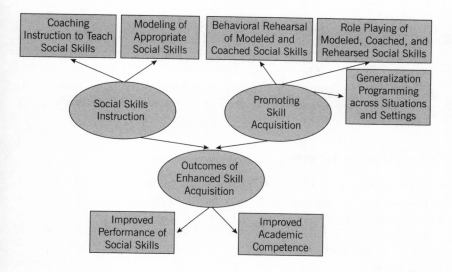

FIGURE 9.1. Theory of change: Acquisition.

(feedback and self-assessment), and Generalize (generalization programming). It is important to note that in each phase, while one strategy provides the basis for instruction, other strategies may be concurrently used to augment learning. For example, in the *Tell* phase, while coaching is the focal point of the lesson, elements of modeling may be used to illustrate examples of the featured skill, and social problem solving can help students discuss and understand the importance of learning the skill.

The outcomes of this six-step instructional model lead to improved acquisition and performance of social skills and their generalization to other settings and social situations. In addition, based on the earlier discussion of social skills as acad*emic enablers*, improved social skill performance is expected to lead to improved academic performance because it enables students to benefit from academic instruction (Caprara et al., 2000; DiPerma & Elliott, 2002; Malecki & Elliott, 2002; Wentzel, 2009).

The SSIS-IG remediation program for social skills acquisition deficits is delivered in a small-group setting (four to five children) conducted by a group leader experienced in working with small groups of children. The SSIS-IG is implemented for two sessions per week for 45 minutes per session (90 minutes per week) over a period of approximately 12 weeks. Approximately two social skills per week are targeted for instruction. The program takes advantage of well-established and effective teaching models, including situated learning, positive peer models, behavioral rehearsal, and specific performance feedback (see theory of change above). In addition to the skills taught, the SSIS-IG offers materials that support home–school communications and student self-assessment to enhance generalization of instructed social skills outside of the school setting.

SKILLS TAUGHT IN THE SSIS-IG

The social skills taught in the SSIS-IG program are derived from the SSIS-RS items (Gresham & Elliott, 2008). The 20 social skills taught in the program are presented in Table 9.2. The conceptual foundation for these skills is based on the notion of *keystone behaviors*. Keystone behaviors are those behaviors that, when changed, are likely to lead to changes in other behaviors not targeted for change. They form a response class, which describes how behaviors are organized into more complex units that become functionally equivalent (Maag, 2006). Instructionally, it is more efficient and effective to identify and teach behaviors at the level of a response class rather than teaching numerous, unrelated separate behaviors. For example, out of 50 separate behaviors that might be targeted for intervention, it may be that only 10–15 behaviors need to be directly taught, if these behaviors were organized into a functionally equivalent response class. The previous discussion of the relationships among social skills, social tasks, and social competence captures this notion of response class. Social tasks such as playing a game, joining a peer group, and having a conversation are all examples of behaviors organized into a response class.

Instructional strategies involve a six-step instructional sequence involving: coaching, modeling, role playing/problem solving, behavioral rehearsal, progress monitoring/feedback, and generalization programming. In the *coaching phase*, the group leader presents and defines the social skill, discusses its importance, and outlines the steps in performing the target social behavior. Coaching teaches general principles of social interaction, allows for integration of behavioral sequences in performing a social skill, sets appropriate goals for accomplishing social interactions, and enhances students' awareness of the impact of their social behavior on others (Gresham & Nagle, 1980; Oden & Asher, 1977). Appendix 9.2 contains a complete scripted lesson for one of the 20 skills taught in the SSIS-IG (Getting along with others).

TABLE 9.2. Social Skills Taught in the SSIS-IG

Communicative behaviors

  1. Taking turns in conversations
  2. Saying "Please" and "Thank you"

Cooperative behaviors

  3. Paying attention to others
  4. Following directions
  5. Paying attention to your work

Assertion behaviors

  6. Expressing feelings
  7. Asking for help
  8. Standing up for others

Responsibility behaviors

  9. Respecting other people's things
10. Doing the right thing
11. Doing your part in a group

Empathy behaviors

12. Making others feel better
13. Doing nice things for others

Engagement behaviors

14. Asking others to do things with you
15. Getting along with others
16. Introducing yourself to others

Self-control behaviors

17. Making compromises
18. Staying calm when criticized
19. taying calm when disagreeing
20. Staying calm when pushed or hit

The *modeling phase* depicts positive and negative social behaviors using pictures, video clips, and role play as well as discussion of alternatives to accomplish the social-behavioral objective. It utilizes principles of vicarious learning and observational learning as described by Bandura (1977, 1986) in his classic work on social learning (social-cognitive) theory. Modeling is one of the most efficient and effective methods of teaching social skills because it does not require that every behavioral component be individually taught in a sequence. Much of the research in social skills interventions utilizes modeling as an essential treatment strategy (Bierman & Powers, 2009; Cook et al., 2008; Gresham, Van, & Cook, 2006; Walker et al., 2004).

The *role-playing* and *social problem-solving phase* directs students to review the social skills definition, describe its importance, review the skill step components, and then enact the social skill in a role-play situation. Social problem solving teaches students how to resolve interpersonal conflicts and problems using a general strategy (general case programming) rather than specific skills. It involves many of the techniques and strategies used in coaching, modeling, and behavioral rehearsal phases.

The *behavioral rehearsal phase* requires students to practice the skills presented in the social skills lessons in contexts outside of the setting of the lesson. This phase incorporates behavioral rehearsal, which is the repeated practice of social skills that enhances retention of the concepts and processes. Behavioral rehearsal is important for the acquisition of social behavior (Bandura, 1977).

The *progress monitoring/feedback phase* requires students to reflect on their own progress. The group leader encourages this reflection using the Social Skills Progress Chart. In addition, the group leader monitors and documents student progress and provides specific performance feedback to students during the lessons.

The *generalization phase* requires students to apply their skills in a variety of settings and social situations, and the group leader encourages students to practice outside the group situation. Generalization might be defined as the occurrence of relevant behaviors under different nontraining conditions without the specific scheduling of those same events or conditions.

Gresham (2011) reported preliminary outcome data on the efficacy of the SSIS-IG. Students were selected based on teacher ratings using the Performance Screening Guide of the SSIS (Gresham & Elliott, 2008). Students receiving PSG ratings of 1 (Very Limited) or 2 (Limited) improvement were placed into the SSIS-IG Tier 2 intervention. Outcome data for all students were collected both before and after the intervention using the SSIS-RS. Biweekly direct classroom observations were collected to examine the percentage of time students were academically engaged in classroom activities. Direct behavior ratings (DBRs) were also collected to track specific target behaviors from the teacher's perspective. Data on school absences, office discipline referrals, and weekly conduct grades were also collected.

Outcome data for the SSIS-IG intervention showed promising results as indicated by substantial improvements across all outcome measures. Using the SSIS-RS, students had a mean pretest score of 67

(2nd percentile) or 6.7 normal curve equivalent (NCE) and a mean posttest score of 83 (13th percentile, or 26.3 NCE), reflecting a change of 12 percentile ranks (19.3 NCEs). Systematic direct observations of academic engaged time showed a mean pretest score of 4.30 and a mean posttest score of 6.15 (a change of 1.85). Mean weekly conduct grades improved from a pretest of 62% to a posttest of 70% (8% improvement). Treatment integrity for the SSIS-IG averaged 93.29%, demonstrating it can be delivered reliably over the duration of the program.

This chapter has provided information on the empirical knowledge base regarding the systematic teaching and reinforcement of social skills that are associated with school and social success. Recommended instructional and behavior management strategies were illustrated for use in the development of social skills that can complement academic performance and the recruitment of healthy social support networks at school. We believe such instruction is essential for a majority of students with DBDs in school who often try to intimidate school staff and bully and harass peers. Due to the strength of their behavior patterns, a combination of universal and selected intervention approaches will usually be required to achieve socially valid outcomes with this student subpopulation in schooling contexts. However, if delivered with integrity, we think implementing such programs is a wise investment of school resources.

Chapter Summary Points

- Competing problem behaviors such as defiance/noncompliance and antisocial behavior patterns prevent children and youth from acquiring and performing prosocial behaviors.

- Peer relationships are important as children make the transition from home to day care to preschool and school environments.

- Peer relationships are important to young children and assume increasing importance as children get older.

- Children with disruptive behavior patterns are often disliked and rejected by their peers as early as the preschool years.

- Peer rejection by normative peers often leads to association with deviant peers that mediates the association with peer rejection to multiple forms of later maladjustment.

- Coercion and negative reinforcement are key processes whereby peer dislike and rejection increase the risk for developing antisocial and oppositional defiant behavior patterns.

- The lack of prosocial behavior leads to peer rejection and the development of disruptive behavior problems later in a child's life.

- Being accepted by one's peers may operate as a protective factor that prevents a child from developing disruptive behavior problems.

- A potentially effective way of decreasing the deleterious effect of disruptive behavior patterns it to teach positive replacement behaviors.

- The matching law states that if disruptive behaviors are reinforced more frequently than prosocial behavior, they will occur more frequently.

- Replacement behavior training is based on the notion of teaching functionally equivalent behaviors using differential reinforcement of incompatible behaviors.

- Behaviors are considered incompatible if they cannot occur simultaneously.

- Social skills are a specific class of behaviors that an individual exhibits to successfully complete a social task.

- Social tasks are a class of interrelated behaviors that are goal directed, such as having a conversation, playing a game, or making friends.

- Social competence is an evaluative term based on judgments that an individual has successfully performed a social task.

- Social skills function as *academic enablers*, or attitudes and behaviors that allow students to participate in and benefit from academic instruction.

- Disruptive behaviors function as *academic disablers* that interfere or compete with the acquisition and performance of prosocial behaviors.

- Social skills deficits can be either *acquisition deficits* ("can't-do" problems) or *performance deficits* ("won't-do" problems).

- Based on narrative and meta-analytic reviews, the most effective social skills intervention strategies are modeling, coaching, behavioral rehearsal, and procedures based on applied behavior analysis.

- The PATHS curriculum is a universal, or Tier 1, social skills intervention that promotes social-emotional competence and reduces aggressive/disruptive behavior.

- The SSIS-CIP is a universal, or Tier 1, social skills intervention program that teaches 10 social skills critical for classroom success.

- Several randomized controlled trials have shown that modeling and coaching are efficacious interventions to improve peer acceptance and prosocial behaviors.

- The most efficacious social skills intervention strategies for remediating social skills *acquisition deficits* are modeling, coaching, behavioral rehearsal, and performance feedback.

- The most efficacious social skills intervention strategies for remediating social skills *performance deficits* are strategies derived from applied behavior analysis (differential reinforcement, peer mediated interventions, behavioral contracts, and token/point systems).

- The SSIS-IG is a Tier 2, or selected, intervention that teaching 20 social skills important for classroom success and the development of positive peer relationships.

APPENDIX 9.1. Sample Lesson from the SSIS-CIP: Staying Calm with Others

Objective: The student will stay calm and control his or her temper in conflict situations with peers. Specifically, the student will identify persons that make him or her angry and use anger-reduction strategies taught in this unit. The student will focus on skills learned in previous units to be able to stay calm with others.

Tell

1. Introduce the Skill and Ask Questions about It.

Say: "Today we are going to talk about staying calm with other people. Staying calm means we don't get mad at others, we try not to lose our temper, and we try to work things out when we have problems."

Say: "Let's think of some things that we can do to stay calm if we get mad or upset.

- "How do we stay calm? (Take a deep breath, count to 10, tell a teacher, Mom, Dad, etc.)
- "What can we do to show we are staying calm? (Be nice, talk about what is bothering us.)
- "Why do we need to stay calm with others? (So we can talk about things clearly, get along better.)
- "Sometimes we might get mad, but we can learn how to get calm again and to stay calm."

2. Define the Skill and Discuss Key Words (*get along, calm, mad, temper, talk*).

Say: "Staying calm with others means that even if we get mad about something, we try not to lose our temper."

Say: "Look at the picture on the front of your book. What do you see in the picture? (Girl, teacher.) She's telling her teacher about something that is bothering her. See how the girl is talking to the teacher. She's staying calm and telling her what is wrong."

Say: "When we stay calm with other people, we are able to figure out our problems and talk about what makes us mad or upset. It's easier to get along when everybody stays calm and doesn't get mad."

3. Discuss Why the Skill Is Important.

Say: "Staying calm is important. It makes us better at getting along with other people and makes people happy when we are nice to them instead of getting mad.

- "Losing your temper or not staying calm can sometimes make things worse.
- "Things won't get better if you don't stay calm.
- "If you can keep from getting mad, you can make things better when talking with other kids.
- "Listening to others and taking turns when you talk can help you stay calm with others."

4. Identify the Skill Steps; Have Students Repeat Them.

Say: "Now open your book to page 2. Please look for the rainbow. Listen to me. I will tell you the steps to stay calm with others.

- "**Step 1: Feel.** How do you feel when you are mad? Do you see the mad face?
- "**Step 2: Think.** Think about what is making you mad and what you can do to stay calm. Do you see the frog thinking?
- "**Step 3: Talk.** Talk things over instead of getting mad. Share your feelings with someone else. Do you see the dog talking?
- "**Step 4: Do.** Do something that will help you stay calm. If you don't get mad, you can be happy. Do you see the mouth smiling?"

Summarize the Skill Steps

Say: "What are the steps again to stay calm with others?

- "**Step 1: Feel.**
- "**Step 2: Think.**
- "**Step 3: Talk.**
- "**Step 4 Do.**"

Say: "Now draw a line between the picture and the words.

- "Where is the word *feel*? (Have students point to the word.) Step 1 is Feel. Where is the mad face? Draw a line from the mad face to the word *feel*.
- "Where is the word *think*? Step 2 is Think. Where is the frog that is thinking? Draw a line from the frog thinking to the word *think*.
- "Where is the word *talk*? Step 3 is Talk. Where is the dog that is talking? Draw a line from the dog talking to the word *talk*.

- "Where is the word *do*? Where is the smiling mouth? Draw a line from the smiling mouth to the word *do*."

Show

Say: "Please look for the raincloud on page 2. Do you see the picture by the raincloud? What do you see in the picture? (Two boys and a girl.) What are they doing? (Standing in line, pushing, getting mad.) The children are standing in a line. The girl is looking at the two boys. She looks worried. One boy is pushing the other boy. The boy who is being pushed looks mad. Draw a circle around the boy who is being pushed. The boys need to work on talking to each other and staying calm. What steps are missing? What steps are not there? (Step 3: Talk. Step: 4 Do.)"

Show the video clips. Then talk about the skill steps.

Say: "Now let's watch a video and look for some examples of students who are staying calm."

Say: "What are the children doing? (Fighting.) Are they sharing? (No.) Are they getting mad or staying calm? (Getting mad.)"

Play the video again.

Say: "See, the girl comes to help them stay calm by thinking of something else they can do."

Say: "Are the boy and girl staying calm in line? (No.) What steps are missing? (Step 2: Think. Step 3: Talk.)"

Play the video again.

Say: "See, the boy and girl not staying calm in the line."

Model and role-play. Use a couple of these situations to model and role-play as time allows.

Say: "Now I need some volunteers."

Positive Model

Show a positive model of staying calm with others for one of the following situations:

- Demonstrate two or three people playing a game together. One person is not taking turns and not following the rules. Show how to ask him or her nicely to please follow the rules and play the right way. The person apologizes and the game continues.

- Demonstrate sharing a coloring book. One person colors on one page and the other person colors on the page directly next to it. One person starts coloring on the other person's page. Show how to ask him or her to please share the book and each should color on his or her own page. The other person agrees.
- Assign roles. Remind listeners to show as many Skill Steps as possible. Have volunteers demonstrate. Thank them.

Say: "Please show what it looks like when listeners use the Skill Steps to say calm with others."

Negative Model

Show a negative model for one of these situations. For negative models, consider the same situations, but this time do not stay calm, don't do anything nice, don't agree to stop the bad behavior, or don't talk to or comply with the other person.

Do

Say: "Now let's see what it looks like when listeners don't use the Skill Steps to stay calm with others."

Say: "Let's go over what we just talked about.

- "How do we stay calm with others? (Try not to get mad, take a deep breath, count to 10.)
- "What can we do to show we are staying calm? (Play nicely together, share, take turns, do not lose temper.)
- "How do you feel when someone is not sharing and taking turns? (Mad, angry, upset.)
- "Why do we need to stay calm with others? (So we can get along better.)
- "What are the four steps to say calm with other people?"

Say: "What are the four steps again to stay calm with others?

- "Step 1: Feel.
- "Step 2: Think.
- "Step 3: Talk.
- "Step 4: Do."

Monitor Progress

Say: "Now, let's use our books again. Look for the star ('How am I doing?') on page 3. Now you know the four steps to stay calm with others. Now think of how often do you stay calm with others. See the stars? The more you can stay calm when you are with others, the more stars you get. If you often stay calm with others, you get four stars. If you need to practice more, then you will get fewer stars.

"How often do you stay calm with other people? Think about the four steps to staying calm with others: feel, think, talk, and do. Do you use these four steps well? Do you stay calm when you are with other people? If yes, find the four stars. Draw a circle around them. You are doing OK. Sometimes it's hard to stay calm with other people. You just need to practice. If you are in the middle, draw a circle around the two or three stars. You may be doing well or doing better. However, we can all practice to be better at staying calm with other people."

Practice

Staying Calm with Others Exercises

Say: "Now let's find the raincloud on page 2 again. See these lines? For these lines, I will spell two words. Write the letters of these words on these lines.

- "The first word is T-H-E What does this spell? (*The.*) The second word is G-I-R-L. What does this spell? (*Girl.*) Who can read this sentence? (*The girl is looking at the boys.*)"

Say: "For these lines, I will spell two more words, Write the letters of the words on these lines.

- "The first word is O-N-E. What does this spell? (*One.*) The second word is B-O-Y. What does this spell? (*Boy.*) Who can read this sentence? (*One boy is not staying calm.*)"

Generalize

Say: "Let's talk about places where we stay calm with others."

Brainstorm places where we stay calm with others; for example:

- Home
- School
- At a friend's house

Say: "Go to the back page. Look for the soccer ball at the top. Look at the pictures. These are places where we can stay calm with others. What are these pictures? (Classroom, play area, lunch area, home, car/bus.) We can stay calm with others at school and at home.

"This week we are practicing the four steps to help us stay calm with others. The four steps are: feel, think, talk, and do. Today, we all practiced in class. Everyone draw a smiley face in this box next to the picture of the classroom. The box says 'I did it!' Today we all did it in class."

Homework

Say: "Today or tomorrow, at lunch, practice with a friend the four steps: Step 1: Feel. Step 2: Think. Step 3: Talk. Step 4: Do."

APPENDIX 9.2. Sample Lesson from the SSIS-IG: Getting Along with Others

Objective: The student will learn to get along with others and join activities that have already started. Specifically, the student will be able to exhibit verbal and nonverbal behaviors that indicate positive interactions with peers during structured and unstructured activities.

Tell

Coaching is an instructional teaching strategy derived from social learning theory that uses verbal instruction and receptive language skills to teach social behavior. The *Tell* phase uses coaching techniques to present social rules or concepts and introduces the skill in a discussion format.

1. Introduce the Skill and Ask Questions about It.

Discuss what it means to get along with others and how to join an activity that has already started. Ask students to think of examples of times when they have gotten along well with others. Ask questions about the skill.

2. Define the Skill and Discuss Key Words.

Define the skill as being nice to the people around us. Discuss strategies for getting along with others, particularly making eye contact, smiling, introducing yourself, sharing, taking turns, following directions, paying attention to others, and playing fairly.

Introduce the Key Words and discuss how each word relates to getting along with others.

Key Words: *share, nice, join, cooperate, activities, include.*

3. Discuss Why the Skill Is Important.

Discuss what benefits the students may experience from getting along with others (e.g., making a new friend, learning something new, feeling included).

Ask the students to discuss what happens when people don't get along well. Have students relate a time that they did not get along well with others.

4. Identify the Skill Steps; Have the Students Repeat Them.

- **Step 1: Find:** Find what you can do to get along with others.
- **Step 2: Talk:** Tell someone you want to get along or help.

- **Step 3: Show:** Show that you want to get along. Be nice.
- **Step 4: Do:** Do nice things to show you want to get along. Smile.

5. Repeat the Skill Steps.

Have the students recite the steps and the correct sequence for the social skill of getting along with others. Verbal rehearsal is an essential component of behavioral rehearsal.

Show

Modeling is an instructional technique based on social learning theory in which an entire behavior sequence is presented for a social skill. Through modeling, the observer can learn how to integrate specific behavioral actions into a composite behavior pattern. The *Show* phase is based on modeling techniques.

Discuss the pictures on the Skill Steps Cue Card.

Have the students discuss what is happening in the picture and which Skill Steps the students are using.

Show the video clips. Then talk about the Skill Steps.

Video Clip: Positive Model

Setting: Classroom. Tyrese and Jada are seated together at a table. They have one book between them.

> TEACHER: Today we'll be reading in pairs. You'll get 10 minutes to read the first chapter, and then I'm going to ask questions. Okay, everybody open up to Chapter 1.

The students start reading. The book is between them, and they are working together to share holding the book and turning the pages.

Video Clip Negative Model

Setting: Classroom. Pazong and Ian are seated together. They have one book between them.

> TEACHER: Today we're going to read in pairs. You'll have 10 minutes to read the first chapter and then I'll ask questions. OK? So open up to Chapter 1, everybody.

Pazaong and Ian need to start reading, but each starts tugging the book to her or his side of the table.

IAN: I can't see (*pulling it toward his side*).

PAZONG: If you pull it, then I can't see (*pulling it to her side*).

IAN: Well, I saw it first.

PAZONG: It has to be in the middle, because I can't see anything.

Pazong and Ian keep arguing and playing tug of war with the book.

Model and role-play the situations as time allows. First, show a positive model of getting along with others, using as many of the Skill Steps as possible. You may assign roles and use either the following scenarios or your own.

- Two people are playing a game together. They are taking turns and talking nicely with each other.
- Two children are sharing a coloring book. One child colors on one page and the other child colors on the other page directly next to it.
- Two people are playing a game. Another person asks to play, and the two players agree and welcome the new player to the game.
- Play a game of telephone message relay.
- In your group of friends, you say a few nice things to each person to show you like them and care about them.
- During class, you are asked to work together with a classmate you have not worked with before. You find a classmate and ask if you could work together on an assignment.
- You want to clean up the area around the school, but it is a big task and you could use some help.

Second, show the negative model of getting along with others for one of the same situations.

Use the same situations, but don't follow the Skill Steps.

Do

In the *Do* phase, students have the opportunity to mimic behavior that was demonstrated in the *Show* phase. Such overt rehearsal emphasizes the steps and correct sequencing that the students recited in the *Tell* phase and observed in the *Show* phase.

Review and have the students role-play.

- Ask the students to state the skill they are learning, why it is important, and what the Skill Steps are.
- Have the students role-play using the same scenarios from the *Show* phase or creating their own.
- Discuss the role plays and which Skill Steps were used.

Repeat the Skill Steps.
Review the Skill Steps again.

- **Step 1: Find.**
- **Step 2: Talk.**
- **Step 3: Show.**
- **Step 4: Do.**

Practice

Practicing the Skill Steps sequences allows students to refine and hone performances of newly learned social skills. The amount of practice necessary depends on the rate of acquisition and quality of each student's behavioral performances.

1. **Use role play to review periodically.** Ask the students to think of an example of when it is easy (or difficult) to get along with others. Role-play these situations.
2. **Brainstorm ideas to improve the skill.** Have students share ideas to improve getting along with others. Make a list of the group's ideas.
3. **Assign homework.** Have the students practice the Skill Steps at school, at home, and in the community. Each time you meet, ask the students where, with whom, and in which situations they practices the Skill Steps.
   - Have the students observe others, either live or on TV, and evaluate how well those people get along with others.
   - Have the students practice getting along with friends, using the Skill Steps.
   - Have the students practice getting along with someone at home, using the Skill Steps.
   - Have the students practice getting along with others at home and at school, recording for the next 3 days how many times they got along with others.
   - Have the students talk with a family member or a friend about ways to get along with others and record the name of the person they talked with.

Monitor Progress

Feedback is a fundamental component of social skills improvement. Provide specific feedback to each student regarding behavioral performances demonstrated in the *Do* and *Practice* phases. Feedback should address both appropriate and inappropriate behaviors as applicable.

In addition, have the students self-assess using the Social Skills Progress Chart.

- Have them think about the Skill Steps needed to get along with others.
- For Day 1, ask them to think about how well they can use the Skill Steps.
- Under Day 1, they should circle 1 if the can use some; 2 if they can use most; and 3 if they can use all the Skill Steps well.
- Repeat this process each time the unit is reviewed.

Generalize

Generalization is critical in ensuring that a newly learned social skill can be applied across multiple settings and situations. Help the students understand that the social skill of getting along with others can be used in a variety of every-day activities and situations.

1. **Discuss physical presence.** Explain the importance of physical positioning, body language, and tone of voice when getting along with others.
2. **Talk about differences.** Discuss some of the differences among students at school. Invite the students to brainstorm ways they could get along with people who are different.
3. **Discuss problems in using the skill.** Discuss problems that the students might encounter in getting along with others. Discuss appropriate reactions if someone isn't friendly.
4. **Brainstorm situations.**
   - Brainstorm places where the students might get along with others (e.g., home, school, a friend's house, camp).
   - Brainstorm people with whom students might get along (e.g., brother or sister, teacher, neighbors, classmates).
   - Brainstorm situations in which it is very important to get along with others (e.g., working on a project with classmates, with family members, living with other children [camp]).

End-of-Unit Review

- Have the students to give examples of when it was very helpful to get along with others.
- Have the students give examples of when it was very difficult to get along with others.
- Make a group list of tips for getting along with others. Brainstorm ideas to help all students improve the skill of getting along with others.
- Review the unit. Ask what is means to get along with others, why the skill is important, and which Skill Steps to use.

- Review what was learned in this unit. Discuss how much the group improved, which Skill Steps the students know best, and which Skill Steps need more practice.
- Summarize the students' feedback and provide feedback to the group. Provide additional suggestions for *Practice* and *Generalize* activities for the students who need more practice.

Case Study Applications for Best Practices

with Kelsey Hartman and Rachel Olinger Steeves

Case 1: Jacob Green

Student Name: Jacob Green
Age: 11
Grade: 5
Race/Ethnicity: African American
Sex: Male

Background Information

Jacob Green was an 11-year-old male referred by his teacher Mr. Tucker for concerns with work refusal. A review of Jacob's cumulative folder revealed that his pediatrician diagnosed Jacob with oppositional defiant disorder (ODD) and ADHD 1 year earlier. He had never been retained or received supplemental academic interventions. In fact, statewide achievement test scores from the previous year indicated mastery of grade-level skills. However, he earned below-average grades in fourth grade. His fourth-grade teacher indicated on several report cards that Jacob was not completing his work.

Kelsey Hartman, MA, is a graduate student in the Department of Psychology, Louisiana State University, Baton Rouge, Louisiana.
Rachel Olinger Steeves, MA, is a graduate student in the Department of Psychology, Louisiana State University, Baton Rouge, Louisiana.

According to Mr. Tucker, Jacob was only completing approximately half of his schoolwork. He normally returned his homework, however, because of parental involvement. Mr. Tucker was concerned because he believed that the work was not too difficult for Jacob, but that without doing his work, eventually Jacob would fall behind in school due to lack of practice in certain skills. Jacob normally did not verbally or otherwise actively refuse to complete his work; mostly he drew cartoons or other pictures on his work. Failure to complete his work did not seem to occur during any specific subject or type of task. The school psychologist conducted three 15-minute systematic direct observations of Jacob during the school day. Across the observations, Jacob averaged 41% on-task, 56% inattentive, and 3% disruptive behavior. The school psychologist noted that when Mr. Tucker redirected Jacob to the assignment, Jacob appeared to agree by nodding or saying "OK," but he did not return to his work. Observations provided additional evidence to support Mr. Tucker's assessment that Jacob was not disruptive, but rather passively refusing to complete his work.

The school psychologist also administered curriculum-based measurements (CBMs) to assess Jacob's general academic skills in math, reading, and writing. Jacob's performance did not indicate any skill deficits, and Mr. Tucker reported that Jacob appeared to have the skills necessary to complete his work. The school psychologist met with Jacob before school one morning and offered him 10 extra minutes of recess if he finished his schoolwork before lunch; Jacob finished all of his work that morning. Therefore, the school psychologist concluded that Jacob's work refusal was likely not due to a skill deficit, but rather to a lack of motivation.

Target Behaviors

1. **Work avoidance:** Work avoidance is defined as not completing schoolwork or only partially completing schoolwork (e.g., not attempting all items) by the due date and time.
2. **Off-task:** Off-task behavior includes failing to attend to tasks for 3 or more seconds and not listening during teacher instruction, indicated by gazing elsewhere.

Intervention Procedures

The school psychologist implemented a behavioral contract to improve Jacob's work completion. A behavioral contract, or contingency contract, is a written agreement between the teacher and student, specifying the appropriate behaviors expected of the student and the consequences for meeting performance criteria or for nonperformance of those behaviors. The behavioral contract was discussed, agreed upon, and written with the assistance of the school psychologist in a meeting with Jacob and his teacher.

Mr. Tucker explained to Jacob that he was concerned about his academic success because of incomplete or missing assignments. Jacob admitted that he disliked schoolwork and that was why he was not completing his work, but that his mom and dad wanted him to do better in school. The school psychologist asked him whether he believed he could complete his assignments if he tried, and Jacob indicated that his schoolwork was not too difficult. Mr. Tucker and the school psychologist then explained that they wanted to see Jacob finish his schoolwork and get better grades in school. Jacob reluctantly agreed that he wanted to do better in school. The school psychologist explained the behavioral contract and the negotiation process and that the goal was to help him in school.

Then as a team, Mr. Tucker, Jacob, and the school psychologist developed the terms of the contract. They agreed that the appropriate behavior to be expected of Jacob was to complete all of his in-school assignments with at least 70% accuracy by the end of the day. This target behavior and performance criterion were added to the contract. It was decided that targeting work completion would improve academic engagement simultaneously. Next, the school psychologist asked Jacob what reward he would like to work for, and Jacob said that he wanted computer time. Mr. Tucker suggested 10 minutes of free time at the end of the day, and Jacob could choose the activity, such as drawing, computer time, games with a friend, a walk in the hallways with a friend, or a visit to see the school counselor, who Jacob liked. Mr. Tucker even offered to post Jacob's cartoons on the classroom walls if they were drawn during appropriate times. Jacob appeared excited about the choices and agreed to the reward, so it was added to the contract. Finally, the school psychologist discussed the need for a penalty clause to ensure that Jacob completed his schoolwork. They agreed that if Jacob failed to finish one of his assignments he could take it home for homework, but if there were two or more incomplete assignments, he would miss recess the next day and complete his work then. The school psychologist wrote the clause into the contract.

Finally, the school psychologist, Mr. Tucker, and Jacob signed the contract. The school psychologist made copies of the contract for Mr. Tucker and Jacob taped his copy to his desk. The contract read:

"I, Jacob Green, agree to complete all of my in-school assignments every day. If I complete all of my schoolwork with at least 70% accuracy by the end of the school day, I will earn 10 minutes of free time at the end of the day. If I do not complete two or more of my assignments by the end of the school day, I will lose recess the next day and complete my schoolwork during recess."

The behavioral contract was implemented the following day. To determine whether Jacob was making progress, Mr. Tucker recorded the percentage of assignments completed daily. Mr. Tucker also reported daily whether or not Jacob earned a reward and the type of reward if applicable as a means of monitoring treatment integrity.

Results

Under typical classroom management procedures, Jacob completed approximately 61% of his schoolwork. When the behavioral contract was implemented, Jacob immediately began completing most of his work (Figure 10.1). He completed 95% of his work over four weeks, with only six days of less than 100% work completion. Jacob only lost recess one day for failing to complete two of his assignments the previous day.

Mr. Tucker reported that Jacob appeared to be more engaged in class when the behavioral contract was in place, and that Jacob was already showing improvement in his grades due to greater work completion. Jacob's teacher consistently implemented the behavioral contract, and only failed to provide Jacob with his reward one day, when Jacob left school early for a doctor's appointment. Mr. Tucker indicated that he found the behavioral contract to be very effective and thought it was an easy solution to Jacob's work refusal. Mr. Tucker added that his relationship with Jacob had also improved.

Discussion

With implementation of a behavioral contract that specified agreed-upon behavioral expectations and consequences, Jacob's work refusal decreased significantly. Because he completed all of his schoolwork fairly consistently across 4 weeks with the behavioral contract, the school psychologist decided to fade the reward from a daily to a weekly reward. The contract was amended to read that Jacob must complete 100% of his schoolwork four out of five days a week to earn 20 minutes of free

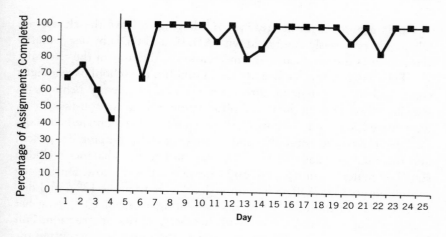

FIGURE 10.1. Percentage of assignments completed by Jacob.

time at the end of the day on Friday. Jacob continued to complete his schoolwork consistently, resulting in better grades.

Case 2: Olivia Jones

Student Name: Olivia Jones
Age: 11
Grade: 4
Race/Ethnicity: African American
Sex: Female

Background Information

Olivia Jones was an 11-year-old female in the fourth grade. She was retained in the first grade due to deficits in reading, but was never referred for special education services. Olivia was referred to the school psychologist by her classroom teacher, Mrs. Franklin, for behavior concerns in the classroom and relationships with her peers. According to Mrs. Franklin, Olivia was seen as a "bully" and engaged in various inappropriate and disruptive behaviors throughout the school day, many of which routinely caused her to be sent to the principal's office. During class, Olivia often required frequent redirections to complete her work and keep her hands to herself. This frequent redirection often resulted in Olivia arguing with her teacher and having to leave the classroom. Olivia was previously diagnosed with ADHD and ODD by her pediatrician, but was not prescribed any medication at the time of the referral.

Following an interview with Mrs. Franklin, the school psychologist conducted three systematic direct observations of Olivia's behavior in the classroom. During the initial observation, Olivia was on-task 27%, inattentive 23%, and disruptive 50% of the time. Disruptive behaviors included talking out, standing and tipping her chair, tapping her pencil, and touching her classmates' materials. Inattentive behaviors included shuffling materials in her desk and staring out the window. During the second observation, Olivia was on-task 39%, inattentive 13%, and disruptive 48% of the time. Most disruption, again involved tipping her chair, talking out, and talking with her peers during instruction. Following the observation, Olivia was sent to the office for disrupting the lesson. Olivia was on-task 57%, inattentive 18%, and disruptive 25% of the time during the final observation. She continued to talk out and argue with Mrs. Franklin during lectures and needed constant redirection.

The school psychologist also conducted CBMs with Olivia in order to determine any areas of academic concern that could be related to the behaviors of concern. Results of the CBM assessments revealed that Olivia was on grade level for mathematics, but was functioning in the frustrational range for reading fluency, indicating that she was performing below grade level.

Target Behaviors

1. **Noncompliance:** Noncompliance includes not doing what her teacher asks within 10 seconds of the first request. This includes refusing to work on class assignments and following her teacher's directions.
2. **Talking out:** Talking out includes impulsively blurting out responses and not raising her hand to participate in class.
3. **Inappropriate peer interactions:** Inappropriate peer interactions includes arguing with peers, making mean comments, kicking or touching peers, making rude nonverbal gestures as ways of seeking attention, and staying calm when criticized.

Intervention Procedures

The school psychologist and Mrs. Franklin chose Check-In/Check-Out (CICO) as the primary intervention used to address Olivia's behavior concerns. CICO is an intervention in which the student is assigned a mentor to check in and out with daily. This mentor is typically a school staff member with whom the student has an existing connection (e.g., the guidance counselor, a previous teacher). Ms. Brown, Olivia's art teacher, served as her mentor for this intervention. Every morning upon arriving at school, Olivia checked in with Ms. Brown, collected her CICO sheet, reviewed her goals for the day, and received positive encouragement about managing her behavior. Olivia then carried her CICO form with her to each class throughout the day and was rated by each of her teachers on the following target behaviors: (1) following directions; (2) raising her hand; (3) keeping hands, feet, and objects to herself; and (4) respecting others by not making mean comments or gestures. A sample of Olivia's CICO form is shown below. At the end of each school day, Olivia brought her form and checked out with Ms. Brown. They reviewed Olivia's progress for the day and discussed things she could have done differently. If Olivia met or exceeded her point goal for the day, then she received a predetermined reward (e.g., extra computer time, candy). Olivia then brought her CICO form home for her mother to review and sign.

Because Olivia's peer interactions were a significant source of frustration and Mrs. Franklin believed that she needed to be taught specific strategies for getting along with others and managing her frustration, Olivia also attended a small social-emotional learning group once per week with four of her same-age peers. Lessons were adapted from the *Strong Kids* curriculum and targeted various aspects of social and self awareness, skills for getting along with others, and anger-management strategies. The skills taught in group combined with the CICO intervention were put in place not only to help Olivia learn the concepts themselves, but also to apply them in her daily interactions with others. In addition to the interventions to address Olivia's behavioral concerns, an individualized repeated-reading academic intervention was also implemented 2 days per week to increase Olivia's reading fluency skills.

To monitor her progress, Mrs. Franklin kept a daily record of the percentage of points Olivia earned for each target behavior on the CICO form. Baseline data were collected for 3 days prior to the implementation of the intervention. In addition, treatment integrity was measured by collecting the CICO forms at the end of each week to determine the percentage of intervention components implemented. Whether each part of the intervention was completed was reviewed (i.e., whether ratings were filled out, goal and number of points written in) and a percentage of necessary components was obtained.

Results

The CICO intervention was implemented for 2 months following baseline data collection. The first 5 weeks of data are shown below. Initially, Olivia was following directions, raising her hand to participate, and respecting her classmates less than 50% of the time. By the end of the fourth week of intervention, all of these behaviors had consistently increased to above 60%. By the end of the second month of intervention, all of these positive replacement behaviors had increased even further, and Olivia seldom required redirection for touching and arguing with her peers (Figure 10.2).

Following the initial 2 months of data collection, Mrs. Franklin reviewed the treatment protocol with the school psychologist and reported high acceptability ratings. She believed the intervention to be successful for Olivia and recommended the social skills curriculum to other teachers with students struggling with related behaviors. Mrs. Franklin also reported that she and Ms. Green enjoyed the CICO intervention and liked the flexibility in amending and altering goals based on the student's behavioral concerns (Figure 10.3). Treatment integrity results showed that Olivia's teachers completed the daily ratings on the

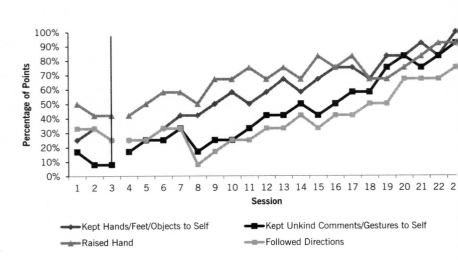

FIGURE 10.2. CICO performance for Olivia.

CICO form 96% of the time, and Ms. Brown completed the necessary steps with Olivia 99% of the time.

Discussion

During the first 4 weeks of CICO and while enrolled in the social skills group, Olivia made slow but steady progress. She started following directions during class and required less redirection for her behavior. She also engaged in less aggressive behavior with her peers. After the first month of intervention, Olivia continued to make progress and remained engaged in the social skills group and in the classroom. Because work completion and following directions were still areas of concern, the CICO goals were amended to include these as target behaviors instead of aggressive behaviors. In a discussion with the school psychologist after the intervention had been modified, Mrs. Franklin reported that

Olivia Date:_____	Follows directions	Respects others			Teacher initials
Key 0 = Not Yet 1 = Good 2 = Excellent	Does what the teacher asks the first time without arguing or talking back	Raises hand to participate or ask questions (did not call out)	Keeps hands, feet, objects to self	Does not say mean comments or make rude nonverbal gestures (glaring, rolling eyes)	
Morning Work	0 1 2	0 1 2	0 1 2	0 1 2	
Math	0 1 2	0 1 2	0 1 2	0 1 2	
Science	0 1 2	0 1 2	0 1 2	0 1 2	
Social Studies	0 1 2	0 1 2	0 1 2	0 1 2	
Reading	0 1 2	0 1 2	0 1 2	0 1 2	
Ancillary	0 1 2	0 1 2	0 1 2	0 1 2	
Today's Goal =	Total Points Earned =				

Comments:

Parent Signature: _____

FIGURE 10.3. Sample CICO daily behavior form for Olivia.

Olivia's classroom behavior and peer relationships had drastically improved and that Olivia was rarely sent to the office anymore. Following the cessation of Olivia's behavioral intervention, she continued to receive individualized reading intervention to further support her reading skill development.

Case 3: Alex Williams

Student Name: Alex Williams
Age: 9
Grade: 4
Race/Ethnicity: Caucasian
Sex: Male

Background Information

Alex Williams was a 10-year-old male who demonstrated significant disruptive behavior in class. His teacher, Mrs. Johnson, contacted the school psychologist for help with Alex's constant "blurting out, throwing things, and walking around the room whenever he wants." During a meeting with the school psychologist, Mrs. Johnson reported that his pediatrician recently diagnosed Jacob with ADHD. His parents were forgoing medication in favor of behavioral treatment at home, but she was unsure how to manage Alex's behavior at school. Alex had already received three office discipline referrals (ODRs) for persistent minor rule violations (e.g., talking out) throughout the day.

Mrs. Johnson indicated that Alex was exhibiting these behaviors frequently on a daily basis. When asked to estimate their frequency, she expressed that he seemed to be disruptive "all the time," and that there was no pattern to the behavior that she could discern. She typically responded with a reprimand and/or redirection. Sometimes she also moved his clip down a color on a traffic-light classroom management system, but it was not effective in changing Alex's behavior. Positive consequences included schoolwide positive behavioral interventions and supports (SWPBIS), which involved providing students with tickets for appropriate behavior to be exchanged at a "store" at the end of the month.

The school psychologist conducted four 15-minute systematic direct observations. On average, Alex was 58% on-task, 9% inattentive, and 33% disruptive. On average across the observations, there were nine instances of talking-out behavior, three instances of out-of-seat behavior, and one instance of throwing objects. The problem behavior seemed to occur more often during independent and group work. The school psychologist observed that Mrs. Johnson often reprimanded Alex, but she rarely asked him to move his clip. Mrs. Johnson did not give Alex any PBIS tickets for appropriate behavior during the observations.

Administration of CBMs revealed that Alex was performing in the low average range in reading and writing, but his scores were around the 50th percentile in math. Mrs. Johnson provided a progress report that showed Alex was earning mostly B's and C's in his classes, and that his skills were average compared to his peers. She expressed that she was in the process of arranging classwide peer tutoring to improve all of her students' reading skills.

Target Behaviors

1. **Talking out:** Talking-out behavior includes instances of speaking without raising his hand and waiting for teacher acknowledgement, except when speaking without raising his hand is acceptable, such as during group work.
2. **Out of seat:** Out-of-seat behavior includes the body breaking contact with the seat or other seating area (e.g., floor), unless the teacher gives students permission to move about the classroom.
3. **Throwing objects:** Throwing objects is defined as throwing any object (e.g., pencil, paper) along a surface or in the air so that it strikes another object or person, but excludes instances of dropping or bumping into objects without the intent to move them.

Intervention Procedures

To address Alex's disruptive behavior, the school psychologist selected a token reinforcement with response cost system. Token reinforcement involves immediately providing tokens contingent on appropriate behavior, which can later be exchanged for rewards. Used in combination with response cost, token reinforcement systems may be more effective in changing behavior quickly. Response cost with tokens involves removing tokens contingent on inappropriate behavior. The token reinforcement with response cost system was customized to Alex and his teacher during a meeting with Mrs. Johnson.

The appropriate behaviors to increase included speaking only with permission, staying in his seat unless given permission to move about, and keeping objects to himself. At the beginning of the day, Mrs. Johnson would remind Alex of the appropriate behaviors and the consequences for following and failing to follow them. Alex would begin each day with three tickets. To provide tickets consistently, Mrs. Johnson agreed to wear a timer in her pocket scheduled to vibrate every 10 minutes. If Alex was engaged in the appropriate behaviors at the end of the interval, he would earn one ticket, which Mrs. Johnson would put in a jar on her desk. She would also provide behavior-specific praise when he earned a ticket, indicating her approval and telling Alex exactly which appropriate behavior(s) he was exhibiting. She was instructed to praise Alex for any instances of appropriate behavior, not only at 10-minute intervals. At any time, if Alex exhibited one of the target behaviors, Mrs. Johnson would remove one of the tickets from the jar, explaining to Alex why he lost a ticket and reminding him of the appropriate behavior(s). At the end of the day, if Alex had at least 10 tickets in the jar, he would earn a reward to be chosen from Mrs. Johnson's treasure chest of small prizes.

The token reinforcement with response cost system was combined with several proactive strategies, including increased supervision and precorrection. Prior to transitions and new activities during the day, Mrs. Johnson would use precorrection to remind the whole class of the behavioral expectations for the transition or activity. She would also increase her supervision or visual monitoring of Alex in order to provide him with praise for appropriate behavior or remove tickets for inappropriate behavior.

Mrs. Johnson and the school psychologist decided to begin the intervention the next day and to implement it daily throughout all classes. Mrs. Johnson monitored Alex's progress by recording the number of tickets Alex had in the jar at the end of the day. Baseline data were collected by tallying the instances of appropriate behavior on the 10-minute interval and any occurrences of inappropriate behavior to provide a hypothetical total number of tickets, taking into account the three free tickets that would be in the jar to begin each day. The record of the number of tickets in the jar, along with a note of what reward was earned if applicable was used to monitor treatment integrity. The school psychologist informed Mrs. Johnson that he would also observe implementation of the intervention on several randomly selected days.

Results

During baseline, Alex would have averaged just two tickets daily if Mrs. Johnson had been providing and removing tickets contingent on

behavior according to the intervention procedures. When Mrs. Johnson began the token reinforcement with response cost system, Alex's
behavior improved immediately and continued to improve over 4 weeks
of intervention. At the end of the day, Alex averaged 14 tickets in the
jar during the intervention phase. He failed to meet his goal two out
of the first three days and one day during the second week. However,
by the final week of intervention, he was earning most of his tickets on
the interval schedule and losing few tickets for inappropriate behavior,
according to his teacher (Figure 10.4). Alex was also consistently earning his reward. Mrs. Johnson provided anecdotal information that Alex
had stopped throwing objects completely and mostly stayed in his seat.
He was still losing several tickets a day for talking out, but this seemed
to occur at a frequency that was normal compared to Alex's peers. Alex
had not received any ODRs since beginning the intervention.

When the school psychologist met with Mrs. Johnson after 4 weeks
of intervention implementation, Mrs. Johnson indicated that she found
the intervention to be acceptable and effective. Mrs. Johnson was consistently completing the record sheet indicating how many tickets Alex had
in the jar at the end of the day and what reward he had earned if applicable, suggesting adequate treatment integrity. When the school psychologist observed Mrs. Johnson's intervention implementation, he noticed
that while Mrs. Johnson was providing tickets on the set schedule, she
was failing to remove tickets consistently for inappropriate behavior.

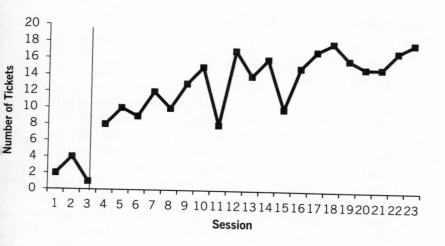

FIGURE 10.4. Tickets earned by Alex.

Performance feedback improved Mrs. Johnson's treatment integrity during subsequent observations.

Discussion

Mrs. Johnson revealed to the school psychologist that she felt the intervention had normalized Alex's behavior as compared to the other students in her class. Given the effectiveness of the token reinforcement with response cost system in decreasing disruptive behavior and increasing appropriate behavior over 4 weeks, Mrs. Johnson was interested in continuing its use with Alex. However, she requested that the time intervals be lengthened to make implementation easier and more sustainable for her. The school psychologist and Mrs. Johnson agreed on 20-minute time intervals with provision and removal of tickets only at those times. They adjusted Alex's goal accordingly and decided to meet again in 4 weeks to evaluate Alex's progress. At that time, they would determine whether to take another step to fade the intervention or terminate it altogether.

Case 4: Ryan Johnson

Student Name: Ryan Johnson
Age: 7
Grade: 1
Race/Ethnicity: African American
Sex: Male

Background Information

Ryan Johnson was a 7-year-old male in the second grade. He had never been retained or received special education services. Ryan was referred by his classroom teacher, Mr. Morris, to the school psychologist for concerns regarding his noncompliance and history of tantrum behaviors in school. According to school staff, Ryan was "needy" and sought adult attention in inappropriate ways through behaviors such as talking out, yelling, crying, getting out of his seat and wandering around the classroom, and interrupting his teacher by knocking classroom materials over. These behaviors occurred multiple times throughout each day, but with varying severity. Mr. Morris expressed that the SWPBIS system they had in place, along with his classroom check system for behavior management, were not enough to support Ryan's needs. When he engaged in severe tantrums, which occurred one to three times per week, Mr. Morris would send Ryan to the office where he received an ODR for his tantrum behaviors. Ryan's pediatrician diagnosed him with ADHD, depression, and ODD. He was prescribed Concerta and Risperdal for associated symptoms of these disorders.

Following an interview with Mr. Morris, the school psychologist conducted three systematic direct observations of his behavior in the classroom. During the initial observation, Ryan was on-task 77% of the time, inattentive 20%, and disruptive 3%. He was inattentive when the teacher did not call on him and engaged in attention-seeking behaviors by talking out, lingering on the carpet, and crawling around at his teacher's feet during transitions. During the second observation, Ryan was on-task 78% of the time, inattentive 13%, and disruptive 9%. Most inattention involved staring or playing with objects at his desk, while most disruptive behavior involved calling out. During the final observation, Ryan was on-task 67%, inattentive 12%, and disruptive 21% of the time. He engaged in a tantrum (i.e., crying, stomping his feet) during the last part of the observation when his teacher did not call on him during a spelling test.

The school psychologist also conducted CBMs with Ryan in order to determine any areas of academic concern that could be related to the behaviors of concern. Results of the CBMs revealed that Ryan was on grade level for all subject areas (i.e., mathematics, reading, and writing). However, despite adequate academic ability, Ryan's grades were suffering because he was not completing his work. He was instead earning C's, D's and F's in many of his class subjects.

Target Behaviors

1. **Tantrums:** Tantrums include instances in which Ryan cries, either at his desk, under his desk, or on the floor. Tantrums also include Ryan eloping, or leaving the classroom, when he is upset and running toward the street.
2. **Noncompliance:** Noncompliance includes not doing what his teacher asks within 10 seconds of the first request. This includes refusing to work on class assignments, follow teacher's directions, and take breaks when upset.
3. **Inappropriate attention seeking:** Inappropriate ways of seeking

attention include not raising hand to ask questions (i.e., talking or blurting out the answer), crying, getting out of his seat to approach his teacher, and wandering around the classroom, knocking things over.

Intervention Procedures

The intervention chosen to target Ryan's behaviors was a school–home note, combined with a supplemental contingency for his tantrum behaviors. The school–home note was a useful intervention for providing consistency and communication between Ryan's teacher and parents. During the day, Ryan received feedback from Mr. Morris about his performance of specific target behaviors. Based on the presenting concerns, his school–home note was broken down into four specific behaviors to address his noncompliance and inappropriate attention-seeking behaviors. These replacement behaviors included: (1) only talked or got out of seat with permission, (2) asked for help when needed, (3) stayed calm when angry or sad, and (4) completed classwork. At the beginning of each day, Mr. Morris reminded him of the positive behaviors he should focus on and set a goal for the day. Throughout the school day during specified class periods, Mr. Morris rated Ryan's behavior for each of the operationally defined replacement behaviors. Ryan received a smiley face (:)) if he performed the target behavior during most of the class activity indicated on the chart. He received a straight face (:|) if he performed the target behavior during only some of the class activity, and a sad face (:() if he performed the behavior rarely or not at all during the class. At the end of each day, Ryan met with his teacher to tally his smiley faces to see if he met his goal. Mr. Morris provided comments and feedback regarding Ryan's performance that day. Ryan then brought his school–home note home to his mother, where he received a predetermined reward from her if he met his goal for the day. If he did not meet his goal, Mr. Morris and his mother reminded him of the behaviors to focus on for the following day.

The supplemental contingency used to target Ryan's tantrum behavior was a modified contingency contract. If Ryan made it through the entire day without engaging in a tantrum (i.e., getting on the floor, crawling under his desk, or leaving the room while crying), he was able to color in a football on his sheet. He could earn one football for each day of the week, and had a predetermined number of footballs he needed to earn (e.g., three or four, based on the severity of his behavior) in order to play football with the school psychologist and a friend on Friday afternoon. A sample school–home note and supplemental contingency like the one used with Ryan is shown below.

In addition to the school–home note and modified contingency contract, Ryan's intervention plan included steps to ensure appropriate responding throughout the day. Ryan's teacher delivered frequent praise for positive behaviors combined with planned ignoring of undesired behaviors. In this way, Ryan received attention for desirable behaviors and did not receive attention for negative behaviors. Mr. Morris also prompted him throughout the day to take breaks, remain calm, and follow instructions.

To monitor Ryan's progress, his teacher completed daily behavior ratings (DBRs) on the target behaviors related to his tantrums, following directions, and work completion. Mr. Morris rated each of these behaviors on a scale from "Never" to "Always." In addition, treatment integrity was measured by collecting the school–home notes at the end of each week. Whether Mr. Morris had filled out the ratings and given his initials each day and whether Ryan's mother had signed the form each evening were the points considered for the measure of integrity.

Results

Prior to intervention implementation, Ryan's teacher assessed each of the three target behaviors for 1 week and also kept a tally of the number of tantrums that Ryan engaged in. During baseline, Ryan engaged in an average of five tantrums per week (or one per day) and rarely used calming strategies, completed his work, or followed his teacher's directions. Mr. Morris continued these ratings throughout the intervention. Results of the intervention over the course of 3 weeks showed it to be effective for reducing Ryan's tantrum behaviors and increasing his compliance to teacher directions and work completion. The graph in Figure 10.5 depicts Mr. Morris' daily ratings of Ryan's behavior and the number of days per week he engaged in tantrums.

Teacher acceptability of the intervention procedures was assessed following the implementation of Ryan's intervention. Mr. Morris indicated that he felt it was effective in reducing Ryan's problem behaviors and would be extremely likely to use it with another student in the future. In addition, he felt he would be likely to recommend this intervention to another teacher for use with students with similar behavioral concerns. Treatment integrity results showed that Mr. Morris completed

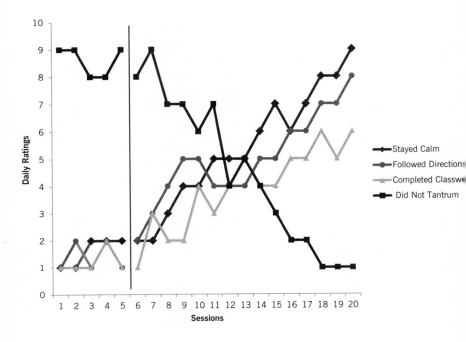

FIGURE 10.5. Ryan's daily behavior ratings.

the steps of the intervention 98% of the time and Ryan's mother signed and returned his form 90% of the time.

Discussion

Following the intervention, discussion with Ryan's teacher and analysis of the data collected revealed that Ryan's tantrums significantly decreased as a result of the intervention, both in frequency and in severity. Instead of crawling under his desk, crying, and running out of the classroom almost every day of the week, Ryan began asking to take breaks and using strategies to help himself calm down when he felt angry. His teacher also reported that he no longer eloped from the classroom or crawled under his desk to gain attention. In addition, Ryan began complying with his teacher's instructions.

Although Ryan's behaviors had changed drastically, Mr. Morris felt that continuing the intervention would be useful for some of his remaining, less severe behaviors. Once his tantrums and noncompliance behaviors appeared to be under control, the intervention was

Ryan Date: _____ Goal: _____ ☺	Only talks or gets out of seat with permission	Asks for help when needed	Stays calm when angry or sad	Completes classwork
DOL/Calendar Math	☺ ☺ ☹	☺ ☺ ☹	☺ ☺ ☹	☺ ☺ ☹
Reading	☺ ☺ ☹	☺ ☺ ☹	☺ ☺ ☹	☺ ☺ ☹
Math	☺ ☺ ☹	☺ ☺ ☹	☺ ☺ ☹	☺ ☺ ☹
Social Studies/Science	☺ ☺ ☹	☺ ☺ ☹	☺ ☺ ☹	☺ ☺ ☹

Teacher Comments:

Parent Signature and Comments:

If Ryan goes the entire day without getting on the floor, crawling under his desk, or leaving the room when he is crying, he gets to color in a football. He can also earn a football if he does not cry at all during the day. When he earns _____ footballs, he gets to play football on Friday afternoon.

FIGURE 10.6. Sample school–home note with supplemental contingency.

modified in order to more explicitly address Ryan's work completion and less severe attention-seeking behaviors (e.g., talking out during lessons). The school–home note in Figure 10.6 was continued to promote Ryan's positive behavior, and the supplemental football contingency was modified to include the newer behaviors of sulking to gain attention that he began to display in place of his tantrums. The school psychologist and Mr. Morris amended the intervention to reflect these updated goals and agreed to meet again in a few weeks to discuss his progress and to determine whether continuing to fade the intervention or terminating it altogether would be the best course of action.

Case 5: Sam Miller

Student Name: Sam Miller
Age: 11
Grade: 5
Race/Ethnicity: Caucasian
Sex: Male

Background Information

Sam was an 11-year-old male in the fifth grade, who was referred by his teacher for argumentative and disruptive behavior. He received testing accommodations and pullout instruction for specific learning disability. According to his teacher, Mrs. Kay, Sam often argued with her when she gave assignments or redirected him to a task. She stated that during independent or group work he "got frustrated," and as his frustration escalated, his disruptive behavior increased in the form of talking out, wandering around the room, or leaving the classroom. He had received three ODRs for verbal aggression and leaving the room without permission. While most of his interactions with adults were negative, he was well liked by his peers. Sam rarely completed and turned in schoolwork and was earning D's and F's in all subjects.

Mrs. Kay indicated that Sam's behavior was more severe during subjects that were difficult for him, particularly reading and social studies. Talking out and argumentative behavior occurred frequently throughout the day and leaving the classroom without permission occurred two or three times a week, which had increased in the weeks prior to the referral. Mrs. Kay's consequences for inappropriate behavior began with two verbal reprimands, then 5 minutes off of recess, and finally an ODR. Leaving the room resulted in an automatic ODR and a note home. Mrs. Kay admitted that due to the number of students in her class, this hierarchy of consequences was inconsistently enforced.

Three 15-minute systematic direct observations were conducted. The first observation was conducted during written work on which they could collaborate. Sam was 55% on-task, 15% disruptive, and 30% inattentive. Toward the end of the observation, he left his desk, wandered around the classroom, and hit a classmate on the head with a pencil. A second observation was conducted during group instruction, where he was 75% on-task, 5% disruptive, and 20% inattentive. The third observation was conducted during group work, and he was 45% on-task, 35% disruptive, and 20% inattentive. During the observation, Sam protested the length of his assignment, left his seat to sharpen his pencil three times, and then tried to hide his worksheet in his desk. The observation was terminated early when Sam swore loudly at Mrs. Kay and received an ODR. Administration of math CBMs indicated he was performing around the 50th percentile in math; reading and writing CBMs were not administered because he was already receiving reading intervention.

Target Behaviors

1. **Verbal aggression:** Verbal aggression includes speaking to his teacher in an argumentative or aggressive tone, raising his voice, and using inappropriate language.
2. **Noncompliance:** Noncompliance includes not following his teacher's instructions within 10 seconds of the first request.
3. **Elopement:** Elopement includes leaving his desk for over 10 seconds, walking around the room, and exiting the classroom without permission.

Intervention Procedures

The school psychologist introduced a Daily Report Card (DRC) and self-management program to address Sam's target behaviors. Sam's DRC was divided into six time periods. For each period he would receive 1 point for adhering to his behavioral expectations. Based on his target behaviors the behavioral expectations were (1) be respectful, (2) follow directions, and (3) stay in seat. He was allowed one warning for each of the three rules before losing the point for the period. At the beginning of each day Mrs. Kay reminded Sam of his behavioral expectations, and after each period, she met with Sam to explain why he did or did not receive a point. If he received a point he was given verbal praise, and if not, the teacher made suggestions for improving his behavior. If Sam achieved his goal number of points at the end of the day, the teacher allowed him to choose a prize from the treasure chest. If he did not achieve his goal, he was reminded of which behaviors to improve on the next day. The initial goal was for Sam to receive 3 points for the day. After 3 consecutive days of receiving at least 3 points, the goal was moved to 4 points, and eventually to 5 points.

In addition to the DRC, Sam was put on a self-management program to help him regulate his feelings of frustration. The self-management technique comprised three sequential steps:

1. **Count to 10:** Sam was instructed to close his eyes, count slowly to 10, and take deep breaths when he began to feel angry or frustrated.
2. **Ask for help:** If the first step did not help, Sam was taught how to appropriately ask for help. Because he appeared to get along better with his peers than with his teacher, the instruction emphasized requesting help from his classmates. To facilitate this step, the teacher moved moderate- to high-achieving peers into his "pod" of desks.
3. **Take a break:** If the first two steps did not relieve Sam's frustration, he was allowed a three-minute break in the room's "Reading Corner." To request a break, Sam raised three fingers in the air. The teacher set a timer for 3 minutes and prompted him to return to work when the timer went off.

Before intervention implementation, Sam was pulled from class and trained on how and when to employ the self-management steps. An anger alternatives card was placed on his desk to remind him of the steps. The school psychologist worked with the teacher to recognize signs of Sam's frustration and how to prompt him to implement the self-management steps. Mrs. Kay prompted Sam sequentially through the steps when he appeared to become upset. The DRC served as a permanent product of this intervention, with the teacher adding the frequency of breaks each day at the bottom of the card. A school psychologist collected the DRCs weekly as a measure of both treatment integrity and progress monitoring.

Results

Before the intervention began, Mrs. Kay completed the DRC for 2 days without showing it to Sam or otherwise implementing the intervention. He would have earned 1 point on both days. During 3 weeks of the DRC and self-management program, the frequency of Sam's disruptive behavior decreased (Figure 10.7). The number of points earned daily steadily increased before leveling out at 5 to 6 points. Sam achieved a 123% increase in points from the first week of intervention to the last week of intervention. The goal number of points increased from three to four on day 10 of the intervention and increased to 5 points on day 14 of the intervention. Overall, he met his goal 76% of days during 3 weeks of intervention.

The number of breaks Sam took increased steadily with the number of points he earned but began decreasing as his points leveled out. This decrease indicated that as he began exhibiting positive replacement behaviors (e.g., counting to 10 and asking for help), he was able to manage his emotions more quickly before he needed a break. Mrs. Kay reported that Sam was asking for help more often from both herself and his peers and that he appeared less frustrated during classwork. While he occasionally protested his work, his tone was nonaggressive. He did not receive any ODRs following implementation of the intervention. Mrs. Kay completed 94% of the DRCs and was observed by the school psychologist to be appropriately prompting Sam's self-management techniques.

Discussion

Before intervention, Sam displayed disruptive behavior likely due to difficulty with classwork. By encouraging self-management skills to

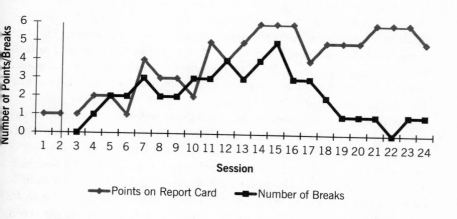

FIGURE 10.7. DRC points and frequency of breaks for Sam.

manage his frustration, Sam was able to approach his schoolwork in a calm and effective manner. He experienced significant decreases in talking-out behavior, argumentative exchanges with his teacher, and no longer left the classroom without permission, thus minimizing the distractions both to himself and other students. During a meeting with the school psychologist, Mrs. Kay said she planned to continue using the DRC, but intended to gradually eliminate the number of breaks allowed per day. Mrs. Kay and the psychologist agreed to meet every 4 weeks to check in on his behavior and discuss adjustments to the intervention.

Case 6: Lucy Smith

Student Name: Lucy Smith
Age: 8
Grade: 3
Race/Ethnicity: African American
Sex: Female

Background Information

Lucy Smith was an 8-year-old third-grade student referred by her classroom teacher to the school psychologist to target noncompliance, work avoidance, and tantrum behaviors. Based on information obtained from Ms. Stevens, Lucy's teacher, she often sought out adult attention through inappropriate and disruptive means, such as kneeling on the floor, leaving the classroom without permission, yelling, and crying. Ms. Stevens described Lucy as an exceptionally bright student. However, her academic performance was suffering, likely due to her behavior and failure to complete assignments. Prior to the referral, Lucy had received counseling for her behavior at her previous school, but had not received any formalized special education services.

The school psychologist conducted three systematic direct observations of Lucy's behavior in the classroom following the interview with her teacher. During the first observation, Lucy left the classroom without permission and lingered in the hallway for more than 15 minutes. Upon returning to the classroom, she was inattentive and took a significant amount of time to return to the task. She was then 39% on-task, 49% inattentive, and 12% disruptive. Similar behaviors were observed in the second observation in which Lucy was 39% on-task, 34% inattentive, and 27% disruptive. The final observation was conducted during an afternoon group activity in which Lucy was on-task 15% of the time, inattentive 37% of the time, and disruptive 48% of the time. She engaged in disruptive and negative attention-seeking behaviors, which clearly interfered with her individual performance, and were also interrupting her peers.

In addition to behavioral observations, the school psychologist administered CBMs to collect additional data on Lucy's academic performance in math, reading, and writing. Based on results from the assessment, Lucy's academic skills were at or above her current grade level in all assessed areas.

Target Behaviors

1. **Tantrums:** Tantrums include inappropriate ways of seeking attention such as eloping (leaving the classroom) when she is upset, pushing her desk into another student, and knocking over materials in the classroom.
2. **Noncompliance:** Noncompliance includes not doing what her teacher asks within 5–10 seconds of the request; for Lucy, this includes passive noncompliance (e.g., continuing a task the teacher requests that she stop) and active noncompliance (e.g., verbally or physically indicating that she will not comply).
3. **Work avoidance:** Work avoidance includes failure to complete academic assignments or to only partially complete assignments.

Intervention Procedures

Based on the information obtained from Ms. Stevens and the school psychologist's assessments, a self-monitoring intervention was chosen to target Lucy's behavior problems. Self-monitoring interventions provide an opportunity for students to observe, rate, and record their own behavior. By doing so, students are made more aware of their misbehavior and the associated consequences. Lucy's self-monitoring chart included goals to target the following replacement behaviors: (1) stays calm when upset, (2) follows teacher directions, and (3) completes classwork. Each morning, Lucy retrieved a new sheet from Ms. Stevens and was assigned a point goal for the day. Lucy then kept the sheet with her throughout the day and monitored and rated her own behavior (i.e., 0, 1, or 2) over 30-minute time intervals. Ms. Stevens kept track of the intervals with the use of a vibrating timer and prompted Lucy to fill out her ratings at the end of every 30-minute period. Ms. Stevens then reviewed Lucy's self-ratings, initialed the sheet, and discussed any inconsistencies that she may have observed at the end of each specific class period. The total possible number of points for each day was 72, and Lucy's initial goal was 58, or approximately 80% of the total. If Lucy met her goal, she received a choice of three reinforcing activities (e.g., free computer time). Her goal was systematically increased as the intervention progressed. An example of a potential self-monitoring form like the one used with Lucy is attached below.

In addition to the self-monitoring intervention, explicit and frequent praise were delivered when Lucy engaged in appropriate behaviors. Disruptive or inappropriate behaviors were ignored, so she did not receive attention for these negative behaviors. The school psychologist also met weekly with Lucy to discuss and model appropriate behaviors and anger-management strategies. Ms. Stevens also provided opportunities for her to practice these strategies in the classroom in between weekly meetings with the school psychologist.

The intervention was implemented daily and progress was monitored by the school psychologist through weekly observations and review of the self-monitoring forms to determine whether modification, fading, or termination of the intervention was necessary. The school psychologist also collected Lucy's charts weekly to monitor implementation and problem-solve any missed steps with her teachers.

Results

Prior to the above intervention being implemented, the school psychologist observed the target behaviors over five 30-minute sessions across 2 weeks. Data collected pre- and postintervention implementation (i.e., total frequency of each target behavior over the observations) are also presented in the graph in Figure 10.8. Results suggested that with the implementation of the intervention, Lucy's inappropriate behaviors decreased. Specifically, the frequency of Lucy's noncompliance, work avoidance, and tantrum behaviors decreased dramatically.

Based on the information obtained through a review of Ms. Steven's treatment integrity, she correctly implemented 94% of the necessary steps of the intervention. Ms. Stevens and Lucy's mother asserted that the intervention was effective and easy to implement.

Discussion

Following the implementation of intervention, analysis of the data collected and discussion with Ms. Stevens revealed that Lucy's tantrums

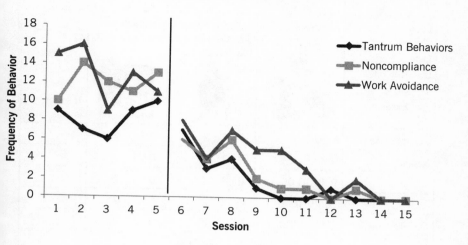

FIGURE 10.8. Observations of Lucy's problem behavior.

significantly decreased. In addition, she engaged in less noncompliant and work-avoidance behaviors. As these behaviors decreased, Lucy's work completion significantly increased and her grades began to steadily improve. Because Lucy demonstrated significant progress with the intervention, Ms. Stevens chose to continue using it as a part of Lucy's daily school routine. However, rather than assessing behaviors at 30-minute intervals, she began recording behaviors at the end of each class period, for alternative behaviors (Figure 10.9). Lucy completed the anger-management curriculum and demonstrated significant gains from the first to final session.

Case 7: Phil Duffy

Student Name: Phil Duffy
Age: 6
Grade: 1
Race/Ethnicity: Caucasian
Sex: Male

Background Information

Phil was a first-grade student referred to the school psychologist by his teacher for displaying aggressive behavior. He received two office

Lucy Date: 0 = Not Yet 1 = Good 2 = Excellent!	Stays calm when upset	Follows directions on the first try	Completes classwork	Teacher initials
Calendar Math	8:30-9:00	0 1 2	0 1 2	
Reading	9:00-9:30	0 1 2	0 1 2	
	9:30-10:00	0 1 2	0 1 2	
	10:00-10:30	0 1 2	0 1 2	
Social Studies	10:30-11:25	0 1 2	0 1 2	
LUNCH AND RECESS				
Math	12:00-12:30	0 1 2	0 1 2	
	12:30-1:00	0 1 2	0 1 2	
Science	1:00-1:30	0 1 2	0 1 2	
Writing	1:30-2:00	0 1 2	0 1 2	
	2:00-2:30	0 1 2	0 1 2	
Ancillary	2:30-3:00	0 1 2	0 1 2	
Dismissal	3:00-3:30	0 1 2	0 1 2	
	Today's Goal:		Total Points:	

Parent Signature: _____

FIGURE 10.9. Sample of self-monitoring sheet for Lucy.

discipline referrals (ODRs) for instances of bullying, including verbal aggression on the bus and in the classroom. According to his teacher, Mrs. Moore, Phil often argued with his peers during group activities about following the classroom rules and the teacher's directions, which he tried to enforce by bossing his peers. He also sometimes called his peers inappropriate names and used vulgar language. His peers frequently engaged in arguments with Phil, instead of ignoring his behavior. Typically Mrs. Moore reprimanded him, but when Phil continued to argue with his peers, he was required to work on the assignment alone. Phil was prescribed Intuniv and Concerta to manage symptoms of ADHD.

The school psychologist conducted three 15-minute systematic direct observations. During one observation of whole-group instruction, Phil was on-task 85% of the time, inattentive 12% of the time, and disruptive 3% of the time. A second observation showed he was on-task 75% of the time, inattentive 20% of the time, and disruptive 15% of the time during circle time. The final observation was conducted during a group activity. Phil was on-task 80% of the time and disruptive 20% of the time. Most disruptions included shouting at and arguing with peers for not following directions given by the teacher.

After reviewing the student's cumulative record and speaking with Phil's teacher, the school psychologist determined there were no academic concerns. He was earning A's and B's in all core subjects.

Target Behavior

Inappropriate peer interactions: Inappropriate peer interactions include not getting along with others, not staying calm during disagreements, verbal aggression, name calling, raising his voice toward peers, negative communication or arguing, and vulgar language toward peers.

Intervention Procedures

The school psychologist introduced the teacher to a DRC intervention for Phil. Mrs. Moore would rate Phil throughout the day on his prosocial behavior, including cooperation with students during group work, using kind words when speaking to others, compromising during disagreements, and remaining calm when disagreeing with others. Based on Mrs. Moore's ratings on the DRC, Phil could earn a reward at the end of the day for demonstrating prosocial behavior.

At the beginning of the day, Mrs. Moore told Phil the goal number of points for the day, gave examples and nonexamples of prosocial behavior, and reminded him that he could earn a reward at the end of the day if he met his goal. The teacher allowed Phil to choose the reward he wanted to work for that day. Phil kept the report card on his desk, and the teacher reminded him at the beginning of each activity of the appropriate behaviors.

Mrs. Moore monitored Phil's behavior during seven time periods. At the end of each time period, Mrs. Moore rated Phil on his prosocial behavior, reviewed his behavior with him, and praised him for appropriate behavior or encouraged him to try again in the next period. Phil earned 1 point if he demonstrated prosocial behavior throughout most

of the time period or 0 points if he engaged in inappropriate peer interactions.

The total number of points possible by the end of the day was 7.
His initial goal was 5 points. At the end of the day, if Phil had earned
at least 5 points, Mrs. Moore praised him, and he earned his reward. If
he did not meet his goal, Mrs. Moore discussed with him how he could
improve his behavior and reminded him that he could earn a reward the
next day.

Along with the DRC, the teacher praised him more often throughout the day when he interacted positively with peers. She also increased
supervision during group activities in order to provide more praise.
Baseline data were collected by having Mrs. Moore complete the DRC
for six days without providing feedback or a reward to Phil. Treatment integrity was monitored by collecting the DRCs, a permanent
product of the intervention, but the school psychologist also checked in
with Mrs. Moore weekly to collect data and monitor progress (Figure
10.10).

Results

With implementation of the DRC intervention, Phil's inappropriate peer
interactions decreased. During baseline, Phil exhibited negative behavior

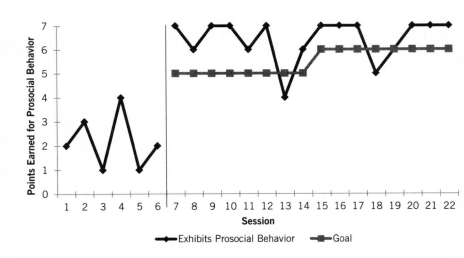

FIGURE 10.10. DRC points for Phil.

toward peers multiple times throughout the day. When his teacher began providing praise and rewarding him for prosocial behavior in a systematic way with the DRC, Phil's prosocial behavior increased immediately so that he was meeting his goal and earning 6 to 7 points consistently. Phil did not meet his goal on two days during intervention. However, given the stability of his improvement in prosocial behavior, the goal was increased. Phil continued to reach his goal in the following week. There were several days that Mrs. Moore failed to complete the DRC, resulting in a treatment integrity score of 85%.

Phil's teacher expressed that the intervention was feasible and easy to implement throughout the day. She reportedly felt more comfortable allowing him to engage in peer activities with the use of the DRC (Figure 10.11). According to Mrs. Moore, the rewards were easy to provide and Phil seemed to enjoy them.

0 = Not Yet 1 = Excellent	Getting along with others (share, take turns, work together, stay calm when disagreeing)	Total teacher rated points	Teacher initials and time of rating
Morning Work (8:20-9:00)	0 1		
Whole Group (9:00-9:45)	0 1		
ELA Centers (9:45-11:00)	0 1		
Ancillary (1:00-1:45)	0 1		
Math (1:45-2:30)	0 1		
Science/Social Studies (2:30-3:00)	0 1		
End of Day (3:00-3:15)	0 1		
Total Points _____ Goal _____		Comments:	

Did you provide a reward? (Circle one)   YES   NO

What was the reward? _____ Date _____

FIGURE 10.11. Sample DRC for Phil.

Discussion

Phil was initially exhibiting verbal aggression and engaging in other negative peer interactions. When Phil's teacher implemented the DRC, which included more frequent reminders of the appropriate behavior, regular feedback and praise, as well as a reward for appropriate behavior, Phil's behavior improved. Mrs. Moore was so impressed with Phil's behavior that she decided to implement the intervention in other settings (e.g., bus time, recess) to promote generalization of the behavior. In addition, Phil's parents were pleased that Phil had received no additional ODRs and informed Mrs. Moore that they were interested in adding a home component to the intervention. They wanted Phil to be able to work toward a larger reward on the weekends. The school psychologist contacted the parents and arranged a meeting to incorporate the home component into the intervention.

Case 8: Mark Blackwell

Student Name: Mark Blackwell
Age: 12
Grade: 6
Race/Ethnicity: Caucasian
Sex: Male

Background Information

Mark was a 12-year-old male with multiple changes in his living situation over the past several years who recently enrolled at a middle school. He had attended a number of schools across several districts and had a history of frequent suspensions for verbally and physically aggressive behaviors, such as cursing at peers and teachers, taunting and threatening to fight peers, throwing things at others, and pushing and hitting peers. When Mark first arrived at his present school, his new teacher reported that he was calm and compliant. However, several weeks later, he was involved in a number of incidences of verbal aggression against teachers and verbal and physical aggression against peers that seemed to be escalating in severity. Mark's behavior resulted in a referral to the school psychologist in an attempt to prevent more severe behaviors and to develop more appropriate behaviors.

The school psychologist began by completing a district record review on Mark, in which she discovered Mark's prior suspensions. She then conducted an interview with his teacher, Ms. Phillips, who denied that Mark had any academic deficits, citing satisfactory work completion and quality, and his near-perfect attendance record. His aggressive behaviors were her primary concern because they severely interfered with his school functioning. According to school staff accounts, Mark's behaviors included variations of physical and verbal aggression against students and adults. Ms. Phillips reported notable events occurring before his problem behaviors, including no one paying attention to Mark, students walking near him, or staff talking to each other. Notable consequences included Ms. Phillips verbally reprimanding Mark, school staff blocking and redirecting his behaviors, or other students becoming visibly upset. Most acts of aggression had so far comprised yelling and cursing at teachers and other students, and throwing things at peers. Ms. Philips reported that she suspected his aggression served to gain attention, although she indicated that Mark was capable of using appropriate methods of soliciting attention from others. At the conclusion of the interview, the school psychologist requested that Ms. Phillips begin collecting frequency data on the number of aggressive acts and appropriate requests for attention per day. The school psychologist also provided Ms. Phillips with a scatterplot chart and requested that she take data on the time and frequency of aggressive behavior occurrences throughout the day for three consecutive days to ascertain the most problematic times of day.

The scatterplot analysis revealed that while behavioral occurrences were observed throughout each day, the highest frequency appeared around late morning, typically during unstructured classroom activities. The school psychologist then proceeded to conduct descriptive antecedent–behavior–consequence (ABC) data collection for 1 hour per day across 2 days, during the late morning. This observational method produced data on the environmental events that often preceded and followed each behavior occurrence. Mark's aggression was most frequently preceded by the absence of attention. The most frequent consequence included verbal reprimands and statements by his teacher or other students.

Results of both the interview and direct observations indicated the function of Mark's behaviors was attention. Furthermore, notes in Mark's cumulative folder from previous teachers also suggested an attention function to his aggression. No documentation was available regarding attempted interventions.

Five days of baseline data showed a slight upward trend in aggressive behaviors, with 10 occurrences during day 1, 12 occurrences during day 2, and 13 occurrences during day 3, 12 occurrences during day 4, and 17 occurrences during day 5. Appropriate requests for attention remained low and steady, ranging from 0 to 3 occurrences. The school psychologist developed an intervention based on all the data collected.

Target Behaviors

1. **Physical aggression:** Any acts of physical contact against another individual with enough force to cause physical harm. Aggressive behaviors include hitting, kicking, slapping, biting, and punching.
2. **Verbal aggression:** Any instance of cursing, negative comments to others, or verbal intimidation directed toward other individuals.

Intervention Procedures

Mark's teacher implemented the following intervention procedures continuously throughout each day with the goal of decreasing his aggressive behaviors and increasing appropriate requests for attention (e.g., vocally requesting attention in a socially appropriate manner, including calling one's name, greeting someone, or requesting help).

The school psychologist introduced a proactive strategy to Ms. Phillips as part of a multicomponent intervention to address Mark's problem behavior. She trained Ms. Phillips to implement noncontingent reinforcement (NCR), or scheduled attention, in which she provided attention to Mark unconditionally every 20 minutes, in the form of social praise, conversation, and so forth. Ms. Phillips placed a vibrating timer set to go off every 20 minutes in her pocket to remind her to provide attention.

When Mark appropriately solicited attention from others by asking for help or calling one's name, his behavior was reinforced with such attention each time it occurred. Inappropriate solicitations (e.g., verbal and physical aggression) were purposefully ignored. In addition, a point system was put into place that consisted of Mark earning a point for each 15-minute interval absent of verbal or physical aggression (i.e., differential reinforcement of zero rates of responding; DR0). Points were removed contingent on any act of aggression. Points could be exchanged at the end of each day for a prize from a treasure chest. A survey was administered to Mark prior to the construction of the treasure chest to learn what kinds of items he preferred.

To reduce the amount of peer attention provided to Mark for his inappropriate behavior, all students within the classroom were placed on an interdependent group contingency point system. When a student was observed by the teacher ignoring Mark's aggressive behaviors, and subsequently reported to the teacher that such behaviors occurred against him or her, the class earned a point. Conversely, the class lost a point if any student provided direct attention to Mark as a result of his aggressive behaviors (e.g., "Hey, don't say that!"). A cumulative goal number of points eventually earned the class a pizza party.

All established crisis prevention protocols remained in place in the event Mark's behaviors became a danger to himself or others. The school psychologist using a behavior checklist measured treatment integrity every 3 days. Treatment acceptability was also measured at the end of the intervention through the *Usage Rating Profile-Intervention*, a treatment acceptability scale administered to Mark's teacher.

Results

Baseline data demonstrated a gradual increasing trend in aggressive behaviors with an average of 13 occurrences (Figure 10.12). Once an intervention was implemented, an immediate change in level occurred, along with a visible decreasing trend. Aggressive behavior was nearly eliminated by the end of the 2-week intervention. Furthermore, a substantial increase in appropriate solicitations of attention was observed as aggressive behaviors decreased. The school psychologist reported average fidelity of treatment implementation at 87%. Results of the treatment acceptability scale completed by Ms. Phillips indicated high acceptability and appropriateness of the treatment. Finally, Ms. Phillips

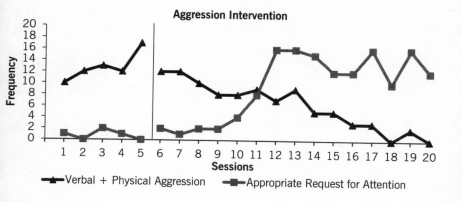

FIGURE 10.12. Frequency of aggressive behavior for Mark.

expressed satisfaction with the results of the intervention, indicating Mark's change in behavior served to reinforce her continuation of the intervention.

Discussion

The primary goals of the intervention were to extinguish Mark's aggressive behaviors and increase appropriate methods of soliciting attention so that he could be successful in school. The multicomponent intervention illustrated the effectiveness of a function-based classroom intervention in achieving such goals. The next step was to gradually fade the intervention by increasing the duration of the planned attention (i.e., NCR) schedule, increasing the interval of the differential reinforcement point system, and beginning to reinforce socially appropriate attention-seeking behaviors intermittently.

References

Achenbach, T., & Rescorla, L. (2000). *Manual for the ASEBA preschool forms and profiles.* Burlington: University of Vermont, Department of Psychiatry.

Achenbach, T., & Rescorla, L. (2001). *Manual for the ASEBA school-age forms and profiles.* Burlington: University of Vermont, Department of Psychiatry.

Ager, C., & Cole, C. (1991). A review of cognitive-behavioral interventions for children and adolescents with behavioral disorders. *Behavioral Disorders, 16,* 276–287.

Alberto, P., & Troutman, A. (2009). *Applied behavior analysis for teachers* (8th ed.). Upper Saddle River, NJ: Pearson/Merrill/Prentice Hall.

American Psychiatric Association. (2013). *Diagnostic and statistical manual of mental disorders* (5th ed.). Arlington, VA: Author.

American Psychological Association. (2004). *Working group on psychoactive medications in children.* Washington, DC: Author.

Anderson, C., & Borgmeier, C. (2010). Tier II interventions within the framework of school-wide behavior support: Essential features for design, implementation, and maintenance. *Behavior Analysis and Practice, 3*(1), 33–45.

Anderson, J., Williams, S., McGee, R., & Silva, P. (1987). DSM-III disorders in preadolescent children: Prevalence in a large sample from the general population. *Archives of General Psychiatry, 44,* 69–76.

Ang, R., & Hughes, J. (2001). Differential benefits of skills training with antisocial youth based on group composition: A meta-analytic investigation. *School Psychology Review, 31,* 164–185.

Arnold, C., Kuller, L., & Greenlick, M. (Eds.). (1981). *Advances in disease prevention* (Vol. 1). New York: Springer.

Azrin, N., & Besalel, V. (1999). *How to use positive practice, self-correction and overcorrection* (2nd ed.). Austin, TX: PRO-ED.

Baer, D. M. (1977). "Perhaps it would be better not to know everything." *Journal of Applied Behavior Analysis, 10*, 167–172.

Baer, D. M., Wolf, M. M., & Risley, T. R. (1968). Some current dimensions of applied behavior analysis. *Journal of Applied Behavior Analysis, 1*, 91–97.

Bandura, A. (1977). *Social learning theory*. Englewood Cliffs, NJ: Prentice Hall.

Bandura, A. (1986). *Social foundations of thought and action: A social cognitive theory*. Englewood Cliffs, NJ: Prentice Hall.

Barkley, R. (2006). *Attention-deficit hyperactivity disorder: A handbook for diagnosis and treatment* (3rd ed.). New York: Guilford Press.

Barkley, R. A. (2007). School interventions for attention deficit hyperactive disorder: Where to from here? *School Psychology Review, 36*(2), 279–286.

Barnett, D., Daly, E., Jones, K., & Lentz, F. E. (2004). Response to intervention: Empirically based special service decisions for increasing and decreasing intensity using single case designs. *Journal of Special Education, 38*, 66–79.

Barrish, H., Saunders, M., & Wolf, M. M. (1969). Good Behavior Game: Effects on individual contingencies for group consequences on disruptive behavior in a classroom. *Journal of Applied Behavior Analysis, 2*, 119–124.

Beelmann, A., Pfingsten, U., & Losel, F. (1994). Effects of training social competence in children: A meta-analysis of recent evaluation studies. *Journal of Clinical Child Psychology, 23*, 260–271.

Bergan, J. (1977). *Behavioral consultation*. Columbus, OH: Merrill.

Bergan, J., & Kratochwill, T. (1990). *Behavioral consultation and therapy*. New York: Plenum Press.

Bernal, M., Klinnert, M., & Schultz, L. (1980). Outcome evaluation of behavioral parent training and client-centered parent counseling for children with conduct problems. *Journal of Applied Behavior Analysis, 13*, 677–691.

Bierman, K. L., & Powers, C. J. (2009). Social skills training to improve peer relations. In K. Rubin, W. Bukowski, & B. Laursen (Eds.), *Handbook of peer interactions, relationships, and groups* (pp. 603–621). New York: Guilford Press.

Blouin, A., Bornstein, R., & Trites, R. (1978). Teen-age alcohol use among hyperactive children: A five-year follow-up study. *Journal of Pediatric Psychology, 3*, 188–194.

Bracht, G., & Glass, G. (1968). The external validity of experiments. *American Educational Research Journal, 5*, 437–474.

Bronfenbrenner, U. (1979). *The ecology of human development: Experiments by design and nature*. Cambridge, MA: Harvard University Press.

Bukowski, W. (1991). *A framework for drug abuse prevention research:*

Methodological issues. Retrieved October 30, 2003, from *www.nida. nih.gov/pdf/monographs/107/pdf.*

Bullis, M., & Walker, H. M. (1994). *Comprehensive school-based systems for troubled youth.* Eugene: University of Oregon, Institute on Violent and Destructive Behavior.

Burns, B., & Hoagwood, K. (2002). *Community treatment for youth: Evidence-based interventions for severe emotional and behavioral disorders.* New York: Oxford University Press.

Busk, P., & Serlin, R. (1992). Meta-analysis for single-case research. In T. Kratochwill & J. Levin (Eds.), *Single-case design and analysis* (pp. 187–212). Hillsdale, NJ: Erlbaum.

Caldarella, P., & Merrell, K. (1997). Common dimensions of social skills in children and adolescents: Taxonomy of positive social behaviors. *School Psychology Review, 26,* 265–279.

Caprara, G., Barbaranelli, C., Pastorelli, C., Bandura, A., & Zimbardo, P. (2000). Prosocial foundations of children's academic achievement. *Psychological Science, 11,* 302–305.

Carr, E. (1994). Emerging themes in functional analysis of problem behavior. *Journal of Applied Behavior Analysis, 27,* 393–400.

Chafouleas, S., McDougal, J., Riley-Tillman, C., Panahon, C., & Hilt, A. (2005). What do daily behavior report cards (DBRCs) measure?: An initial comparison of DBRCs with direct observation for off-task behavior. *Psychology in the Schools, 42,* 669–676.

Chafouleas, S., Riley-Tillman, C., & McDougal, J. (2002). Good, bad, or in-between: How does the daily behavior report card rate? *Psychology in the Schools, 39,* 157–169.

Chamberlain, P., & Patterson, G. R. (1995). Discipline and child compliance in parenting. In M. H. Bornstein (Ed.), *Handbook of parenting* (Vol. 4, pp. 205–225). Hillsdale, NJ: Erlbaum.

Chamberlain, P., & Reid, J. (1998). Comparison of two community alternatives to incarceration of chronic juvenile offenders. *Journal of Consulting and Clinical Psychology, 66,* 624–633.

Chambless, D., & Hollon, S. (1998). Defining empirically supported therapies. *Journal of Consulting and Clinical Psychology, 66,* 7–18.

Chenier, J., Fisher, A., Hunter, K., Patty, E., Libster, L., O'Leary, K., et al. (2011, February). *What works regarding social skills interventions using single subject designs?* Symposium presented at the annual meeting of the National Association of School Psychologists, San Francisco, CA.

Christensen, A., Johnson, S., Phillips, S., & Glasgow, R. (1980). Cost effectiveness in behavioral family therapy. *Behavior Therapy, 11,* 208–226.

Cohen, J. (1988). *Statistical power analysis for the behavioral sciences* (2nd ed.). Hillsdale, NJ: Erlbaum.

Coie, J., & Jacobs, M. (1993). The role of social context in the prevention of conduct disorder [Special issue]. *Development and Psychopathology, 5,* 26–27.

Coie, J., Dodge, K., & Coppotelli, H. (1982). Dimensions and types of social status: A cross-age perspective. *Developmental Psychology, 18,* 557–570.

Coie, J., Dodge, K., & Kupersmidt, J. (1990). Peer group behavior and social status. In S. Asher & J. Coie (Eds.), *Peer rejection in childhood* (pp. 17–59). New York: Cambridge University Press.

Coie, J., Watt, N., West, S., Hawkins, J., Asarnow, J, Markman, H., et al. (1993). The science of prevention: A conceptual framework and some directions for a national research program. *American Psychologist, 48,* 1013–1022.

Coleman, M., Wheeler, L., & Webber, J. (1993). Research on interpersonal problem-solving training: A review. *Remedial and Special Education, 14,* 25–36.

Colvin, G., Kame'enui, E., & Sugai, G. (1993). School-wide and classroom management: Reconceptualizing the integration and management of students with behavior problems in general education. *Education and Treatment of Children, 16,* 361–381.

Colvin, G., & Sugai, G. (1989). *Managing escalating behavior.* Available from Behavior Associates, PO Box 5317, Eugene, OR 97405.

Conduct Problems Prevention Group. (1992). A developmental and clinical model for the prevention of conduct disorder: The Fast Track Program. *Development and Psychopathology, 4,* 509–527.

Conduct Problems Prevention Group. (1999). Initial impact of the Fast Track prevention trial for conduct problems: I. The high risk sample. *Journal of Consulting and Clinical Psychology, 67,* 648–657.

Conduct Problems Prevention Group. (2002). Evaluation of the first three years of the Fast Track prevention trial with children at high risk for adolescent conduct problems. *Journal of Abnormal Child Psychology, 30,* 19–35.

Conners, C. K. (1997). *Conners Rating Scales—Revised manual.* New York: Multi-Health Systems.

Cook, C. R., Gresham, F. M., Kern, L., Barreras, R. B., Thornton, S., & Crews, S. D. (2008). Social skills training with secondary EBD students: A review and analysis of the meta-analytic literature. *Journal of Emotional and Behavioral Disorders, 16,* 131–144.

Cook, C. R., Volpe, R. J., & Delport, J. (2014). Systematic progress monitoring of students with emotional and behavioral disorders: The promise of change-sensitive brief behavior rating scales. In H. M. Walker & F. M. Gresham (Eds.), *Handbook of evidence-based practices for emotional and behavioral disorders: Applications in schools* (pp. 211–228). New York: Guilford Press.

Cooper, J., Heron, T., & Heward, W. (2007). *Applied behavior analysis* (2nd ed.). Upper Saddle River, NJ: Prentice Hall.

Cottle, C., Lee, R., & Heilbrun, K. (2001). The prediction of criminal recidivism in juveniles: A meta-analysis. *Criminal Justice and Behavior, 28,* 367–394.

Crews, S. D., Bender, H., Cook, C., Gresham, F. M., Kern, L., & Vanderwood, M. (2007). Risk and protective factors of emotional and/or behavioral disorders in children and adolescents: A mega-analytic synthesis. *Behavioral Disorders, 32,* 64–77.

Crick, N., & Dodge, K. (1994). A review and reformulation of social-information processing mechanisms in children's social adjustment. *Psychological Bulletin, 115,* 74–101.

Crone, D., Hawken, L., & Horner, R. (2010). *Responding to problem behavior in schools: The Behavior Education Program* (2nd ed.). New York: Guilford Press.

Crone, D., & Horner, R. (2003). *Building positive behavioral support systems in schools: Functional behavioral assessments.* New York: Guilford Press.

Crone, D., Horner, R., & Hawken, L. (2004). *Responding to problem behavior in schools: The Behavior Education Program.* New York: Guilford Press.

Darch, C., & Kame'enui. E. (2004). *Instructional classroom management: A proactive approach to behavior management* (2nd ed.). Upper Saddle, NJ: Merrill/Prentice Hall.

Darwin, C. (1859). *Origin of species.* Available through Wikipedia.

De Los Reyes, A., & Kazdin, A. (2005). Informant discrepancies in the assessment of childhood psychopathology: A critical review, theoretical framework, and recommendations for further study. *Psychological Bulletin, 131,* 483–509.

Del'Homme, M., Sinclair, E., & Kasari, C. (1994). Preschool children with behavioral problems: Observation in instructional and free play contexts. *Behavioral Disorders, 19,* 221–232.

Denton, C., & Vaughn, S. (2010). Preventing and remediating reading difficulties: Perspectives from research. In M. Shinn & H. Walker (Eds.), *Interventions for achievement and behavior problems in a three-tier model including RTI* (pp. 469–500). Bethesda, MD: National Association of School Psychologists.

Dinsmoor, J. (1995). Stimulus control: Part I. *The Behavior Analyst, 18,* 51–68.

DiPerma, J., & Elliott, S. N. (2000). *Academic Competence Evaluation Scale.* Minneapolis, MN: Pearson Assessments.

DiPerma, J., & Elliott, S. N. (2002). Promoting academic enablers to improve student achievement: An introduction to the miniseries. *School Psychology Review, 31,* 293–297.

Dishion, T. (1990). The peer context of troublesome child and adolescent behavior. In P. Leone (Ed.), *Understanding troubled and troubling youth: Multidisciplinary perspective* (pp. 128–153). Newbury Park, CA: Sage.

Dishion, T., & Andrews, D. (1995). Preventing escalation in problem behaviors with high-risk, young adolescents: Immediate and one-year outcomes. *Journal of Consulting and Clinical Psychology, 63,* 1–11.

Dishion, T., Patterson, G., Stoolmiller, M., & Skinner, M. (1991). Family, school, and behavioral antecedents to early adolescent involvement with antisocial peers. *Developmental Psychology, 27,* 172–180.

Dishion, T., & Stormshak, E. (2007). *Intervening in children's lives: An ecological family-centered approach to mental health care.* Washington, DC: American Psychological Association.

Dodge, K. (1986). A social information processing model of social competence in children. In M. Perlmutter (Ed.), *Minnesota Symposium on Child Psychology* (Vol. 18, pp. 77–125). Hillsdale, NJ: Erlbaum.

Dodge, K,. Dishion, T., & Lansford, J. (Eds.). (2006). *Deviant peer influences in programs for youth: Problems and solutions.* New York: Guilford Press.

Drummond, T. (1993). *The Student Risk Screening Scale.* Grants Pass, OR: Josephine County Mental Health Program.

Dryfoos, J. (1990). *Adolescents at risk: Prevalence and prevention.* New York: Oxford University Press.

Dunlap, G., & Fox, L. (2014). Supportive interventions for young children with social, emotional, and behavioral delays and disorders. In H. M. Walker & F. M. Gresham (Eds.), *Handbook of evidence-based practices for emotional and behavioral disorders: Application in schools* (pp. 503–533). New York: Guilford Press.

DuPaul, G., Laracy, S., & Gormley, M. (2014). Interventions for students with attention-deficit/hyperactivity disorder: School and home contexts. In H. M. Walker & F. M. Gresham (Eds.), *Handbook of evidence-based practices for emotional and behavioral disorders: Applications in schools* (pp. 292–306). New York: Guilford Press.

Eber, L., Malloy, J. M., Rose, J., & Flamini, A. (2014). School-based wraparound for adolescents: The RENEW model. In H. M. Walker & F. M. Gresham (Eds.), *Handbook of evidence-based practices for emotional and behavioral disorders: Applications in schools* (pp. 378–393). New York: Guilford Press.

Eddy, J., Reid, J., & Curry, V. (2002). The etiology of youth antisocial behavior, delinquency, and violence in a public health approach to prevention. In M. Shinn, H. Walker, & G. Stoner (Eds.), *Interventions for academic and behavior problems: II. Preventive and remedial approaches* (pp. 27–51). Bethesda, MD: National Association of School Psychologists.

Elliott, S. N. (1988). Acceptability of behavioral treatments in educational settings. In J. C. Witt, S. N. Elliott, & F. M. Gresham (Eds.), *Handbook of behavior therapy in education* (pp. 121–150). New York: Plenum Press.

Elliott, S. N., & Gresham, F. M. (2007). *Social Skills Improvement System:*

Classwide Intervention Program Teacher's Guide. Minneapolis, MN: Pearson Assessments.

Elliott, S. N., & Gresham, F. M. (2008). *Social Skills Improvement System: Intervention Guide.* Minneapolis, MN: Pearson Assessments.

Embry, D. D. (2002). The Good Behavior Game: A best practice candidate as a universal behavioral vaccine. *Clinical Child and Family Review, 5,* 273–297.

Erchul W., & Sheridan, S. (Eds.) (2014). *Handbook of research in school consultation* (2nd ed.). New York: Routledge.

Evans, I., Meyer, L., Kurkjian, J., & Kishi, G. (1988). An evaluation of behavioral interrelationships in child behavior therapy. In J. C. Witt, S. N. Elliott, & F. M. Gresham (Eds.), *Handbook of behavior therapy in education* (pp. 189–216). New York: Plenum Press.

Eyberg, S. M., Nelson, M. M., & Boggs, S. R. (2008). Evidence-based psychosocial treatments for children and adolescents with disruptive behavior. *Journal of Clinical Child and Adolescent Psychology, 37,* 215–237.

Fairbanks, S., Sugai, G., Guardino, D., & Lathrop, M. (2007). Response to intervention: Examining classroom behavior support in second grade. *Exceptional Children, 73,* 288–310.

Fawcett, S. (1991). Social validity: A note on methodology. *Journal of Applied Behavior Analysis, 24,* 235–239.

Feil, E., Frey, A., Small, J., Seeley, J., Golly, A., & Walker, H. (2014). *The efficacy of a home–school intervention for preschoolers with challenging behaviors: A randomized controlled trial of Preschool First Step to Success.* Manuscript under review.

Filter, K., McKenna, M., Benedict, E., Horner, R., Todd, A., & Watson, J. (2007). Check in/check out: A post-hoc evaluation of an efficient, secondary-level targeted intervention for reducing problem behavior in schools. *Education and Treatment of Children, 30,* 69–84.

Flay, B., Biglan, A., Boruch, R., Castro, F., Gottfredson, D., Kellam, S., et al. (2005). Standards of evidence: Criteria for efficacy, effectiveness, and dissemination. *Prevention Science, 6*(3), 151–175.

Forehand, R., Middlebrook, J., Rogers, T., & Steffe, M. (1983). Dropping out of parent training. *Behaviour Research and Therapy, 21,* 663–668.

Forness, S., Kim, J., & Walker, H. M. (2012). Prevalence of students with EBD: Impact on General Education. *Beyond Behavior, 21*(2), 3–10.

Forness, S., Walker, H., & Serna, L. (2014). Establishing an evidence base: Lessons learned from implementing randomized controlled trials for behavioral and pharmacological interventions. In H. M. Walker & F. M. Gresham (Eds.) *Handbook of evidence-based practices for emotional and behavioral disorders: Applications in schools* (pp. 567–583). New York: Guilford Press.

Fraser, M. (Ed.). (1997). *Risk and resilience in childhood: An ecological perspective.* Washington, DC: NASW Press.

Fraser, M., & Galinsky, M. (1997). Toward a resilience-based model of practice. In M. Fraser (Ed.), *Risk and resilience in childhood: An ecological perspective* (pp. 265–275). Washington, DC: NASW Press.

Frey, A., Small, J., Forness, S., Feil, E., Seeley, J., & Walker, H. (2014). *First Step to Success: Applications to preschools at risk of developing autism spectrum disorders*. Manuscript under review.

Gage, N., Lewis, T., & Stichter, J. (2012). Functional behavioral assessment-based interventions for students with or at risk for emotional and/or behavioral disorders in school: A hierarchical linear modeling meta-analysis. *Behavioral Disorders, 37,* 55–77.

Godbold, E., Vance, M., Chenier, J., Rodriguez, J., Menesses, K., Libster, L., et al. (2010, February). *Evidence-based social skills interventions: What really works*. Symposium presented at the annual meeting of the National Association of School Psychologists, Chicago, IL.

Gorman-Smith, D. (2006). *How to successfully implement evidence-based social programs: A brief overview for policy makers and program providers*. Washington, DC: Coalition for Evidence-Based Policy.

Greenberg, M., Domitrovich, C., & Bumbarger, B. (2001). The prevention of mental disorders in school-age children: Current state of the field. *Prevention and Treatment, 4,* 191–213.

Greenberg, M., Speltz, M., & DeKylen, M. (1993). The role of attachment in the early development of disruptive behavior problems. *Development and Psychopathology, 5,* 191–213.

Gresham, F. M. (1981a). Assessment of children's social skills. *Journal of School Psychology, 19,* 120–134.

Gresham, F. M. (1981b). Social skills training with handicapped children: A review. *Review of Educational Research, 51,* 139–176.

Gresham, F. M. (1985). Utility of cognitive-behavioral procedures for social skills training with children: A review. *Journal of Abnormal Child Psychology, 13,* 411–433.

Gresham, F. M. (1986). Conceptual issues in the assessment of social competence in children. In P. Strain, M. Guralnick, & H. Walker (Eds.), *Children's social behavior: Development, assessment, and modification* (pp. 143–180). New York: Academic Press.

Gresham, F. M. (1991). Conceptualizing behavior disorders in terms of resistance to intervention. *School Psychology Review, 20,* 23–36.

Gresham, F. M. (1998). Social skills training: Should we raze, remodel, or rebuild? *Behavioral Disorders, 24,* 19–25.

Gresham, F. M. (2002). Responsiveness to intervention: An alternative approach to the identification of learning disabilities. In R. Bradley, L. Danielson, & D. Hallahan (Eds.), *Identification of learning disabilities: Research to practice* (pp. 467–520). Mahwah, NJ: Lawrence Erlbaum.

Gresham, F. M. (2004). Current status and future directions of school-based behavioral interventions. *School Psychology Review, 33,* 326–343.

Gresham, F. M. (2005). Response to intervention: An alternative means of identifying students as emotionally disturbed. *Education and Treatment of Children, 28,* 328–344.

Gresham, F. M. (2007). Evolution of the response-to-intervention concept: Empirical foundations and recent developments. In S. Jimmerson, M. Burns, & A. VanDerHeyden (Eds.), *Handbook of response to intervention: The science and practice of assessment and intervention* (pp. 10–24). New York: Springer.

Gresham, F. M. (2010). Evidence-based social skills interventions: Empirical foundations for instructional approaches. In M. Shinn & H. Walker (Eds.), *Interventions for achievement and behavior problems in a three-tier model including RTI* (pp. 337–362). Bethesda, MD: National Association of School Psychologists.

Gresham, F. M. (2011). Social behavior assessment and intervention: Observations and impressions. *School Psychology Review, 40,* 275–283.

Gresham, F. M. (2014). Treatment integrity within a three-tiered model. In H. M. Walker & F. M. Gresham (Eds.), *Handbook of evidence-based practices for emotional and behavioral disorders* (pp. 446–456). New York: Guilford Press.

Gresham, F. M., & Elliott, S. N. (1990). *Social Skills Rating System.* Minneapolis, MN: Pearson Assessments.

Gresham, F. M., & Elliott, S. N. (2008). *Social Skills Improvement System: Rating Scales Manual.* Minneapolis, MN: Pearson Assessments.

Gresham, F. M., & Elliott, S. N. (2014). Social skills assessment and training in emotional and behavioral disorders. In H. M. Walker & F. M. Gresham (Eds.), *Handbook of evidence-based practices for emotional and behavioral disorders* (pp. 152–172). New York: Guilford Press.

Gresham, F. M., Elliott, S. N., & Kettler, R. (2011). Base rates of social skills acquisition, performance deficits, strengths, and problem behaviors: An analysis of the Social Skills Improvement System-Rating Scales. *Psychological Assessment, 22,* 809–815.

Gresham, F. M., Gansle, K., Noell, G., Cohen, S., & Rosenblum, S. (1993). Treatment integrity of school-based behavioral intervention studies: 1980–1990. *School Psychology Review, 22,* 254–272.

Gresham, F. M., & Gresham, G. N. (1982). Interdependent, dependent, and independent group contingencies for controlling disruptive behavior. *Journal of Special Education, 16,* 101–110.

Gresham, F. M., & Lambros, K. M. (1998). Behavioral and functional assessment. In T. S. Watson & F. M. Gresham (Eds.), *Handbook of child behavior therapy* (pp. 3–22). New York: Plenum Press.

Gresham, F. M., Lane, K. L., & Lambros, K. M. (2000). Comorbidity of conduct problems and ADHD: Identification of "fledgling psychopaths." *Journal of Emotional and Behavioral Disorders, 8,* 83–93.

Gresham, F. M., Lane, K. L., McIntyre, L., Olson-Tinker, H., Dolstra, L., MacMillan, D., et al. (2001). Risk factors associated with the co-occurrence of hyperactivity–impulsivity–inattention and conduct problems. *Behavioral Disorders, 26,* 189–199.

Gresham, F. M., & Lochman, J. E. (2009). Methodological issues in research using cognitive-behavioral interventions. In M. Mayer, R. Van Acker, J. Lochman, & F. M. Gresham (Eds.), *Cognitive-behavioral interventions for emotional and behavioral disorders* (pp. 58–81). New York: Guilford Press.

Gresham, F. M., & Lopez, M. F. (1996). Social validation: A unifying concept for school-based consultation research and practice. *School Psychology Quarterly, 11,* 204–227.

Gresham, F. M., MacMillan, D., Beebe-Frankenberger, M., & Bocian, K. (2000). Treatment integrity in learning disabilities intervention research: Do we really know how treatments are implemented? *Learning Disabilities Research and Practice, 15,* 198–205.

Gresham, F. M., MacMillan, D. L., Bocian, K., Ward, S., & Forness, S. (1998). Comorbidity of hyperactivity-impulsivity-inattention + conduct problems: Risk factors in social, affective, and academic domains. *Journal of Abnormal Child Psychology, 26,* 393–406.

Gresham, F. M., & Nagle, R. J. (1980). Social skills training with children: Responsiveness to modeling and coaching as a function of peer orientation. *Journal of Consulting and Clinical Psychology, 48,* 718–729.

Gresham, F. M., & Noell, G. H. (1993). Documenting the effectiveness of consultation outcomes. In J. Zins, T. Kratochwill, & S. Elliott (Eds.), *Handbook of consultation services for children* (pp. 249–276). San Francisco: Jossey-Bass.

Gresham, F. M., Reschly, D. J., & Shinn, M. (2010). RTI as a driving force in educational improvement: Research, legal, and practice perspectives. In M. Shinn & H. M. Walker (Eds.), *Interventions for achievement and behavior problems in a three-tier model including RTI* (pp. 47–78). Bethesda, MD: National Association of School Psychologists.

Gresham, F. M., Sugai, G., & Horner, R. (2001). Interpreting outcomes of social skills training for students with high-incidence disabilities. *Exceptional Children, 67,* 331–344.

Gresham, F. M., Van, M., & Cook, C. R. (2006). Social skills training for teaching replacement behaviors: Remediation of acquisition deficits for at-risk children. *Behavioral Disorders, 30,* 32–46.

Gresham, F. M., Watson, T. S., & Skinner, C. H. (2001). Functional behavioral assessment: Principles, procedures, and future directions. *School Psychology Review, 30,* 156–172.

Gumpel, T. P. (2007). Are social competence difficulties caused by performance or acquisition deficits?: The importance of self-regulatory mechanisms. *Psychology in the Schools, 44,* 351–372.

Haley, J. (1976). *Problem solving therapy.* San Francisco: Jossey-Bass.

Hanf, C. (1969). *A two-stage program for modifying maternal controlling during mother–child interaction.* Paper presented at the meeting of the Western Psychological Association, Vancouver, BC, Canada.

Hanf, C. (1970). *Shaping mothers to shape their children's behavior.* Unpublished manuscript, University of Oregon Medical School.

Hawken, L. (2006). School psychologists as leaders in the implementation of a targeted intervention: The Behavior Education Program (BEP). *School Psychology Quarterly, 21,* 91–111.

Hawken, L., MacLeod, K., & Rawlings, L. (2007). Effects of the Behavior Education Program (BEP) on problem behavior with elementary school students. *Journal of Positive Behavioral Interventions, 9,* 94–101.

Hawken, L., Vincent, C., & Schuman, J. (2008). Response to intervention for social behavior: Challenges and opportunities. *Journal of Emotional and Behavioral Disorders. 16,* 213–225.

Hawkins, R. (1991). Is social validity what we are interested in? *Journal of Applied Behavior Analysis, 24,* 205–213.

Hayes, S., Nelson, R., & Jarrett, R. (1987). The treatment utility of assessment: A functional approach to evaluating assessment quality. *American Psychologist, 42,* 963–974.

Henggeler, S. W., & Lee, T. (2003). Multisystemic treatment of serious conduct problems. In A. Kazdin & J. Weisz (Eds.), *Evidence-based psychotherapies for children and adolescents* (pp. 301–322). New York: Guilford Press.

Henggeler, S., Melton, G., & Smith, L. (1992). Family preservation using multisystemic therapy: An effective alternative to incarcerating serious juvenile offenders. *Journal of Consulting and Clinical Psychology, 60,* 953–961.

Henggeler, S. W., Pickrel, S., Brondino, M., & Crouch, J. (1996). Eliminating (almost) treatment dropout of substance abusing or dependent delinquents through home-based multisystemic therapy. *American Journal of Psychiatry, 153,* 427–428.

Hennekens, C., & Buring, J. (1987). Measures of disease frequency and association. In S. Mayrent (Ed.), *Epidemiology in medicine* (pp. 54–98). Boston: Little, Brown.

Herman, K., Reinke, W., Frey, A., & Shepard, S. (2014). *Motivational interviewing in schools.* New York: Springer.

Herrnstein, R. (1961). Relative and absolute strength of a response as a function of the frequency of reinforcement. *Journal of the Experimental Analysis of Behavior, 4,* 267–272.

Herrnstein, R. (1970). On the law of effect. *Journal of the Experimental Analysis of Behavior, 13,* 243–266.

Hinshaw, S. (1992). Externalizing behavior problems and academic underachievement in childhood and adolescence: Causal relationships and underlying mechanisms. *Psychological Bulletin, 111,* 127–155.

Hollinger, J. (1987). Social skills for behaviorally disordered children as preparation for mainstreaming: Theory, practice, and new directions. *Remedial and Special Education, 8,* 17–27.

Horner, R., & Billingsley, F. (1988). The effects of competing behavior on the generalization and maintenance of adaptive behavior in applied settings. In R. Horner, G. Dunlap, & R. Koegel (Eds.), *Generalization and maintenance: Lifestyle changes in applied settings* (pp. 197–220). Baltimore, MD: Brookes.

Horner, R. H., Carr, E. G., Halle, J., McGee, G., Odom, S., & Wolery, M. (2005). The use of single-subject research to identify evidence-based practice in special education. *Exceptional Children, 71,* 165–179.

Horner, R., Sugai, G., Smolkowski, K., Todd, A., Nakasato, J., & Esperanza, J. (2009). A randomized control trial of school-wide positive behavior support in elementary schools. *Journal of Positive Behavioral Interventions, 11,* 133–144.

Horner, R., Sugai, G., & Todd, A. (1994). *Effective behavioral support in schools.* Field initiated research proposal submitted to the U.S. Department of Education. Eugene: Education and Community Supports, University of Oregon.

Hughes, R., & Wilson, P. (1988). Behavioral parent training: With or without participation of the child. *Child and Family Behavior Therapy, 10,* 11–23.

Hymel, S., & Asher, S. (1977, April). *Assessment and training of isolated children's social skills.* Paper presented at the biennial meeting of the Society for Research in Child Development, New Orleans, LA.

Irvin, L., Tobin, T., Sprague, J., Sugai, G., & Vincent, C. (2004). Validity of office discipline referral measures as indices of school-wide behavioral status and effects of school-wide behavioral interventions. *Journal of Positive Behavior Interventions, 6*(3), 131–147.

Issaacson, W. (2007). *Einstein: His life and universe.* New York: Simon & Schuster.

Iwata, B., Dorsey, M., Slifer, K., Bauman, K., & Richman, G. (1982/1994). Toward a functional analysis of self-injury. *Journal of Applied Behavior Analysis, 27,* 3–20.

Iwata, B., & Smith, R. (2007). Negative reinforcement. In J. Cooper, T. Heron, & W. Seward (Eds.), *Applied behavior analysis* (2nd ed., pp. 291–303). Upper Saddle River, NJ: Pearson/Prentice Hall.

Jacobson, N., Follette, W., & Revenstorf, D. (1984). Psychotherapy outcome research: Methods for reporting variability and evaluating clinical significance. *Behavior Therapy, 15,* 336–352.

Jacobvitz, D., Sroufe, L., Stewart, M., & Leffert, N. (1990). Treatment of attentional and hyperactivity problems in children with sympathoimetic drugs: A comprehensive review. *Journal of the American Academy of Child and Adolescent Psychiatry, 29,* 677–688.

Jensen, P., & Cooper, J. (2002). *Attention deficit hyperactivity disorder: State of the science.* New York: Civic Research Institute.

Jessor, R., Van Den Bos, J., Vanderryn, J., Costa, F., & Turbin, M. (1995). Protective factors in adolescent problem behavior: Moderator effects and developmental change. *Developmental Psychology, 31,* 923–933.

Jimmerson, S., Burns, M., & VanDerHeyden, A. (2007). *Handbook of response to intervention: The science and practice of assessment and intervention.* New York: Springer.

Johns, A., Patrick, J., & Rutherford, K. (2008). Best practices in district-wide positive behavior support implementation. In A. Thomas & J. Grimes (Eds.), *Best practices in school psychology* (Vol. 3, pp. 721–734). Bethesda, MD: National Association of School Psychologists.

Jones, E., & Nisbett, R. (1972). The actor and observer: Divergent perceptions of the causes of behavior. In E. Jones, D. Kanouse, H. Kelly, R. Nisbett, S. Valins, & B. Weiner (Eds.), *Attribution: Perceiving the causes of behavior* (pp. 79–94). Morristown, NJ: General Learning Press.

Juel, C. (1988). *Learning to read and write: A longitudinal study of 54 children from first through fourth grades.* Paper presented at the annual conference of the American Educational Research Association, New Orleans, LA.

Kamphaus, R., & Reynolds, C. (2007). *BASC–2 Behavioral and Emotional Screening System (BASC–2 BESS).* San Antonio, TX: Pearson Assessments.

Kandel, E., Mednick, S., Kirkegaard-Sorenson, L., Hutchings, B., Knop, J., Rosenberg, R., et al. (1988). IQ as a protective factor for subjects at high risk for antisocial behavior. *Journal of Consulting and Clinical Psychology, 56,* 224–226.

Kauffman, J. (1999). How we prevent prevention of emotional and behavioral disorders. *Exceptional Children, 65,* 448–468.

Kauffman, J. M. (2014). On following the scientific evidence. In H. M. Walker & F. M. Gresham (Eds.), *Handbook of evidence-based practices for emotional and behavioral disorders: Applications in schools* (pp. 1–5). New York: Guilford Press.

Kazdin, A. E. (1977). Assessing the clinical or applied significance of behavior change through social validation. *Behavior Modification, 1,* 427–452.

Kazdin, A. E. (1981). Acceptability of child treatment techniques: The influence of treatment efficacy and adverse side effects. *Behavior Therapy, 12,* 493–506.

Kazdin, A. E. (1982). *Single-case research designs.* New York: Oxford University Press.

Kazdin, A. (1987). Treatment of antisocial behavior in childhood: Current status and future directions. *Psychological Bulletin, 102,* 187–203.

Kazdin, A. (1991). Prevention of conduct disorder. In *The prevention of mental disorders: Progress, problems, and prospects.* Washington, DC: National Institute of Mental Health.

Kazdin, A. (1993). Psychotherapy for children and adolescents: Current progress and future research directions. *American Psychologist, 48,* 644–657.

Kazdin, A. (2003a). Clinical significance: Measuring whether interventions make a difference. In A. E. Kazdin (Ed.), *Methodological issues and strategies in clinical research* (3rd ed., pp. 691–710). Washington, DC: American Psychological Association.

Kazdin, A. (2003b). Problem-solving skills training and parent management training for conduct disorder. In A. Kazdin & J. Weisz (Eds.), *Evidence-based psychotherapies for children and adolescents* (pp. 241–262). New York: Guilford Press.

Kazdin, A. (2004). Evidence-based treatments: Challenges and priorities for practice and research. *Child and Adolescent Psychiatry Clinics of North America, 13*(4), 923–940.

Kazdin, A. E. (2005). *Parent management training: Treatment for oppositional, aggressive, and antisocial behavior in children and adolescents.* New York: Oxford University Press.

Kazdin, A., Siegel, T., & Bass, D. (1992). Cognitive problem-solving skills training and parent management training in the treatment of antisocial behavior in children. *Journal of Consulting and Clinical Psychology, 60,* 733–747.

Kazdin, A., & Wassell, G. (2000). Therapeutic changes in children, parents, and families resulting from treatment of children with conduct problems. *Journal of the American Academy of Child and Adolescent Psychiatry, 39,* 414–420.

Kazdin, A., & Weisz, J. (2003). Context and background of evidence-based psychotherapies for children and adolescents. In A. Kazdin & J. Weisz (Eds.), *Evidence-based psychotherapies for children and adolescents* (pp. 3–20). New York: Guilford Press.

Kellam, S. (2002, October). *Prevention science, aggression, and destructive outcomes: Long term results of a series of prevention trials in school settings.* Presentation to the National Press Club, Washington, DC.

Kellam, S., Mayer, I., Rebok, G., & Hawkins, W. (1998). Effects of improving achievement on aggressive behavior and of improving aggressive behavior on achievement through two preventive interventions: An investigation of causal paths. In B. P. Dohrenwend (Ed.), *Adversity, stress, and psychopathology* (pp. 486–505). New York: Oxford University Press.

Kelley, M. L. (1990). *School-home notes: Promoting children's classroom success.* New York: Guilford Press.

Kennedy, C. H. (2005). *Single-case designs for educational research.* Boston: Allyn & Bacon.

Kerr, M., & Nelson, C. M. (2010). *Strategies for addressing behavior problems in the classroom* (6th ed.). Upper Saddle River, NJ: Pearson Education.

Konopasek, D., & Forness, S. (2014). Issues and criteria for the effective use of psychopharmacological interventions in schooling. In H. M. Walker & F. M. Gresham (Eds.), *Handbook of evidence-based practices for emotional and behavioral disorders: Applications in schools* (pp. 457–475). New York: Guilford Press.

Kratochwill, T. R., Hitchcock, J., Horner, R. H., Levin, J. R., Odom, S. L., Rindskopf, D. M., et al. (2010). Single-case design technical documentation. Retrieved from What Works Clearinghouse website *http://ies.ed.gov/ncee/wwc/pdf/wwc_scd.pdf.*

Kupersmidt, J., Coie, J., & Dodge, K. (1990). The role of peer relationships in the development of disorder. In S. Asher & J. Coie (Eds.), *Peer rejection in childhood* (pp. 274–308). New York: Cambridge University Press.

Kupersmidt, J., & Patterson, C. (1991). Childhood peer rejection, aggression, withdrawal, and self-perceived competence as predictors of self-reported behavior problems in preadolescence. *Journal of Abnormal Child Psychology, 19,* 427–449.

Kusche, C., & Greenberg, M. (1994). *The PATHS curriculum.* Seattle, WA: Developmental Research and Programs.

LaGreca, A. M., & Santogrossi, D. S. (1980). Social skills training with elementary school students: A behavioral group approach. *Journal of Consulting and Clinical Psychology, 48,* 220–227.

Lahey, B., Loeber, R., Stouthamer-Loeber, M., Christ, M., Green, S., Russo, M., et al. (1990). Comparison of DSM-III and DSM-III-R diagnoses for prepubertal children: Changes in prevalence and validity. *Journal of the American Academy of Child and Adolescent Psychiatry, 29,* 620–626.

Lahey, B., Piacentini, J., McBurnett, K., Stone, P., Hartdagen, S., & Hynd, G. (1987). Psychopathology in the parents of children with conduct disorder and hyperactivity. *Journal of the American Academy of Child and Adolescent Psychiatry, 27,* 163–170.

Lalli, J., Vollmer, T., Prograr, P., Wright, C., Borrero, J., Dency, D., et al. (1999). Competition between positive and negative reinforcement in the treatment of escape behavior. *Journal of Applied Behavior Analysis, 32,* 285–296.

Landrum, T., & Lloyd, J. (1992). Generalization in social behavior research with children and youth who have emotional or behavioral disorders. *Behavior Modification, 16,* 593–616.

Landrum, T., Tankersley, M., & Kauffman, J. (2003). What is special about special education for students with emotional or behavioral disorders? *Journal of Special Education, 37,* 148–156.

Lane, K., Bruhn, A., Eisner, S., & Kalberg, J. (2010). Score reliability and validity of the Student Risk Screening Scale: A psychometrically sound, feasible tool for use in urban middle schools. *Journal of Emotional and Behavioral Disorders, 18,* 211–224.

Lane, K., Kalberg, J., Parks, R., & Carter, E. (2008). Student Risk Screening Scale: Initial evidence for score reliability and validity at the high school level. *Journal of Emotional and Behavioral Disorders, 16,* 178–190.

Lane, K., Menzies, H., Oakes, W., & Kahlberg, J. (2012). *Systematic screenings of behavior to support instruction: From preschool to high school.* New York: Guilford Press.

Lane, K., Oakes, W., Ennis, R., Cox, M., Schatschneider, C, & Lambert, W. (2013). Additional evidence for the reliability and validity of the Student Risk Screening Scale at the high school level: A replication and extension. *Journal of Emotional and Behavioral Disorders, 21,* 97–115.

Lane, K., Oakes, W., Menzies, H., & Germer, K. (2014). Screening and identification approaches for detecting students at risk. In H. M. Walker & F. M. Gresham (Eds.), *Handbook of evidence-based practices for emotional and behavioral disorders* (pp. 129–151). New York: Guilford Press.

Leff, S., Waanders, C., Waasdorp, E., & Paskewich, B. (2014). Bullying and aggression in schools. In H. M. Walker & F. M. Gresham (Eds.), *Handbook of evidence-based practices for emotional and behavioral disorders: Applications in schools* (pp. 277–291). New York: Guilford Press.

Litow, L., & Pumroy, D. (1975). A brief review of classroom group oriented contingencies. *Journal of Applied Behavior Analysis, 8,* 341–347.

Lochman, J. E., Barry, T., & Pardini, D. (2002). Anger control training for aggressive youth. In A. Kazdin & J. Weisz (Eds.), *Evidence-based psychotherapies for children and adolescents* (pp. 263–281). New York: Guilford Press.

Lochman, J., Coie, J., Underwood, M., & Terry, R. (1993). Effectiveness of a social relations intervention program for aggressive and nonaggressive rejected children. *Journal of Consulting and Clinical Psychology, 61,* 1053–1058.

Lochman, J. E., & Gresham, F. M. (2009). Intervention development, assessment, planning, and adaptation: The importance of developmental models. In M. Mayer, R. Van Acker, J. Lochman, & F. M. Gresham (Eds.), *Cognitive-behavioral interventions for emotional and behavioral disorders* (pp. 29–57). New York: Guilford Press.

Lochman, J., & Wells, K. (1996). A social-cognitive intervention with aggressive children: Prevention efforts and contextual implementation issues. In R. Peters & R. McMahon (Eds.), *Prevention and early intervention: Childhood disorders, substance use, and delinquency* (pp. 111–143). Thousand Oaks, CA: Sage.

Lochman, J., Whidby, J., & FitzGerald, D. (2000). In P. Kendall (Ed.), *Child and adolescent therapy* (2nd ed., pp. 31–87). New York: Guilford Press.

Loeber, R. (1988). Behavioral precursors and accelerators of delinquency.

In W. Buikhuisen & S. Mednick (Eds.), *Explaining criminal behavior* (pp. 51–67). Leiden, NY: Brill.

Loeber, R. (1991). Antisocial behavior: More enduring than changeable? *Journal of the American Academy of Child and Adolescent Psychiatry, 30,* 393–397.

Loeber, R., & Dishion, T. (1983). Early predictors of male adolescent delinquency: A review. *Psychological Bulletin, 94,* 68–99.

Loeber, R., & Farrington, D. (Eds.). (1998). *Serious and violent juvenile offenders: Risk factors and successful interventions.* Thousand Oaks, CA: Sage.

Loeber, R., & Keenan, K. (1994). Interaction between conduct disorder and its comorbid conditions: Effects of age and gender. *Clinical Psychology Review, 14,* 497–523.

Loeber, R., & LeBlanc, M. (1990). Toward a developmental criminology. In M. Tonry & N. Morris (Eds.), *Crime and justice: A review of research* (Vol. 12, pp. 375–473). Chicago: University of Chicago Press.

Lynam, D. (1996). Early identification of chronic offenders: Who is the fledgling psychopath? *Psychological Bulletin, 120,* 209–234.

Lyon, G. R. (2002, November). *The current status and impact of U.S. reading research.* Keynote address to the National Association of University Centers for Excellence in Developmental Disabilities, Bethesda, MD.

Maag, J. W. (2005). Social skills training for youth with emotional and behavioral disorders and learning disabilities: Problems, conclusions, and suggestions. *Exceptionality, 13,* 155–172.

Maag, J. W. (2006). Social skills training for students with emotional and behavioral disorders: A review of reviews. *Behavioral Disorders, 32,* 5–17.

Maggin, D., Briesch, A., & Chafouleas, S. (2013). An application of the What Works Clearinghouse Standards for evaluating single-subject research. *Remedial and Special Education, 34*(1), 44–58.

Malecki, C. M., & Elliott, S. N. (2002). Children's social behaviors as predictors of academic achievement: A longitudinal analysis. *School Psychology Quarterly, 17,* 1–23.

March, R., & Horner, R. (2002). Feasibility and contributions of functional behavioral assessment in schools. *Journal of Emotional and Behavioral Disorders, 10,* 158–170.

Martella, R., Marchand-Martella, N., Woods, B., Thompson, S., Crockett, C., Northrup, E., et al. (2010). Positive behavior support: Analysis of consistency between office discipline referrals and teacher recordings of disruptive classroom behaviors. *Behavioral Development Bulletin, 10,* 25–32.

Martens, B. K., DiGennaro Reed, F., & Magnuson, J. D. (2014). Behavioral consultation: Contemporary research and emerging challenges. In W. P. Erchul & S. M. Sheridan (Eds.), *Handbook of research in school consultation* (2nd ed., pp. 180–209). New York: Routledge.

Martens, B. K., & Lambert, T. L. (2014). Conducing functional behavioral assessments for students with emotional and behavioral disorders. In H. M. Walker & F. M. Gresham (Eds.), *Handbook of evidence-based practices for emotional and behavioral disorders: Applications in schools* (pp. 243–257). New York: Guilford Press.

Mastropieri, M., & Scruggs, T. (1985–1986). Early intervention for socially withdrawn children. *Journal of Special Education, 19*, 429–441.

Mathur, S., & Rutherford, R. (1991). Peer-mediated interventions promoting social skills for children and youth with behavioral disorders. *Education and Treatment of Children, 14*, 227–242.

McCurdy, B., Kunsch, C., & Reibstein, S. (2007). Secondary prevention in the urban school: Implementing the Behavior Education Program. *Preventing School Failure, 51*, 12–19.

McFall, R. (1982). A review and reformulation of the concept of social skills. *Behavioral Assessment, 4*, 1–35.

McIntosh, K., Frank, J., & Spaulding, S. (2010). Establishing research-based trajectories of office discipline referrals for individual students. *School Psychology Review, 39*, 380–394.

McIntosh, R., Vaughn, S., & Zaragoza, N. (1991). A review of social interventions for students with learning disabilities. *Journal of Learning Disabilities, 24*, 451–458.

McKevitt, B., & Braaksma, A. (2008). Best practices in developing a positive behavior support system at the school level. In A. Thomas & J. Grimes (Eds.), *Best practices in school psychology* (Vol. 3, pp. 735–747). Bethesda, MD: National Association of School Psychologists.

McMahon, R. J. (1999). Parent training. In S. Russ & T. Ollendick (Eds.), *Handbook of psychotherapies with children and adolescents* (pp. 153–180). New York: Kluwer Academic/Plenum Press.

McMahon, R., & Forehand, R. (2003). *Helping the noncompliant child: Family-based treatment for oppositional behavior* (2nd ed.). New York: Guilford Press.

Messick, S. (1995). Validity of psychological assessment: Validation of inferences from persons' responses and performances as scientific inquiry into score meaning. *American Psychologist, 50*, 741–749.

Michael, J. (2007). Motivating operations. In J. Cooper, T. Heron, & W. Seward (Eds.), *Applied behavior analysis* (2nd ed., pp. 374–391). Upper Saddle River, NJ: Pearson Prentice Hall.

Minuchen, S. (1974). *Families and family therapy*. Cambridge, MA: Harvard University Press.

Moffitt, T. (1990). Juvenile delinquency and attention deficit disorder: Boys' developmental trajectories from age 3 to age 15. *Child Development, 61*, 893–910.

Moffitt, T. (1993). Adolescence-limited life-course persistent antisocial behavior: A developmental taxonomy. *Psychological Review, 100*, 674–701.

Moffitt, T. (2003). Life-course persistent and adolescence-limited antisocial behavior: A 10-year research review and research agenda. In B. Lahey, T. Moffitt, & A. Caspi (Eds.), *Causes of conduct disorder and juvenile delinquency* (pp. 49–75). New York: Guilford Press.

MTA (Multimodal Treatment Study of Children with ADHD) Cooperative Group. (1999). A 14-month randomized clinical trial of treatment strategies for attention-deficit/hyperactivity disorder. *Archives of General Psychiatry, 56,* 1073–1086.

MTA Cooperative Group. (2004). National Institute of Mental Health multimodal treatment study of ADHD follow-up: 24-month outcomes of treatment strategies for attention-deficit/hyperactivity disorder. *Pediatrics, 113,* 754–761.

Myles, B., & Simpson, R. (1996). Impact of facilitated communication combined with direct instruction on academic performance of children with autism. *Focus on Autism and Other Developmental Disabilities, 11,* 37–52.

Nash, J., & Bowen, G. (2002). Defining and estimating risk and protection: An illustration from the school success profile. *Child and Adolescent Social Work Journal, 19,* 247–261.

Nathan, P., Stuart, S., & Dolan, S. (2000). Research on psychotherapy efficacy and effectiveness: Between Scylla and Charybdis? In A. E. Kazdin (Ed.), *Methodological issues and strategies in clinical research* (3rd ed., pp. 505–546). Washington, DC: American Psychological Association.

National Reading Panel. (2000). Teaching children to read: An evidence-based assessment of the scientific research literature on reading and its implications for reading instruction. Retrieved from *www.nichd.nih.gov/publications/pubskey.cfm?from=nrp.*

Nelson, R., Benner, G., Reid, C., Epstein, M., & Currin, D. (2002). The convergent validity of office discipline referrals with the CBCL-TRF. *Journal of Emotional and Behavior Disorders, 10,* 181–188.

Nevin, J. (1988). Behavioral momentum and the partial reinforcement effect. *Psychological Bulletin, 103,* 44–56.

Newman, J., & Wallace, J. (1993). Divergent pathways to impulsive behavior: Implications for disinhibitory psychopathology in children [Special issue]. *Clinical Psychology Review, 13,* 699–720.

Nezu, A., & Nezu, C. (2008). Treatment integrity. In D. McKay (Ed.), *Handbook of research methods in abnormal and clinical psychology* (pp. 351–366). Thousand Oaks, CA: Sage.

Oden, S. L., & Asher, S. R. (1977). Coaching children in social skills for friendship making. *Child Development, 48,* 495–506.

Offord, D., Boyle, M., & Racine, Y. (1989). Ontario Child Health Study: Correlates of disorder. *Journal of the American Academy of Child and Adolescent Psychiatry, 28,* 856–860.

Olmeda, R., & Kauffman, J. (2003). Sociocultural considerations in social skills research with African American students with emotional and behavioral disorders. *Journal of Developmental and Physical Disabilities, 15*, 101–121.

O'Neill, R., Albin, R., Storey, K., Horner, R., & Sprague, J. (2014). *Functional behavior analysis and program development* (3rd ed.). New York: Cengage Learning.

Oshinsky, D. M. (2005). *Polio: An American story*. New York: Oxford University Press.

Parker, J., & Asher, S. (1987). Peer relations and later personal adjustment: Are low-accepted children at risk? *Psychological Bulletin, 102*, 357–389.

Parker, R., Hagan-Burke, S., & Vannest, K. (2007). Percentage of all non-overlapping data (PAND): An alternative to PND. *The Journal of Special Education, 40*, 194–204.

Patterson, G. R. (1974). Interventions for boys with conduct problems: Multiple settings, treatments, and criteria. *Journal of Consulting and Clinical Psychology, 42*, 471–481.

Patterson, G. R. (1982). *Coercive family process*. Eugene, OR: Castaldia Press.

Patterson, G. (2002). The early development of coercive family process. In J. Reid, G. Patterson, & J. Synder (Eds.), *Antisocial behavior in children and adolescents: A developmental analysis and model for intervention* (pp. 45–64). Washington, DC: American Psychological Association.

Patterson, G. R., & Bank, L. I. (1989). Some amplifying mechanisms for pathologic processes in families. In M. R. Gunnar & E. Thelen (Eds.), *Systems and development: The Minnesota symposia on child psychology* (pp. 167–209). Hillsdale, NJ: Erlbaum.

Patterson, G. R., Chamberlain, P., & Reid, J. (1982). A comparative evaluation of a parent-training program. *Behavior Therapy, 13*, 638–650.

Patterson, G., Reid, J., & Dishion, T. (1992). *Antisocial boys*. Eugene, OR: Castalia.

Patterson, G. R., Reid, J. B., Jones, R. R., & Conger, R. E. (1975). *A social learning approach to family intervention: Families with aggressive children* (Vol. 1). Eugene, OR: Castalia.

Perepletchikova, F. (2014). Assessment of treatment integrity. In L. Hagermoser Sanetti & T. R. Kratochwill (Eds.), *Treatment integrity: A foundation for evidence-based practice in applied psychology* (pp. 131–158). Washington, DC: American Psychological Association.

Peterson, L., Homer, A., & Wonderlich, S. (1982). The integrity of independent variables in behavior analysis. *Journal of Applied Behavior Analysis, 15*, 477–492.

Rae-Grant, N., Thomas, H., Offord, D., & Boyle, M. (1989). Risk, protective factors and prevalence of behavioral and emotional disorders in children and adolescents. *Journal of the American Academy of Child and Adolescent Psychiatry, 28*, 262–268.

Reid, J. (1993). Prevention of conduct disorder before and after school entry: Relating interventions to developmental findings. *Development and Psychopathology, 5,* 311–319.

Reid, J. B., & Eddy, J.M. (2002). Interventions for antisocial behavior: Overview. In J. Reid, G. Patterson, & J. Synder (Eds.), *Antisocial behavior in children and adolescents: A developmental analysis and model for intervention* (pp. 195–202). Washington, DC: American Psychological Association.

Reid, J., Patterson, G., & Synder, J. (2002). *Antisocial behavior in children and adolescents: A developmental analysis and model for intervention.* Washington, DC: American Psychological Association.

Reynolds, C., & Kamphaus, R. (2004). *Behavioral assessment system for children* (2nd ed.). Minneapolis, MN: Pearson Assessments.

Rosenshine, B. (2008). Systematic instruction. In T. Good (Ed.), *21st century education: A reference handbook* (Vol. 1, pp. 235–243). Thousand Oaks, CA: Sage.

Rosenthal, R., & Rosnow, R. (1991). *Essentials of behavioral research: Methods and data analysis* (2nd ed.). New York: McGraw-Hill.

Rosenthal, R., Rosnow, R., & Rubin, D. (2000). *Contrasts and effect sizes in behavioral research.* Cambridge, UK: Cambridge University Press.

Rutter, M. (1979). Protective factors in children's responses to stress and disadvantage. In J. Rolf (Ed.), *Primary prevention of psychopathology: Vol. 3. Social competence in children* (pp. 49–74). Hanover, NH: University Press of New England.

Rutter, M. (1982). Prevention of children's psychosocial disorders: Myth and substance. *Pediatrics, 70,* 883–894.

Rutter, M. (1985). Resilience in face of adversity: Protective factors and resistance to psychiatric disorder. *British Journal of Psychiatry, 147,* 598–611.

Sameroff, A., & Seifer, R. (1990). Early contributors to developmental risk. In S. Weintraub (Ed.), *Risk and protective factors in the development of psychopathology* (pp. 52–66). New York: Cambridge University Press.

Sameroff, A., Seifer, R., Barocas, R., Zax, M., & Greenspan, S. (1987). Intelligence quotient scores of 4-year-old children: Social-environmental risk factors. *Pediatrics, 79,* 343–350.

Schloss, P., Schloss, C., Wood, C., & Kiehl, W. (1986). A critical review of social skills research with behaviorally disordered students. *Behavior Disorders, 12,* 1–14.

Schneider, B. (1992). Didactic methods for enhancing children's peer relations: A quantitative review. *Clinical Psychology Review, 12,* 363–382.

Schneider, B., & Byrne, B. (1985). Children's social skills training: A meta-analysis. In B. Schneider, K. Rubin, & J. Ledingham (Eds.), *Children's peer relations: Issues in assessment and intervention* (pp. 175–190). New York: Springer-Verlag.

Schuhmann, E., Foote, R. Eyberg, S., Boggs, S., & Angina, J. (1998). Efficacy of parent–child interaction therapy: Interim report of a randomized trial with short-term maintenance. *Journal of Clinical Child Psychology, 27,* 34–45.

Schwartz, I., & Baer, D. (1991). Social validity assessments: Is current practice state of the art? *Journal of Applied Behavior Analysis, 24,* 189–204.

Sechrest, L., McKnight, P., & McKnight, K. (1996). Calibration of measures for psychotherapy outcome studies. *American Psychologist, 51,* 1065–1071.

Seeley, J., Severson, H., & Fixen, A. (2014). Empirically based targeted prevention approaches for addressing externalizing and internalizing behavior disorders within school contexts. In H. M. Walker & F. M. Gresham (Eds.), *Handbook of evidence-based practices for emotional and behavioral disorders: Applications in schools* (pp. 307–323). New York: Guilford Press.

Severson, H., & Walker, H. (2002). Proactive approaches for identifying children at risk for sociobehavioral problems. In K. Lane, F. M. Gresham, & T. O'Shaughnessy (Eds.), *Interventions for children with or at risk for emotional and behavioral disorders* (pp. 33–53). Boston: Allyn & Bacon.

Shadish, W. R., Cook, T. D., & Campbell, D. T. (2002). *Experimental and quasi-experimental designs for generalized causal inference.* Boston: Houghton Mifflin.

Shinn, M., & Walker, H. M. (2010). *Interventions for achievement and behavior problems including RTI.* Bethesda, MD: National Association of School Psychologists.

Shure, M. (1997). Interpersonal cognitive problem solving: Primary prevention of early and high-risk behaviors in preschool and primary years. In G. Albee & T. Gullotta (Eds.), *Primary prevention works.* Thousand Oaks, CA: Sage.

Sinclair, E. (1993). Early identification of preschoolers with special needs in Head Start. *Topics in Early Childhood Education, 13,* 12–18.

Sinclair, E., Del'Homme, M., & Gonzalez, M. (1993). Systematic screening for preschool behavioral disorders. *Behavioral Disorders, 18,* 177–188.

Skinner, B. F. (1953). *Science and human behavior.* New York: MacMillan.

Smith, S., Lochman, J., & Daunic, A. (2005). Managing aggression using cognitive-behavioral interventions: State of the practice and future directions. *Behavioral Disorders, 30,* 227–240.

Smolkowski, K., Strycker, L., & Seeley, J. (2014). The role of research in evaluation of interventions for school-related behavioral disorders. In H. M. Walker & F. M. Gresham (Eds.), *Handbook of evidence-based practices for emotional and behavioral disorders: Applications in schools* (pp. 552–567). New York: Guilford Press.

Snyder, J. (2002). Reinforcement and coercion mechanisms in the development of antisocial behavior: The family. In J. Reid, G. Patterson, &

J. Snyder (Eds.), *Antisocial behavior in children and adolescents: A developmental analysis model for intervention* (pp. 101–122). Washington, DC: American Psychological Association.

Snyder, J., & Stoolmiller, M. (2002). Reinforcement and coercion mechanisms in the development of antisocial behavior: The family. In J. Reid, G. Patterson, & J. Snyder (Eds.), *Antisocial behavior in children and adolescents: A developmental analysis and model for intervention* (pp. 65–100). Washington, DC: American Psychological Association.

Stage, S., & Quiroz, D. (1997). A meta-analysis of interventions to decrease disruptive classroom behavior in public education settings. *School Psychology Review, 26,* 333–368.

Stamler, J. (1978). Lifestyles, major risk factors, proof, and public policy. *Circulation, 58,* 3–19.

Stouthamer-Loeber, M. Loever, R., Farington, D., Zhang, Q., Van Kammen, M., & Maguin, E. (1993). The double edge of protective and risk factors for delinquency: Interrelations and developmental patterns. *Development and Psychopathology, 5,* 683–701.

Strain, P., Kohler, F., & Gresham, F. M. (1998). Problems in logic and interpretation of quantitative synthesis of single case research: Mather and colleagues as a case in point. *Behavioral Disorders, 24,* 74–85.

Substance Abuse and Mental Health Services Administration. (2012). *Nonresearcher's guide to implementing evidence-based programs.* Washington, DC: National Registry of Evidence-Based Programs and Practices. Available from *www.nrepp.samhsa.gov.*

Sugai, G., & Horner, R. (1997). Discipline and behavior support: Preferred processes and practices. *Effective School Practices, 17,* 10–22.

Sugai, G., & Horner, R. (1999). Discipline and behavioral support. *Effective School Practices, 17,* 10–22.

Sugai, G., & Horner, R. (2002). The evolution of discipline practices: School-wide positive behavior supports. *Child and Family Behavior Therapy, 24,* 23–50.

Sugai, G., & Horner, R. (2008). What we know and need to know about preventing behavior problems in schools. *Exceptionality, 16,* 67–77.

Sugai, G., & Horner, R. (2009). Responsiveness to intervention and school-wide positive behavior supports: Integration of multi-tiered system approaches. *Exceptionality, 17,* 223.

Sugai, G., Horner, R., & Gresham, F. M. (2002). Behaviorally effective school environments. In M. Shinn, H. Walker, & G. Stoner (Eds.), *Interventions for academic and behavior problems: II. Preventive and remedial approaches* (pp. 313–350). Bethesda, MD: National Association of School Psychologists.

Sugai, G., Sprague, J., Horner, R., & Walker, H. M. (2000). Preventing school violence: The use of office discipline referrals to assess and monitor school-wide discipline interventions. *Journal of Emotional and Behavioral Disorders, 8,* 94–101.

Synder, J., & Stoolmiller, M. (2002). Reinforcement and coercion mechanisms in the development of antisocial behavior: The family. In J. Reid, G. Patterson, & J. Synder (Eds.), *Antisocial behavior in children and adolescents: A developmental analysis and model for intervention* (pp. 65–100). Washington, DC: American Psychological Association.

Tellegen, A. (1985). Structures of mood and personality and their relevance to assessing anxiety, with an emphasis on self-report. In A. H. Tuma & J. D. Maser (Eds.), *Anxiety and anxiety disorders* (pp. 681–706). Hillsdale, NJ: Erlbaum.

Templeton, J. (1990). Social skills training for behavior-problem adolescents: A review. *Journal of Partial Hospitalization, 6*, 49–60.

Tingstrom, D., Sterling-Turner, H., & Wilczynski, S. (2006). The Good Behavior Game: 1969–2002. *Behavior Modification, 30*, 225–253.

U.S. Department of Health and Human Services. (1999). *Mental health medications*. Bethesda, MD: Author.

Vollmer, T. (2002). Punishment happens: Some comments on Lerman and Vordan's review. *Journal of Applied Behavior Analysis, 35*, 469–473.

Walker, H. M., Colvin, G., & Ramsey, E. (1994). *Antisocial behavior in school: Strategies and best practices*. Pacific Grove, CA: Brooks/Cole.

Walker, H. M., Horner, R., Sugai, G., Bullis, M., Sprague, J., Bricker, D., et al. (1996). Integrated approaches to preventing antisocial behavior patterns among school-age children and youth. *Journal of Emotional and Behavioral Disorders, 4*, 193–256.

Walker, H. M., Irvin, L., Noell, J., & Singer, G. (1992). A construct score approach to the assessment of social competence: Rational, technological considerations, and anticipated outcomes. *Behavior Modification, 16*, 448–474.

Walker, H. M., Kavanagh, K., Stiller, B., Golly, A., Severson, H., & Feil, E. (1998). First Step: An early intervention approach for preventing antisocial behavior. *Journal of Emotional and Behavioral Disorders, 6*, 66–80.

Walker, H. M., & McConnell, S. (1995). *Walker–McConnell Scale of Social Competence and School Adjustment*. Florence, KY: Thomson Learning.

Walker, H. M., Nishioka, V., Zeller, R., Severson, H., & Feil, E. (2000). Causal factors and potential solutions for the persistent under-identification of students having emotional or behavioral disorders in the context of schooling. *Assessment for Effective Intervention, 26*, 29–40.

Walker, H. M., Ramsey, E., & Gresham, F. M. (2004). *Antisocial behavior in school* (2nd ed.). New York: Cengage Learning.

Walker, H. M., Seeley, J., Small, J., Severson, H., Graham, B., Feil, E., et al. (2009). A randomized control trial of the First Step to Success early intervention: Demonstration of program efficacy outcomes in a diverse urban school district. *Journal of Emotional and Behavioral Disorders, 17*, 197–212.

Walker, H. M., & Severson, H. (1990). *Systematic screening for behavior disorders*. Longmont, CO: Sopris West.

Walker, H. M., & Severson, H. (2002). Developmental prevention of at-risk outcomes for vulnerable antisocial children and youth. In K. Lane, F. M. Gresham, & T. O'Shaughnessy (Eds.), *Interventions for children with or at-risk for emotional and behavioral disorders* (pp. 177–191). Boston: Allyn & Bacon.

Walker, H. M., Severson, H., & Feil, E. (1995). *Early screening project: A proven child find process*. Longmont, CO: Sopris West.

Walker, H. M., Severson, H., & Seeley, J. (2010). Universal, school-based screening for the early detection of behavioral problems contributing to later destructive outcomes. In H. M. Walker & M. Shinn (Eds.), *Interventions for achievement and behavior problems in a three-tier model including RTI* (pp. 677–703). Bethesda, MD: National Association of School Psychologists..

Walker, H. M., Severson, H., Seeley, J., Feil, E., Small, J., Golly, A., et al. (2014). The evidence base of the First Step to Success early intervention for preventing emerging antisocial behavior patterns. In H. M. Walker & F. M. Gresham (Eds.), *Handbook of evidence-based practices for emotional and behavioral disorders: Applications in schools* (pp. 518–537. New York: Guilford Press.

Walker, H. M., & Shinn, M. (2010). Systemic, evidence-based approaches for promoting positive student outcomes within a multitier framework: Moving from efficacy to effectiveness. In M. Shinn & H. M. Walker (Eds.), *Interventions for achievement and behavior problems in a three-tier model including RTI* (pp. 1–26). Bethesda, MD: National Association of School Psychologists.

Walker, H. M., & Sprague, J. (1999). Longitudinal research and functional behavioral assessment issues. *Behavioral Disorders, 24,* 331–334.

Walker, H. M., Stiller, B., Golly, A., Kavanagh, K., Severson, H., & Feil, E. (1997). *First Step to Success: Helping young children overcome antisocial behavior*. Longmont, CO: Sopris West.

Waschbush, D. (2002). A meta-analytic examination of comorbid hyperactive–impulsive–inattention problems and conduct problems. *Psychological Bulletin, 128,* 118–150.

Webster-Stratton, C., & Hammond, M. (1997). Treating children with early-onset conduct problems: A comparison of child and parent training interventions. *Journal of Consulting and Clinical Psychology, 65,* 93–109.

Webster-Stratton, C., & Hancock, I. (1998). Training for parents of young children with conduct problems: Content, methods, and therapeutic processes. In C. E. Schaefer & J. M. Briesmeister (Eds.), *Handbook of parent training* (pp. 98–152). New York: Wiley.

Webster-Stratton, C., Hollingsworth, T., & Kolpacoff, M. (1989). The long-term effectiveness and clinical significance of three cost-effective training programs for families with conduct-problem children. *Journal of Consulting and Clinical Psychology, 56,* 558–566.

Webster-Stratton, C., Reid, M., & Hammond, M. (2001). Social skills and problem-solving training for children with early-onset conduct problems: Who benefits? *Journal of Child Psychology and Psychiatry, 42,* 943–952.

Webster-Stratton, C., Reid, M., & Hammond, M. (2004). Treating children with early-onset conduct problems: Intervention outcomes for parent, child, and teacher training. *Journal of Clinical Child and Adolescent Psychology, 33,* 105–124.

Weiss, G., Kruger, E., Danielson, V., & Elman, M. (1975). Effects of long-term treatment of hyperactives with methlphenidate. *Canadian Medical Association Journal, 112,* 159–165.

Weisz, J. (2004). *Psychotherapy for children and adolescents.* New York: Cambridge University Press.

Wentzel, K. R. (2005). Peer relationships, motivation, and academic performance at school. In A. Elliot & C. Dweck (Eds.), *Handbook of competence and motivation* (pp. 279–296). New York: Guilford Press.

Wentzel, K. R. (2009). Peers and academic functioning at school. In K. H. Rubin, W. M. Bukowski, & B. Laursen (Eds.), *Handbook of peer interactions, relationships, and groups* (pp. 531–547). New York: Guilford Press.

Wentzel, K. R., & Looney, I. (2007). Socialization in school settings. In J. E. Grusec & P. D. Hastings (Eds.), *Handbook of socialization: Theory and research* (pp. 382–403). New York: Guilford Press.

Wentzel, K. R., & Watkins, D. E. (2002). Peer relationships and collaborative learning as contexts for academic enablers. *School Psychology Review, 31,* 366–377.

White, J., Moffitt, T., & Silva, P. (1989). A prospective replication of protective effects of IQ in subjects at high risk for juvenile delinquency. *Journal of Consulting and Clinical Psychology, 57,* 719–724.

Wolf, M. M. (1978). Social validity: The case for subjective measurement or how applied behavior analysis is finding its heart. *Journal of Applied Behavior Analysis, 11,* 203–214.

Yeaton, W., & Sechrest, L. (1981). Critical dimensions in the choice and maintenance of successful treatments: Strength, integrity, and effectiveness. *Journal of Consulting and Clinical Psychology, 49,* 156–167.

Yell, M. (2009). Teaching students with EBD I: Effective teaching. In M. Yell, N. Meadows, E. Drasgow, & J. Shriner (Eds.), *Evidence-based practices for educating students with emotional and behavioral disorders* (pp. 320–341). Upper Saddle River, NJ: Pearson Education.

Yell, M., Meadows, N., Drasgow, E., & Shriner, J. (2009). *Evidence-based practices for educating students with emotional and behavioral disorders.* Upper Saddle River, NJ: Pearson Education.

Zaragoza, N., Vaughn, S., & McIntosh, R. (1991). Social skills interventions for children with behavior problems: A review. *Behavioral Disorders, 16,* 260–275.

Zigler, E., Taussig, C., & Black, K. (1992). Early childhood intervention: A promising preventative for juvenile delinquency. *American Psychologist, 47,* 997–1006.

Index

social skills interventions and, 209
validity and, 26
Rate of reinforcement, 149–150. *See also*
Reinforcement
Ratio schedules of reinforcement, 146, 159.
See also Schedule of reinforcement
Reductive non-punishment-based procedures,
118, 124–127, 129
Refusals, 3. *See also* Noncompliance
Reinforcement. *See also* Negative
reinforcement; Positive reinforcement
case studies, 239–242, 241*f*, 260–264,
263*f*
competing problem behaviors and, 196
contingencies of reinforcement, 137–138
differential reinforcement, 124, 126–127
functional behavioral assessment (FBA)
and, 71–72
matching law and, 16–17
multicomponent interventions and, 163
overview, 18, 132
parent training and, 136, 137–139, 142,
144–151, 152, 159
peer rejection and, 215
punishment-based procedures and,
119–124
reductive non-punishment-based
procedures and, 124–127
social validation and, 92
time-out procedures and, 122–123
Reinforcement schedules. *See* Schedule of
reinforcement
Reinforcers, 144–145. *See also*
Reinforcement; Rewards
Rejection. *See* Peer rejection
Reliability of a test, 51–52, 59–60
Renegotiation, 3. *See also* Noncompliance
Replacement behavior training (RBT)
overview, 195–196, 198, 215–217
positive replacement behaviors, 199–203
social skills interventions and, 203–215,
211*f*, 213*t*
Replication, 30, 45
Reprimands, verbal, 120
Research evidence, 24–25, 45, 99. *See also*
Evidence-based practices
Resistance to change, 83, 97
Response chains, 143–144, 159
Response class, 143, 159
Response cost, 123–124, 129, 239–242, 241*f*
Response to intervention (RTI). *See*
also Interventions; Multi-tiered
intervention approaches; Primary
(Tier 1) prevention; Secondary (Tier 2)
intervention approaches; Tertiary (Tier
3) intervention approaches
as an example of evidence-based practice,
23
intensity of intervention and, 102–103
intervention selection and, 103–105

overview, 81–89, 97, 128
primary prevention strategies and,
187–189
program evaluation and, 50
types of, 105–107
Responsibility behaviors, 213*t*
Rewards, 14, 112–113, 132. *See also*
Reinforcement
Risk factor exposure model, 117
Risk factors
assessment and, 54–58, 57*t*
competing problem behaviors and,
195–196
early identification and screening of DBDs
and, 59–60
First Step to Success (FSS) and, 111
functional behavioral assessment (FBA)
and, 117
identifying, 183–184
mega-analysis of, 184–186, 185*t*, 186*t*
multicomponent interventions and, 176
multisystemic therapy (MST) and, 165
overview, 55, 74–75, 133–134, 180–181,
182–183
primary prevention strategies and, 178,
192, 193
school failure and, 78
Risk-factor model, 6, 8–9, 181, 182, 193
Role plays
parent training and, 136, 152, 154, 175
Social Skills Improvement System
Classwide Intervention Program (SSIS-
CIP) and, 208
Social Skills Improvement System
Intervention Guide (SSIS-IG), 210–211,
211*f*, 212, 214, 225–226
Rule-breaking behavior, 3

S

Schedule of punishment, 149–150. *See also*
Punishment
Schedule of reinforcement, 125–126, 145–
147, 159. *See also* Reinforcement
Scheduled attention, 260–264, 263*f*
Schedules, 151
School performance, 3. *See also* Academic
achievement
School readiness, 77–78
School records, 49
School setting. *See also* Assessments
multisystemic therapy (MST) and, 166
overview, 77–78, 97, 127
risk and protective factors and, 193
selecting an evidence-based practice and,
34–37, 46
School-based interventions. *See also*
Interventions
Behavior Education Program (BEP),
107–110, 111*t*
conceptualization of, 100–102

replacement behavior training (RBT) and, 199–200
Social Skills Improvement System Classwide Intervention Program (SSIS-CIP), 207–209
Social Skills Improvement System Intervention Guide (SSIS-IG), 210–215, 211f, 213t
Social Skills Rating System (SSRS), 202–203
Social skills training, 171
Social tasks, 199–200
Social validity, 32, 89–96, 98. See also Evidence-based practices; Validity
Social-cognitive skills, 133–134, 205
Social-ecological theory, 165
Socioeconomic status, 13, 55, 193
Special education, 97
Specificity, 60, 60f, 75
Spontaneous recovery, 125
S-R learning theory, 100, 101, 128
Standard-protocol approaches to RTI, 105, 107, 128. See also Response to intervention (RTI)
Standards, 28–29
Statistical analysis, 87–88
Statistical conclusion validity, 27, 35, 45. See also Validity
Stepping-stone model, 6, 9–10
Stimulus control, 138–139
Strength of treatment, 84, 97
Student Risk Screening Scale (SRSS), 63–64, 65f, 75
Subjective evaluations, 95, 98
Substance abuse, 8
Substance Abuse and Mental Health Services Administration (SAMHSA), 33–34, 39
Subtype model, 6, 10–11
Sustaining gains, 43–44, 137
Systematic direct observations (SDOs). See also Assessments; Direct observations; Observation in assessment
case studies, 234, 238–239, 243
direct behavior ratings (DBRs) and, 69–70, 71f
overview, 69, 75
Systematic Screening for Behavior Disorders (SSBD)
First Step to Success (FSS) and, 111–112
overview, 61–66, 65f, 75
response to intervention (RTI) and, 104–105
Systemic direct observation, 49. See also Assessments; Observation in assessment

T

Talking-out behavior, 233–238, 236f, 237f, 238–242, 241f
Tangible reinforcers, 144. See also Reinforcement

Tantrums, 242–248, 246f, 247f, 252–255, 255f, 256f
Teachers, 61, 61–62, 162, 169–170, 195–196
Temperamental factors, 6, 9–10, 12, 13, 133–134, 159. See also Causality
Tertiary (Tier 3) intervention approaches. See also Multi-tiered intervention approaches
evidence-based practices and, 100
intensity of intervention and, 103
intensive school-based interventions, 114–118
overview, 81, 128, 188
punishment-based procedures and, 119–124
school-based interventions, 118–127, 128, 129
Test–retest reliability, 59–60. See also Reliability of a test
Theory of change model, 210, 211f
Therapist competence, 84–85
Therapy. See Counseling; Psychotherapy
Three-term contingency, 136, 138, 159, 175
Threshold method, 22
Throwing objects, 238–242, 241f
Time-out procedures, 121–123, 129
Time-out ribbon, 122, 123
Token systems
case studies, 239–242, 241f
parent management training and, 175
parent training and, 155
replacement behavior training (RBT) and, 199t
Topographical response class, 143, 159
Treatment adherence, 84–85
Treatment decision tests, 47. See also Assessments
Treatment differentiation, 84–85, 97
Treatment effectiveness, 86–89, 98
Treatment integrity, 84–86, 93, 97
Treatment planning, 136, 136–137
Treatment strength, 84, 97
Treatment validity. See also Validity
functional behavioral assessment (FBA) and, 116–117
intervention decisions and, 49
overview, 74
response to intervention (RTI) and, 105
Trend, 30, 45, 86, 87
Types of disruptive behavior disorders (DBDs), 2–3, 4t. See also Antisocial behavior pattern; Defiant/disrespectful behavior pattern; Disruptive behavior disorders (DBDs) in general